CHILD PSYCHIATRIC TREATMENT

Child Psychiatric Treatment : A Practical Guide

Philip G. Ney & Deanna L. Mulvihill

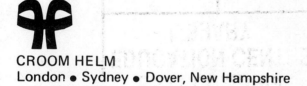

CROOM HELM
London • Sydney • Dover, New Hampshire

© 1985 Philip G. Ney and Deanna Mulvihill
Croom Helm Ltd, Provident House, Burrell Row,
Beckenham, Kent BR3 1AT
Croom Helm, Australia Pty Ltd, First Floor, 139 King Street,
Sydney, NSW 2001, Australia

British Library Cataloguing in Publication Data

Ney, Philip G.
    Child psychiatric treatment.
    1. Child psychiatry
    I. Title   II. Mulvihill, Deanna
    618.92'89   RJ499

    ISBN 0-7099-1823-2
    ISBN 0-7099-1824-0 Pbk

Croom Helm, 51 Washington Street, Dover, New Hampshire 03820, USA

Library of Congress Cataloging in Publication Data

Ney, Philip G. (Philip Gordon)
    Child psychiatric treatment.

    Includes index.
    1. Child psychiatry. 2. Child psychopathology.
I. Mulvihill, Deanna.   II. Title. (DNLM: 1. Child
Psychiatry – methods. 2. Mental Disorders – in infancy
and childhood. 3. Mental Disorders – therapy
WS 350 N571c)
RJ499.N47   1984   618.92'89   84-20048
ISBN 0-7099-1823-2
ISBN 0-7099-1824-0 (Pbk.)

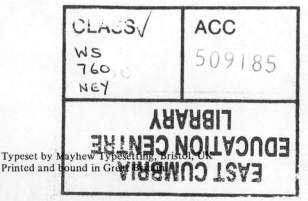

Typeset by Mayhew Typesetting, Bristol, UK
Printed and bound in Great Britain

CONTENTS

FOREWORD

This is a remarkable book. It is not often that we are offered a new and comprehensive way of looking at the treatment of children's problems, yet this is just what Philip Ney and Deanna Mulvihill do offer us. As the title implies, this is a practical book, born of long experience, about how to help children and their families. Yet it is much more than a 'how to' book. As well as suggesting many kinds of things we can do to help disturbed children and their families, the authors also take a critical look at the present state of child psychiatric services and the limitations of many of the traditional ways of dealing with troubled children. Thus before getting down to the details of their techniques and programmes, the authors examine the dilemmas facing those who work in this field, dealing with the large numbers which seem to be a part of the present-day scene. Traditional treatment methods, while certainly valuable in certain situations and for certain problems, also have serious limitations. This applies especially to residential treatment, which is expensive and of limited availability, as well as carrying the risk of institutionalising children and separating them — emotionally as well as physically — from their families.

On first consideration an inpatient programme which is based on the principle of admitting all children for the same length of time — whatever their diagnoses and however severe their problems — seems strange to say the least. Yet the authors put forward an excellent rationale for this procedure, as well as describing it in detail. Nevertheless, most of the material in the book is suitable for use in a wide variety of treatment programmes — inpatient, daypatient or even outpatient, with or without particular time limitations.

The natural place for a child to grow up is within the family. It is therefore pleasing to see that the concept of 'family restoration' is central to the authors' approach. It makes little sense to follow a programme which is not geared specifically to uniting, or usually reuniting, the child with a specific family (normally his or her own natural family); hence the authors' insistence that the discharge placement must be agreed before the child is admitted. Institutional 'drift', in which the child remains in an institution for longer than planned while 'placement' is awaited, is one of the very real dangers of inpatient treatment.

Having taken a general look at child psychiatric treatment needs, and the strains and stresses to which those attempting to meet these needs are exposed, the authors then describe specific treatment techniques. While these are certainly not all original, I believe that never before have so many specific techniques designed for particular indications been brought together in one place and described so succinctly and clearly. In all, 44 individual techniques are discussed, and something creative and constructive is provided for virtually every child psychiatric disorder. They are graded according to the degree of skill needed by those employing them. These are followed by descriptions of 14 group techniques, also graded according to the skill level required. If the book contained nothing else, these two sections would be of immense value to anyone attempting to develop comprehensive treatment programmes for children and their families.

But there is much more. Techniques need to be part of overall programmes, and ten programmes are presented, covering child abuse, anorexia, autism, depression, encopresis, fire-setting, incest, school phobia, weight control and conversion reactions. Many of us who have to develop treatment programmes for children and families will certainly find these useful. It is also possible to combine the various techniques in alternative ways in order to provide programmes for other problems.

Treating children without dealing also with their families has serious limitations. The authors suggest that child treatment should be combined with training sessions for the parents and a five-week programme of such sessions is described in detail, together with five follow-up lessons. The book concludes with some sample discharge summaries and a comprehensive description of how the units the authors have run are organised.

I cannot believe that anyone interested in the treatment of disturbed children and their families will fail to find this book utterly fascinating. More important, it must stimulate their thinking on some very basic questions concerning the treatment of children and provide them with a whole range of ideas from which they will be able to select those that suit them and the families they are treating. I doubt whether anyone will want to use every technique described here, and they may not adopt the specific programmes exactly as they are set out in this book. Indeed, the authors invite us to select from, modify and develop the ideas they present. It may also be that a fixed 12-week programme, including five inpatient weeks, may not be practical or appropriate in many settings — although it may indeed be especially valuable in situations where third party insurers fund only limited treatment periods. No, this is not a cookbook, but rather an inspirational one, an example of creative thinking and comprehensive treatment planning. It is a fresh look at age-old problems. The authors are to be congratulated on the clear, humane way they have broached their subject. Their care and concern for children and parents shine through the book, yet there is no sentimentality about it; it is just a down-to-earth practical approach and one designed to use scarce treatment resources in a cost-effective and creative way.

It is a pleasure to have been asked to write this foreword to what is surely a major, and long overdue, addition to the child psychiatric literature.

Philip Barker, MB, BS, FRCP(Ed), FRCPsych., FRCP(C),
Professor of Psychiatry and Paediatrics,
University of Calgary.

PREFACE

Many years ago, or so it seems, a young psychiatrist stood at the nurses' station of a general hospital psychiatric unit, and tried desperately to deal with the pointed questions of three nurses who had him backed into a corner and wouldn't let him out. He tried to give reasonable answers but he had not received the proper training, nor, as far as he was aware, had anybody else in his position as consultant child psychiatrist. Fortunately, having come from a large family where bantering and teasing were the rule, he had learned to think on his feet. Even so, his knowledge of the individual adolescent patient plus a good idea of the diagnosis and dynamics, didn't help him in answering the nurses' persistent, 'All right, then what do we do?'

It was painfully evident that the nurses were not only intelligent, perceptive people, but they were determined to put their talents to good use, given direction and encouragement. The young psychiatrist quickly found that such responses as 'talk to them' or 'observe them' or 'use your intuition', got nowhere fast. Having used some lame excuse to ponder the question, he hurriedly beat a retreat. This and similar encounters made the psychiatrist realise that what was needed was an array of useful techniques which could be applied in various combinations to the whole range of child psychiatric problems and they would have to be techniques which would not need prolonged training to learn. It was not a sudden revelation but a gradual dawning from his desperate need to find ways out of tight corners imposed by determined nurses or desperate children.

The techniques in this book were developed by the authors but have become refined by criticism and helpful comments through the daily interaction with eager, determined staff. It has always been a co-operative effort and much of the credit should go not only to the staff, but to the children and families. If these techniques are valuable, and grateful parents seem to believe so, then staff members, too many to be named, should feel appreciated.

My first opportunity to establish a unit and organise a programme came in 1965, when the Director of a training school for retarded children allocated a space and some of his best staff to establish an experimental unit for autistic children. I learned how eager staff became, when they had encouragement, not only to understand the clinical problems but participate in the evolution of treatment programmes.

They became loyal, determined innovative therapists who produced some very good results with severely disturbed children.

I next worked with a wide variety of professionals to establish a 60-bed unit for children and adolescents at the Adler Zone Center, in Champaign, Illinois. It was a brave experiment in which everybody was given equal opportunity to admit and treat children, regardless of their professional background. I found, unfortunately, that in many of the crunches, 'the child psychiatrist' was asked to manage the situation, although he was not given any greater responsibility or authority.

Returning to Canada I decided to locate in Victoria where a new psychiatric facility provided the opportunity to set up a unit for disturbed children and their families. Unfortunately, the only place was on the sixth floor of the psychiatric facility. This area was originally allocated to 'order in council' or forensic patients. After three and a half years of negotiating, the unit was modified to accommodate children, the programme organised and the unit was reasonably staffed. The idea of predetermined admissions and discharges was a hard one to sell, not only to the hospital administration, colleagues and government, but also to the staff.

We all began with some trepidation but, after ten years, the programme has proved itself and now continues with much the same format. My colleagues in psychiatry, Dr Rick Arnot, Dr Wallace Grant and Dr Harold Penner, have given plenty of support and corrective feedback. I am glad now that, from the very beginning, we were determined to evaluate the effectiveness of the programme with daily measures of the children's behaviour and follow-up of the children and their families one year later.

During a sabbatical from the University of British Columbia, I was invited to help develop a psychiatric unit at the University of Hong Kong, Queen Mary Hospital. We had cramped facilities but a willing staff and administration. A day programme was established and is now, with the capable direction of Dr Felice Lieh Mak and Dr Ernest Luk, providing a good service to a wide variety of patients. Although the local population was somewhat sceptical, eventually the community warmed to the idea of treating children and families together. The staff, having had little training in treating child psychiatric patients, did learn many of the techniques now contained in this book.

I have known many good nursing staff, but the head nurses that I have worked with on the Children's Unit stand out as first rate professionals. Mrs Mavis Martin worked many long hours with me helping to put together the initial proposal for the Children's Unit at the Royal

Jubilee Hospital. Mrs Martin gave leadership to our staff for seven years before becoming a supervisor. Mrs Deanna Mulvihill, who left a head nurse's position at the Children's Hospital of Eastern Ontario, replaced Mrs Martin and has worked with me to write up these techniques. Mrs Mulvihill also assisted in the training of staff and the opening of the Unit in Christchurch. Miss Lau Ping Che and Miranda Ho worked patiently and persistently in Hong Kong to develop nursing skills and a favourable attitude from the administration. Mrs Margaret Greenslade has carefully encouraged nursing staff and added her considerable clinical acumen to the application of these techniques, on Ward 24 at the Christchurch Public Hospital. There are other credits, too many to mention, but they include many fine psychologists, social workers, occupational therapists, nurses, childcare workers, administrators and psychiatric registrars. The teachers seconded to our units have been the best in the school districts. A special thank you to Dr Bill Mills, Dr Rick Hanna, Mr Gary Wickett, Miss Wendy Cammish and Mrs Margot Ney, who have given encouragement and valuable help in the writing of this book.

I was given the opportunity by the University of Otago and the Canterbury Hospital Board, to establish a child psychiatric unit at the Christchurch Hospital. Dr David Andrews patiently helped us achieve modifications of the physical space which was a fairly typical paediatric unit. Miss Margret Darby has helped collect very good staff from a variety of sources. Though we had only a brief training period the staff threw their hearts into the challenge and quickly learned the techniques, then worked with me to modify them.

Now the more experienced staff teach the newcomers. Other professionals from the community have come to learn how the unit deals with desperately ill children. We all hope that the emphasis on programmes built on definable, measurable techniques for children hospitalised for a predetermined period of time, will begin a small revolution in psychiatric care.

The techniques and programmes in this book are an attempt to treat the psychodynamic, transactional, behavioural, social and existential problems of troubled families. It is a medical and educational process with families learning from insight, instruction and experience. It's expecting a great deal to accomplish any significant change in all these areas in 10 weeks, but it does happen. Often there is enough change that the family needs no further treatment, sometimes it is an accelerated portion of a longer period of treatment in the family and occasionally it is one in a series of admissions.

Although these techniques were described in the context of an in-patient unit, they are as useful in outpatient settings. We hope you find them practical and useful for a wide variety of problems. We would feel flattered if you modify them for your situation and let us know what works best.

We would also add that, for ease of reading, we have used 'he' throughout when referring to a child, rather than 'he/she'.

In times of economic stress, hospital boards too often consider cuts to child psychiatric units first. We hope board members will remember that children suffer as much as adults, and that psychiatric illness is as painful and debilitating as any other. If there is lasting benefit from our efforts and value in this book, we thank god who gives to all people their strength and understanding.

1 OVERVIEW

The Problem

There is good reason to believe that the prevalence of severe, emotional, behavioural and psychiatric disorders among children is increasing. The best evidence indicates that child abuse is more frequent. We are beginning to realise how frequent depression is among adults and there is no reason to believe that depression is any less frequent among children. After all, they have similar biochemistry, constitutional predisposition, intensity of life stresses and for them losses are probably more important.

During the last two decades the number of admissions to residential treatment centres for children with emotional, behavioural and psychiatric disorders has markedly increased. Many reports (1, 3) indicate a great need for more child psychiatric services. Yet the efficiency of inpatient care has not been systematically assessed. There is considerable controversy regarding the optimal site for treatment and the most effective treatment methods (3, 6, 7). Most follow-up studies are subjective and difficult to evaluate (2).

The study by Winsberg et al. (14) attempted randomly to assign children either to inpatient or outpatient care. They sought to measure the effectiveness of the programme in terms of behavioural change, educational process, maternal psychiatric symptoms and role functioning in family adjustment. Unfortunately, they were unable to adhere to their original design because some of those assigned to outpatient treatment required urgent hospitalisation. However, they did conclude that some children for whom extended inpatient treatment was recommended, could be maintained in the community with special care and intervention.

Blinder et al. (4) found that of 117 patients (mean age 9.7 years) admitted over a two-year period, 72 per cent returned home, 10 per cent were placed in foster homes and 7 per cent entered programmes for residential treatment. The average length of stay for these children was 51 days. Shafii et al. (12) reported that of the 145 children and adolescents they admitted in one year, 82 per cent were discharged to their homes or previous residence, 18 per cent required other placement and 15 per cent were readmitted. The average length of stay of

1

these children (2-year-olds to 16-year-olds) was 24 days.

There is increasing community pressure for assessment and treatment of children but inpatient programmes have a number of built-in difficulties:

(a) Because there has been so little research on residential treatment of children, psychiatrists have difficulty determining which treatment is appropriate for which diagnosis for what period of time.

(b) In-depth assessment seldom provides useful guidance in determining which child will respond well to residential treatment.

(c) Multi-professional assessment centres too often provide diagnosis without appropriate treatment.

(d) Elaborate recommendations often do not work because no one has taught parents or teachers how to apply them after the child is discharged.

(e) A diagnosis applied to children once institutionalised is more often appropriate for the peculiar behaviours they show within that unusual setting than it is for behaviour typical of their home environment.

(f) Community workers often feel that they are insufficiently involved in planning the inpatient treatment of children whom they know very well.

(g) After many hours of hard-won patient confidence, community counsellors and social workers may resent their charges being taken from their care, even when they are prepared to admit the child's condition is worsening.

(h) Many families feel insufficiently involved in planning the treatment programme and have little opportunity to be involved in therapy.

(i) If the child is hospitalised for an indefinite period, family groupings tend to coalesce extruding the irritating child. Consequently there is increasing pressure to have the child placed in a foster home or institution.

(j) Without a well-integrated, consistently-applied programme there is a struggle to maintain a therapeutic milieu. Much staff effort goes into controlling behaviour and there is little time or energy available for individual or group treatment.

(k) Treatment staff from different professions instead of working as a team may waste time contesting what part of the child or family is their prerogative to treat.

(l) Treatment programmes have become increasingly expensive but staff time and facilities have not been effectively utilised.

(m) Problems of staff burn-out are accentuated by feelings that individual abilities have not been well utilised.

(n) Many improvements in the child during hospitalisation do not generalise into the home setting because little time has been spent working on those problems that more typically occur in the child's natural environment.

With these problems in mind we have worked with some very talented colleagues from a variety of disciplines to provide efficient use of staff and effective treatment of families. We believe the techniques and programmes that have evolved are useful for a wide variety of settings in addition to child psychiatric units.

The Unit

The Family Units at the Royal Jubilee Hospital (RJH), Victoria, BC, Canada and the one at Christchurch Public Hospital, Christchurch, New Zealand, have some unique features. Children are admitted to hospital on a predetermined date for a pre-established period of five weeks. Following hospitalisation, the treatment techniques are carried out for an additional five weeks in the family's home. Then contact is terminated. If continuing help is required, it will have been organised with the programme staff by a community agency.

By structuring the programme around fixed dates of admission, discharge and final termination, and by limiting the duration of treatment to ten weeks, our hope has been to reduce the disruption that the family might otherwise suffer. In addition, the structured programme is more efficient in terms of expensive hospital time than an unstructured programme, with no loss in effectiveness (9).

The staffing at both hospitals is similar. There is: a Unit Coordinator (part-time psychiatrist), two or three consulting psychiatrists, head nurse, eight nurses, nine child and family workers, one social worker, two psychologists (Christchurch), a teacher (seconded from the local school board), occupational therapist, ward clerk, dietary and house-keeping staff. Additional staffing can include up to two registrars in training and one teacher's aide. Although this sounds like a very rich patient–staff ratio, it should be remembered these staff are working with two children before admission, ten children admitted and ten children in follow-up. Very frequently as much time is spent with other family members, so in effect the staff is dealing with 80–100 people at any one time.

Most of the children have been referred to the unit by a general practitioner. To date, no referral has been rejected regardless of the severity of the condition or the presenting complaints. However, if the child is not a member of an intact family, we require that his discharge placement be determined before admission and that those who will care for him (usually foster or group-home parents), agree to work intensively with our staff during his stay in hospital.

To maximise use of the time devoted to treatment, as much information as possible must be gathered before the child's admission. Therefore, two weeks before admission, each member of the child's treatment team makes an individual assessment of the child and the family in their usual environment. The nurse, or child and family counsellor, has been assigned as a primary worker. This person will remain with the child throughout assessment, inpatient treatment and follow-up, and be responsible for their continuing treatment and for co-ordinating the child's programme. The primary care worker acts much like a primary care physician in the community, calling upon consultants as they are needed. It is felt that a consultation model (the primary care worker chooses whom amongst all the other staff to consult with and when), provides the primary care worker with greater responsibility and impetus to act in a professional manner, than a supervision model (the junior staff are required to meet regularly with senior staff), which tends to foster dependency, indecision and hierarchy building.

The information obtained during the pre-admission assessment is presented at the planning conference held the day of admission. This conference is attended by the child and his family, the treatment team members, representatives of other social agencies that may have been involved and the general practitioner, if he is available. The referred child, his parents and siblings are asked what they consider the problems to be and what changes they would like the staff to help them make. After hearing the staff's assessment the whole group works together to itemise the problems, isolate the key conflicts, establish treatment goals, and decide on the techniques to be used and assign the tasks to various therapists. The treatment plan may be modified by information presented at daily conferences held to review each family's progress during admission, but most goals are adhered to.

The teacher's pre-admission assessment of the child is done during a visit to the child's school, when he will observe the child's classroom and playground behaviour. The child's behaviour problems and possible learning disabilities are discussed with the classroom teacher. Additional data are obtained from the principal, school counsellor, school psychologist and former teachers who may have knowledge of this child's learning strengths and weaknesses, his social and personal characteristics, and the family's educational concern. Later the child and family are interviewed to discover their interests and worries about his school progress.

It is essential for the continuing health of a child that a family be maintained as a healthy, cohesive unit. Good evidence indicates that children need continuous care by two parents. There are many deleterious effects to children being placed outside their homes and they usually take their conflicts with them wherever they go. For these reasons, every effort is made to treat the whole family and return the child to his home. Treatment of the child's problems can only be successful if the home environment is changed. To do this requires the analysis and correction of the key conflicts, changing problem behaviours, teaching communication and parenting skills, establishing community contacts, etc. To determine what is happening in the family, and how severely the child is affected, requires at least two pre-admission home visits, interviews, questionnaires, educational, psychological and sensory-motor testing, a review of reports provided by community agencies, talks with community therapists, a physical examination and a medical investigation. If a community agency is recommending a foster home placement we do not become involved with assessment or treatment until it is decided who the foster parents will be and if they will work with us. We usually advise a referring agency to give our programme a try before giving up on a family.

Following admission we work hard to make the critical transition during the first few weeks as successful as possible by continuing the same techniques, modified for home and school settings. All the staff who have been involved with the family's treatment will continue seeing the child and his family two or three times a week for the following five weeks. We have found that the continuing involvement of the primary care worker is essential. This person has established a close relationship with the child and the child counts on him during the crisis that inevitably occurs, usually three or four weeks after admission. There is often a short honeymoon period, usually the first two weeks after discharge, then some of the problems temporarily reappear. If the family overreacts and begins to think that really nothing has changed, they suddenly become very negative towards the child. The child needs to know that his primary care worker will stand by him and the family must understand, with the support given by other staff members, that this is probably a temporary phenomenon. A realisation of these factors guided the government and hospital administration into deciding to fund our unit for enough staff to cover pre-admission assessments and follow-up therapy, something that was unique in both countries at the time it first began.

It is assumed, with good justification, that if parents could see themselves as successful parents, they would feel warmer towards their children and spend more time at being parents. With proper methods of communicating and management, those parents who humiliate and batter would find they would no longer have to abuse their children. When there is no longer a continuing hostility between the child and his parent, the child feels more inclined to please his parent, who responds in turn with greater warmth.

There are very few places in the world with enough child psychiatrists to assess and consult on severe child psychiatric problems, let alone treat them, but almost every family has a physician who would take a greater interest in children with emotional problems if he felt he had better back-up resources. Many community professionals who are treating very disturbed families and children could continue if they were confident of a treatment resource they could use when things became too difficult. General practitioners have responded to our invitation to remain involved while the child and his family are treated on our unit. Some attend family training, others spend time consulting with the physicians on the unit or participating in treatment. Social workers and teachers come to observe and learn whatever we find is successful in a particular case. Hopefully, if we can put enough time and effort into training community practitioners, they will feel more inclined to continue their treatment; or if the child is hospitalised, be more ready to pick up where we stop and continue the use of some of the techniques we have found successful.

If we are a community resource we must be able to receive referrals from any source. Many referrals have come from school counsellors, ministers, courts or social workers. To keep the medical lines of communication clear, they are asked to contact the family physician for a medical referral. Family physicians usually agree and almost always provide very helpful, additional information which often begins with the birth of the referred child. Community professionals are expected to continue their treatment while the child is hospitalised and we make offices available for them. They are invited to attend conferences, watch our staff, and ask as many questions as they like. Insights gained from these discussions are used to treat or guide other families.

The unit screening committee seeks to establish the proper mix of patients. Too many depressed, active, psychotic or retarded children have a bad effect on the milieu and many of the programmes. To date, the programme has not turned away a single patient who was too severely ill. The only ones who have been turned down for admission have been those few who have recovered while awaiting admission or those whose treatment could be tried on an outpatient basis first. The waiting list usually varies from one to three months in length.

The unit screening committee of five to six staff generally approve all referrals from reputable sources. We feel we are a community resource and it is up to the community to learn how best to use us. Since we are unable to assess a patient or family situation as accurately as a physician or social worker who have known the family for a long time, and since we cannot assess their ability to treat, we will accept their evaluation of the situation. This confidence in community professionals has seldom been abused.

When planning the unit we hypothesised that a programme geared to correct the problems as they occur in the community would be more efficient and more relevant than any programme that first admits, then diagnoses and plans treatment. This hypothesis is substantiated by the results to date (10). However, more time needs to be spent in making assessments in the community. The primary care staff have repeatedly reported that the few pre-admission home visits they were able to make are extremely valuable. Though a home visit might take twice as long as an interview on the unit, the staff usually discover as much as four times more, valuable information. The unit operates on the assumption that it is less costly to investigate the problem of a child in his family prior to admission than during admission.

When the RJH Unit was being planned 14 years ago we decided that since we were unable to predict which children would do well and which should be discharged when, it might be an idea to have an arbitrary length of admission for all children. Based on my previous experience (PGN) it appeared five weeks would be a reasonable guess at the time required for effective treatment of most problems. We believe that an interval of time at the end of the five-week follow-up period, during which there was no treatment from any resource, would be the best way of determining how well the family had been helped. However, any family which wasn't functioning well at the end of the twelve-week period, could request that the child be considered for re-admission. Over a 10-year period we found our re-admission rate ran between 6 and 7 per cent. Very few were re-admitted for a third time although one autistic child who was making slow but steady progress was admitted almost annually.

Second admissions have been useful in helping a child and family firmly establish some of the changes that occurred during second admissions or also used in instances where a child has been moved to a foster home following a breakdown of his own. The new admission would require the involvement of the foster parents who would also be involved in parent training. The second admissions were usually of the more severely ill children, including autistic, retarded, epileptic, psychotic or depressed children. Although we have been engaged in a longitudinal study seeking to discover the best prognostic indicators, our hypothesis that we are unable to predict which child is going to succeed seems to be correct. There have been many surprises. In fact, it is hard not to believe the staff's opinion that the more disturbed a child is the greater will be our success.

The five-week admission is sometimes a phase in the child's total treatment that begins and ends in the community. Thus it is important that the community therapists are involved in the child's treatment while he is hospitalised. Their contribution to the unit's programme is co-ordinated with that of the hospital staff at the admission conference. They are encouraged to intensify their treatment from the usual once a week contact to at least two or three times a week during the hospitalisation to help accelerate any change. They are given office space and some secretarial help.

In situations where the child is first brought to the attention of a social worker or physician in the community, who, after examination, deems it necessary to have the child hospitalised, the referral is made to the unit. Once the screening committee has decided on a date and a primary therapist is assigned, that person is involved in the child's evaluation and treatment right through to the end of follow-up. In situations where social workers, public health nurses, counsellors or physicians are the primary therapist in the community, it is important that they have a major role in planning the treatment programme. Any transfer of responsibility should take place in the community well before and after the inpatient component of the treatment.

The Programme

In the majority of instances the five-week treatment programme is definitive. The short intensive treatment usually does not require prolonged therapies. In some ways it is the psychiatric corollary of the surgical model of treatment. The therapist limits his intervention to only that area which is disturbed or diseased. He tries hard to avoid disturbing normal tissue, cuts quickly and cleanly and gets out of the operative site as soon as possible. In this psychiatric programme, the therapist works to ensure that his intervention does not weaken healthy relationships and does not create unnecessary dependencies upon professional people.

There are fairly discrete phases of the treatment programme:

1. Crisis. There is often an ongoing problem which, because of the events, becomes a crisis, during which the family decides to seek professional help.

2. Assessment and Consideration. When a professional has interviewed the family and upon his recommendation the family consider hospitalisation, there is usually an immediate positive response, 'Yes, this sounds like just the thing, please tell me more.'

3. Ambivalent. When the family goes home to think more about the proposal to admit their child they become very ambivalent, 'He is liable to think we don't love him.' At this time it is important that the referring agency carefully works through the family's mixed feelings and looks at all the options. 'Johnny is probably aware of your mixed feelings, but from my understanding he quite realises that it would be in all of your best interests.' It is helpful for the family to visit the ward and possibly have the parents attend one training seminar.

4. Decisions. The family finally make a decision that they will go along with the recommendation and accept the date assigned for admission. At this point, the anxiety diminishes considerably and symptoms often tend to disappear. The family think that because things are suddenly getting better, that there may not be a need for hospitalisation after all.

5. Planning Conference. This conference involves staff and community professionals who are usually, by this time, quite well known to the family, but it is a large and somewhat intimidating group of people. We make attempts to ensure it is a reasonably relaxed and friendly occasion, but people are there obviously to work hard at putting together a treatment programme, symbolised by having a table in the middle of the group. The parents are usually very anxious and somewhat inhibited but it is surprising how well they can talk and with some encouragement, participate very well in the planning. Because many phenomena are crowded together it is a little bit like an initiation.

6. First Week − Separation Relief. The parents feel considerable relief at no longer having the irritating child on their hands. After recouping their energies, the relief makes them begin to think that maybe they don't want the child back at all and the best thing would be to have him placed in a foster home. The child on the unit is usually anxious, but his curiosity, enjoyment of the good things involved, e.g. swimming pool, and the close relationship with his therapist and the relief of being away from his parents, tend to outweigh all other feelings.

7. Second Week. During this period the parents begin to realise how much work is involved in getting down to changing themselves and their family. They also begin to feel guilty at enjoying the child's absence and to overcome this, they often start bringing elaborate gifts for the child. The child in the unit, during the second week, begins to feel sad and misses his parents. He shows evidence of a pseudo-depression and it reminds us how wise it is to diagnose a child before admission. During this time the child is saying goodbye to his parents and becoming increasingly attached to his primary therapist. This is facilitated by nurturing.

8. Weeks Three and Four. This is a period when most of the hard work is done and the largest gains are made. During the first weekend home, the parents are amazed at how much change has taken place in their child and they become very hopeful, but at the same time, they suspect that it cannot last. The child is good partly because he is trying so hard to please his parents. During the second weekend home, there is a more realistic view of the parents and children when small problems may reoccur. It provides a testing ground of all that the child and parents have learned and an opportunity to refine the guidelines and consequences.

9. Fifth Week. During this time the child is involved in saying goodbye to the unit, although he knows that his primary therapist will continue with him during post-discharge follow-up. Changes are being consolidated, but often the child expresses fears that his family haven't changed and that problems will reoccur. During this time the parents, in their anxiety, go through a brief period of pessimism. They are reassured by staff who use the child's accumulated records to demonstrate how much has changed in the child and the parents themselves.

10. Discharge Conference. This is another critical time which, if all goes well, provides many good feelings for the parents, children and staff. The staff are encouraged to be realistic in their report but try to emphasise the positive aspects.

11. Follow-up, Weeks One and Two. This is a honeymoon period when any change that has occurred provides the children and their parents with considerable enjoyment. The parents, trying hard to make sure things will work, go out of their way to give the child good things and give him much positive feedback.

12. Follow-up, Weeks Three and Four – Testing. During this time the child is less on guard, may show some evidence of an old problem, which may create a panic in the parents. 'Look, he still does it! I knew nothing really changed.' It is important that the staff be able to respond quickly to these minor crises. It is during this time also that the staff are saying goodbye.

13. Follow-up, Week Five. During this time a new beginning for the whole family is occurring. The staff complete their goodbyes and deal with the anxieties the parents feel in being cut loose.

14. Post Follow-up. During this time, all contact with the therapists on the unit is terminated and the family sinks or swims. Often, without any contact with professionals, they begin to realise how many strengths they have and though they may have to struggle, they find that they swim very well, thank you. During this time a family physician or social agency is asked to keep a distant eye on the family, but not to intervene unless absolutely necessary. If things do go wrong, the family are requested to contact first their family physician, who has a complete report with recommendations. At this point his ability to pick up what the therapists have done and use the same techniques, reassures the family that they can probably carry on.

The Christchurch Hospital Unit provides nine beds for pre-programmed admission and one for emergency admissions. Children who are acutely psychotic, suicidal, dangerous fire lighters, etc., can have an immediate 48-hour hospitalisation. During that time, the child can be roughly assessed. This time also provides an opportunity for the social worker or psychiatrist to make arrangements for alternative accommodation, if placement outside the home is necessary. Following the child's discharge from the emergency bed, any additional assessment will be made before he is referred for a period of pre-programmed hospitalisation. Parents and professionals clearly understand the bed must be emptied every 48 hours and under no circumstances may a child stay longer. This ensures that the bed is always available for emergency situations and no back-door admissions occur.

This unit works on a system in which parents gradually assume more care of their children during their hospitalisation. The primary care staff work out a detailed programme outlining the goals for the parents and fit it into the child's weekly schedule. The parents have a copy of this.

Times are allotted when parents are expected to be on the unit for training and observing and these times are scheduled on the child's timetable. The staff begin by introducing the parents to the ward routine, other staff members and giving them some opportunity to observe their child from behind a one-way mirror. By explaining, modelling, instructing, rehearsing and testing, the staff teach parents some of the techniques that should continue at home. Before children are encouraged to assert themselves, it is important to determine just what type of assertion the parents will tolerate. Some parents cannot stand children who are too uppity, brash or impertinent but the level fluctuates during treatment. They become more tolerant as time progresses.

The Child and Family Unit at Christchurch Hospital has a double bed used for parents primarily for the nurturing programme. Like the child's nurturing programme, parents spend three days in bed and during that time they are helped to regress, develop an awareness of their childlike needs and deal with some of the traumatic incidents in their life. Their children often first express concern about the parents' health, then become increasingly anxious also to nurture their parents. They are allowed to, in small but significant ways.

Because of the intense interaction, volunteers are sometimes used to nurture the parents. These are volunteers who are carefully selected and who are willing to continue involvement with the parents after the child has been discharged from follow-up. They act as models, supports and help introduce the family to community supports and recreation.

During the child's two weekend passes home parents have an opportunity to test their ability and apply the knowledge they have recently gained. They are given weekend guidelines which include little forms on which they are expected to make observations and sometimes count behaviours. Following the weekend, there is a debriefing session where the parent and primary care worker discuss how things went, what needs to be changed and what areas of the treatment programme need emphasis during the last two weeks. The programmes have had a large percentage of parents who batter their children. These parents have benefited greatly from understanding the dynamics of the pathological interaction, a more objective assessment of their children and better ways of interacting and communicating with them.

Out-of-town parents have posed a problem of accessibility and involvement. We expect up to 25 per cent of the children admitted to be from towns in rural areas. Our ability to help these children is limited by the fact that their parents cannot afford the money or the time, and distances are considerable. However, we found it remarkable how much effort parents will put into being present, some travelling 400 or 500 miles each weekend to be involved in their child's programme. We have proposed a hospital-run motel or facility which would permit parents an opportunity to stay near the ward at a reasonable rate. Many have taken two weeks of their annual holiday and stayed in local hotels or motels. During the two weeks they receive more intensive therapies, including insight-oriented psychotherapy, learning communication skills, behaviour management and transactional analysis.

It is proven to be very valuable for staff to differentiate between training or teaching sessions and listening and understanding sessions. To some extent it is necessary to split staff and often the primary care staff find themselves doing the teaching or training techniques while more senior staff are involved in insight-oriented psychotherapy. It is possible, however, that one staff member can do both if it is made clear to the child when one or the other is happening. This can be facilitated by making sure that listening sessions take place in quite different offices from the training sessions.

The school teaching staff work towards providing a satisfactory quality of instruction which complements the philosophy and objectives of the treatment programme. Schooling is provided five days each week during normal school hours. Priorities of treatment or school are sorted out at the admission conference or week to week at the ward rounds. The teachers complete a general education assessment to determine the level of academic achievement. Instruction and assignments are provided which are suited to individual pupils grade level placement and ability. For those children who have struggled with learning difficulties, observational and psychometric data are utilised to determine the possibility of a specific learning disability. We have found that a large percentage of children who are thought to have learning disabilities, in fact have depression which undercuts their motivation, or anxiety which interferes with their concentration. The teacher tries out a variety of techniques and whatever he finds successful is demonstrated to the child's usual teacher, who willingly visits from time to time.

Many children have an aversive, conditioned response to school and nothing seems to motivate them. These children do very well on teaching machines where the corrective feedback, though immediate and accurate, is impersonal and never pejorative. The primary care staff act as ego auxiliary, supporting the child, feeding back to him emotional responses and training him in how to deal with the pressure of schoolwork.

When the patient is discharged a prescriptive report is forwarded to the school in which there are recommendations modifying the child's learning environment. The unit teachers are careful not to write reports that could not possibly be carried out in a class of 35 children. During the five-week follow-up period, the unit teacher visits the school to observe the child's behaviour and to discuss with his teacher how the recommendations are working. As at home, there is often a honeymoon period followed by a few crises; it is important, therefore, that the unit teacher be available by telephone to advise and reassure the child's home teacher. Having made school visits the unit teacher sometimes advises the child be placed in a different programme, but wherever possible the child is kept in his local school and with his peers.

On the Friday preceding discharge, the child, his family and various community professionals meet the ward staff for the discharge conference. At this time, the primary care staff remind everyone of the key conflicts and objectives, before reviewing the child's progress, technique by technique. Each of the other staff involved reports on changes, being as objective as possible, but highlighting the progress made. As in the admission conference, attendance is determined by the parents or guardians. If they do not want some of the more personal material discussed in front of the child's teachers or principal they are politely asked to leave.

At the discharge conference the reports include performance on psychological assessments, occupational therapy batteries, blood tests, EEGs, etc. We have found that being frank with parents about their child's functioning enables them to be more realistic and objective in their expectations. Parents hardly ever misinterpret the findings and place greater pressure on the child. The parents are given frank feedback about themselves and the child is informed regarding his physical, emotional and biochemical status. The parents and family are given every opportunity to ask any question they wish. When these are all answered as forthrightly as possible, the group make plans for the follow-up period and duties are assigned. The discharge conference has proved to be a warm, emotionally-charged, critical point, that fixes many impressions in the minds of everyone there. Often it ends with a spontaneous tribute from the parents to the hard work and patience of the staff.

In order to continue the effect of the treatment programme, specific written directions are provided for the child, the family, the family physician and the school. The hospitalised child has his own report which includes a brief statement of the problems he has encountered at his level of understanding, together with reminders and advice. The parents are given a more detailed prescription including a set of tested guidelines and consequences. They are reminded about what they have learned, observations about their child, tips on communication and detailed advice on family management. A detailed medical report is written for the referring physician. It contains an abbreviated history of the present illness, psychiatric evaluation, psychological, occupational and school reports, together with lab. results and a copy of the guidelines written for the parents and for the child. If it is indicated, the physician may, using his own judgement, share pertinent information with other professionals, but the hospital does not usually allow written medical reports to be shared with other community professionals. They are informed, however, that we will discuss matters with them.

The school staff provide counsellors and teachers with a detailed teaching prescription, including a summary of the child's behavioural difficulties at school, changes made during treatment, test results, teaching techniques that have worked and advice for his future schooling. His ability on tests, his various weaknesses and strengths, are detailed so that his teachers, school counsellors or principal, can organise a programme as similar as possible to the one that worked on the unit. During follow-up, reference is often made to the prescriptions.

The teacher, primary care staff or physician often ask, 'Were you able to stick with the recommendations and if not, let's examine why not?'

During the five-week follow-up, the child is visited by the primary care staff. The visit includes the child reporting on how he is adapting. The therapist may rehearse some of the techniques used during the hospitalisation. The primary care staff are also available on the telephone during their shift or the child may phone the secondary staff during the other shifts. Generally, the primary care staff make two visits in the first week, three during the second and third weeks and one on each of the last two weeks. It is very important that the child properly disengages from the primary care staff to whom he has become very attached. This process has begun during the child's discharge and carries on through the follow-up period.

The Results

It has been an important component of the programme of the Child and Family Unit, to monitor the programme's effectiveness. To do this we have taken measures before, immediately after and at one year's follow-up. Using this information, we have made changes in the programme. To date it appears we have been reasonably effective, effective enough to warrant a continuation of the basic components of the therapeutic regime.

All admissions were given the Peterson-Quay (11) inventory of child behaviour problems. Twelve months later the same checklist was mailed out to all families along with a supplementary questionnaire developed by the unit staff. During 1979 there were 102 admissions, i.e. two per week. Boys outnumbered girls by more than 2:1. The most typical male patient would be a Grade 3 boy with anxiety and school adjustment problems. The most typical female patient would be a depressed, post-pubertal girl. The age distribution of boys and girls is a bimodel curve.

Of the 102 admissions, five had been admitted previously including one autistic boy who was admitted five times. Only first-time admissions were included in the present survey. Three families who admitted more than one child were excluded. Most of the children came from the Greater Victoria area but 42 per cent were from small towns and rural areas. In addition to the checklist, questionnaires of child and family function were mailed to 94 families one year after the child's discharge.

Table 1.1: Most Frequent Diagnoses of 1979 Admissions

Diagnosis	Boys	Girls
Behaviour disorder of childhood/adolescence	20	7
Depressive neurosis	16	6
Anxiety neurosis	5	2
Adjustment reaction of childhood/adolescence	3	2
Hyperkinetic syndrome	4	—
Mental retardation	3	1
Unsocialised conduct disorder	3	—
School phobia	—	2
Autism	2	—
Runaway reaction	2	—
Other or not given	15	9
Total	73	29

Table 1.2: Results: Mean P-Q Scores Prior to Admission and One Year After Discharge

Scale	Pre-admission	Follow-up	P
Unsocialised aggression/psychotherapy	21.26	12.44	.001
Neuroticism	12.56	7.78	.001
Inadequacy/immaturity	6.26	3.93	.005
Socialised delinquency	2.22	1.63	.05

A second questionnaire was mailed three weeks later to 34 families who had not responded to the first mailing. In all, 46 questionnaires were received, another 15 were returned by the Post Office. About one-third of the families surveyed had moved during the year since discharge. The return rate was 58 per cent and only 24 per cent of the sample were unaccounted for.

The most severely disturbed children were admitted and no child was excluded from admission because he or she was too severely ill. There was some disparity in diagnosis between the four child psychiatrists admitting patients, mainly due to a difference in diagnostic criteria, but all types of disorder were treated. Mixed anxiety, neurotic and behaviour disorders were the most common diagnosis in both sexes but depressive disorders were increasingly more frequently diagnosed (5).

The Peterson-Quay behaviour problem checklist used scores on four factor analytic scales with acceptable standards of reliability and validity. Mean pre-admission and follow-up scores indicate improvement

Figure 1.1: Age at Admission (to last birthday) 1979 Admissions

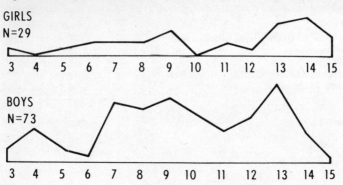

Figure 1.2: Parental Ratings of Unit Effectiveness

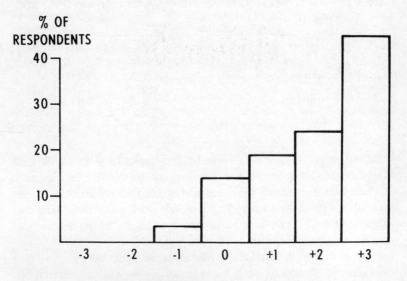

in all four parameters. Probability values were derived from one-tailed T tests for related means.

At one year's follow-up, 28 per cent of children had changed school classes since discharge. In many cases this was the result of an explicit recommendation by the Family Unit teachers. Of the respondents, 24 per cent indicated the referred child had been sent home from school at least once during the year following discharge. Four per cent had been sent home five times or more and 2 per cent of families indicated the referred child had been expelled permanently from school.

Twenty per cent of the children had been in trouble with the police since discharge but only two children had three or more contacts with the police, 13 per cent reported no change, 7 per cent reported a decrease.

Following discharge the majority of families had contact with various treatment resources, usually the referring physicians. Nine per cent of the families responded they had broken up in some sense, two children went to foster homes, one to a group home and one went to live with relatives. In some cases these moves were recommended. No respondents indicated they would definitely like their child to be re-admitted but 15 per cent were not certain.

To the question, how did the family find the treatment programme, the largest group of respondents (40 per cent) chose the most positive alternative on a seven point scale, 'very helpful'. The mean reading was 1.9 or 'moderately helpful'. In addition, most families took the opportunity to make qualitative comments about the overall effectiveness of the programme, e.g. 'Behaviour problems worsened for approximately two months after discharge', 'Extreme anger on child's part from visit to the Family Unit, but all is well now', 'He still requires psychological help of a very intensive nature and constant supervision', 'I feel he needs a great amount of help yet he feels better about being admitted', 'Is there any way his stepfather could sit in on your once a week discussions?', 'The time with you was very helpful to us and continues to be as long as we can remember what we learned'.

To date more than 900 children have been admitted to the unit and an evaluation of their progress has been carried out. Of the first 350 children that we treated (aged between 13 months and 15 years), we found that the length and the mean number of readmissions had decreased from 28 per cent to 6 per cent since the time-limit programme was introduced in 1972 (9). Although we accepted for treatment all types of the most severe problems, 98 per cent of the children went back to the homes they had on admission and on six months' follow-up, 94 per cent of the children were still there. Over the nine years for 900 admissions the readmission rate has remained constant at 7 per cent.

The survey is only quasi-experimental but uses each patient as his own control. Changes in behaviour in the interim between admission and one-year follow-up could be due to maturation or other influences. However, parents generally attribute positive behaviour change to the Family Unit programme. The magnitude of changes is remarkable. 'Unsocialised aggression/psychopathy' includes a variety of disinhibitive behaviours including fighting, poor responsibility and non-compliance to adult authority. The 'neuroticism' scale measures behaviour mediated by anxiety including depression, fearfulness and social withdrawal. The third scale 'inadequacy/immaturity', refers to a syndrome comprised of passivity, short attention span and underachievement in school. The fourth scale 'socialised delinquency', is not particularly appropriate for the Family Unit population, referring as it does to subculturally induced anti-social behaviours of adolescents. Nevertheless, statistically significant improvement was reported on this dimension, as well as those which are more readily recognisable among patients in the unit.

The increasing demand for treatment may be a result of the increasing awareness of psychiatric problems. The apparent increase in depression may indicate that children are not responding well to the increasing rates of divorce and family break-up. Since long periods of psychiatric care do not seem to benefit many children and the costs are becoming increasingly high, the programme for this 10-bed unit attempted to concentrate treatment into a short period and provide equal opportunity to the many children who needed intensive care. Since it seems almost impossible to predict which children will respond well to a psychiatric, inpatient treatment and which children will do well on discharge, treatment was terminated or handed to a community agency after an arbitrary period. There is no good evidence that we possess the criteria to make accurate prognoses. Thus an unnecessarily long period of hospitalisation may indicate the staff's difficulty in detaching from their patient more than it does the child's need for treatment. Lewis *et al*. (7) point out that the disruptive effect of breaking the child–therapist bond is so great, staff may need to continue involvement with the family through and beyond adolescence.

The predetermined period of hospitalisation appears to have advantages over indeterminant hospitalisation. Knowing exactly how long the child will remain with them, staff are able to involve themselves personally to an optimum degree. Not fearing they will be suddenly detached from their child at the whim of the attending physician, they allow themselves to become quickly involved in a meaningful relationship. Knowing that the parents are waiting to receive the child back, they are less resentful of the parents' intrusion.

The child is able to maintain his family and community attachments knowing that he will soon return to them, much like a period of time at summer camp. This removes a great anxiety from the child, allowing him to participate more actively in the change process. Each patient is encouraged to remain in contact by writing to his friends and inviting them to join him on the unit for floor hockey, etc. Since his friends have also been seen in a psychiatric setting they are less likely to tease the patient when he rejoins them at school.

Knowing when the child will leave and return to them, families tend to remain attached. Rather than extrude the child and sigh with relief when that noxious little particle is no longer irritating them, the families are more likely to continue working at the problem together. Rather than closing ranks which exclude the child, they remain open to receive him back. Since they know the unit will not take the child until they have committed themselves to involvement, at first they may participate grudgingly. Later, finding they also benefit, families readily attend family training, child observing and psychotherapy sessions regularly.

With an increasing backlog of children who require treatment, there is a tendency in some inpatient units to select only the most severely ill. When only the worst are treated the outcome hardly justifies the hospitalisation. Treatment programmes which attempt to select those children who should benefit, may be selecting only those children who improve with any kind of treatment. When equal emphasis is given to the dynamic, transactional, behavioural, chemical and cognitive aspects of the child's problem, using techniques that are prescribable and measurable, there seems to be a reasonably good outcome. Though they both treat the full range of the most severely disturbed children, with a 2 per cent to 5 per cent rate of referrals to foster care and a 7 per cent to 8 per cent readmission rate after a 33-day inpatient stay, the Royal Jubilee and the Christchurch Hospital Family Restoration Units compare quite well with other (4, 8, 12, 13) inpatient units.

References

1. Adams, P.L. 'Children and paraservices of the community mental health centers', *J. Am. Acad. Child Psychiatry* (1975), 14: 18-31.
2. Barker, P. *The Residential Psychiatric Treatment of Children* (John Wiley & Sons, New York, 1974)
3. Berlin, I.N. 'Some methods for reversing the myth of child treatment in community mental health centers', *J. Am. Acad. Child Psychiatry* (1975) 14: 76-94
4. Blinder, P.J., Young, W.M., Fireman, K.P. and Miller, S.J. 'The children's psychiatric hospital unit in the community: concept and development', *Am. J. Psychiatry* (1978), 135: 848-51
5. Colbert, P., Newman, B., Ney, P.G. and Young, J. 'Learning disabilities as a symptom of depression in children', *J. Learn. Disab.* (1982), 15: 333-6

6. Harbin, H.T. 'A family-oriented psychiatric inpatient unit', *Family Process* (1979), 18: 281-91
7. Lewis, M., Lewis, D.O., Shanok, S.S. *et al*. 'The undoing of residential treatment: a follow-up study of 51 adolescents', *J. Am. Acad. Child Psychiatry* (1980), 19: 160-8
8. Lynch, M., Steinberg, D. and Ounsted, C. 'Family unit in a children's psychiatric hospital', *Brit. Med. J.* (19 April 1975), 2: 127-9
9. Ney, P.G. and Mills, W.A. 'A time-limited treatment programme for children and their families', *Hosp. Comm. Psychiatry* (1976), 27: 878-9
10. Ney, P.G., Mulvihill, D. and Hanna, R. 'The effectiveness of child psychiatric inpatient care', *Can. J. Psych.* (in press)
11. Peterson, D.R., Quay, H.C. and Cameron, G.R. 'Personality and background factors in juvenile delinquency as inferred from questionnaire responses', *J. Consult. Psychology* (1959), 23: 395-9
12. Shafii, M., McCue, A., Ice, J.F. and Schwab, J.J. 'The development of an acute short-term inpatient child psychiatric setting: A pediatric-psychiatric model', *Am. J. Psychiatry* (1979), 136: 427-30
13. Traffert, D.A. 'Child psychiatric unit in a psychiatric hospital', *Arch. Gen. Psychiatry* (1969), 21: 745-52
14. Winsberg, B.G., Bialer, I., Kupietz, S. *et al*. 'Home vs hospital care of children with behaviour disorders; a controlled investigation', *Arch. Gen. Psychiatry* (1980), 37: 413-18

2 THE PHILOSOPHY OF THE FAMILY RESTORATION PROGRAMME

Introduction

The programme philosophy at the child and family psychiatric unit of the Family Restoration Programme has been developed over a 14-year period. Out of his 20-year experience in child psychiatry this author (PGN) has had the opportunity to plan the programme of four child psychiatric units and participate in the formation of two others. The practical techniques elaborated in this book are designed to deal with the real problems occurring when nurses and other front line staff put into practice treatment objectives for the multi-faceted problems of psychiatrically ill children and their parents.

Increasing Demand for Treatment

Problem

The World Health Organisation has stated that the increase in suicide in adolescents is epidemic. Whether there is a real increase in the number of psychiatrically ill children, or whether our increasing awareness makes us more sensitive to the number of disturbed children previously undiagnosed, is a point yet to be decided by research. Yet if loss is the important determinant of depression, the fact that approximately 50 per cent of American children are losing one parent during their early lives, would make us support that there is an increasing number of depressed children.

As discussed in the Overview, in addition to the increasing demand for treatment there is a growing awareness that long-stay treatment is not necessarily beneficial. Although long-stay treatment might be indicated in a few children, there is no evidence that duration of the inpatient stay is related to a beneficial outcome. Unfortunately, as inpatient care becomes increasingly expensive, so there is increasing pressure on hospitals to provide more efficient care.

Clinicians have considerable difficult in predicting which children will benefit from inpatient care. It is also hard to decide when a child should be discharged. Psychiatrists wish to be reasonably sure that children will stay sufficiently well not to require hospitalisation, but there are few guidelines. There are no good data available to predict accurately which child will sink and which child will swim after discharge. Physicians tend to prognosticate on the basis of their expectations, these expectations being more determined by response to treatment than by diagnosis or objective assessment.

The increasing demands, the inability to predict which children will benefit from inpatient care and the question of when children should be discharged are factors which produce a backlog of patients needing treatment. Since it is not possible to treat all children who might benefit from inpatient care, there is a tendency either to treat the most disturbed or to treat the ones most likely to get well. If only the worst are treated, inpatient care may be seen to be ineffective. If only the most likely to improve are treated, it is possible that we are expending an expensive resource on children who would have improved with outpatient treatment.

Programme

A cornerstone to the philosophy of The Family Restoration Programme is that we will accept every child, regardless of how severely ill he or she is. This means that firestarters, psychotic and autistic children, epileptic children and those with severe behavioural difficulties, children with severe emotional problems, intellectual or physical disabilities and children with a variety of psychosomatic illnesses and emotional problems, may all be admitted. The admission criteria has been empirical. Generally the decision is made by the referring source. We seldom question a well-known family physician, school counsellor or social worker: they can best judge their capabilities and the extent of the child and family pathology. Having their judgement questioned by an admission assessing person who has only seen the child once, may be insulting.

Our general admission criteria are:

(1) Treatment failures: those children who failed to progress or who are becoming worse in spite of treatment.
(2) Children with a high level of personal psychic pain and distress which cannot be alleviated by other methods.
(3) Children with severe disorders, i.e. suicide, acute depression, psychosis, etc.
(4) Children who are experiencing or who are at risk of physical, emotional or sexual abuse or neglect.
(5) Children and families where there needs to be an increase in the

intensity of treatment to provide discernible progress.
(6) Emergencies.
(7) Children who are causing family disintegration.

All children are admitted for precisely the same amount of time, regardless of their age, sex, diagnosis or apparent prognosis. The unit takes an empirical approach and provides all children with an equal opportunity. Rather than discharging the child when he may appear to be ready for discharge, all children are discharged after five weeks of inpatient treatment. Each of these children then receives five weeks of follow-up, at their home, from ward staff. When this ends, our care terminates.

This empirical model recognises there is little science to the prediction of psychiatric illness. However, staff members are asked to try and guess whether the child will succeed or fail following discharge. Because the children are followed up for this five-week interval, then checked at one year after discharge, we are accumulating data which will make it possible to predict which children will do better with which treatment techniques.

Net Effect

Since all severely ill children are accepted, staff are not influenced by factors of race, sex, intellect or socio-economic status in choosing when to admit or discharge. Because staff know exactly how long the child will be hospitalised they are better able to attach and detach. Knowing how long the child is with them, they do not hesitate to become attached. Knowing when the child is to be discharged, they can start saying goodbye at an appropriate time. The staff know that regardless of how unready for discharge the child appears to be, he will certainly leave them on a definite date. This tends to force them to look for child and family strengths.

Children's discharges are not delayed by the protective attitude of staff. Since the staff are less possessive and protective of their charges, they require that parents play a greater part in the treatment process. Parents are seen with less scepticism and are given greater opportunities to demonstrate their strengths.

Because the child knows when he is to be discharged, he has fewer uncertainties with which to deal. The child knows that his good or bad behaviour will not influence the date of discharge. Since he knows when he will be returning to his school and peers it is easier for him to maintain contact with them. Instead of trying to calculate how to react he can get on with serious psychotherapy. He does not have to go through a process of mourning such as he might if he were not sure how long he would be in hospital.

Because the family knows exactly when the child will return to them, they tend not to close ranks, but leave space open for the child. Too often in the past the child has been treated as a foreign body. When he is gone from their midst, the family sighs with relief. That relief becomes the reason with which they justify their intention to keep the child out of the home. All the time the child is cared for by hospital staff the family become increasingly adept at rationalising their desire to let the child go. 'He does so much better in hospital. Obviously he should not live with us. Don't you think you should find him some nice family where he would be happier?'

Increasing Demand for Assessment

Problem

When society is unable to deal with its difficult members, there is a tendency to hand out labels and then to isolate those who are labelled. When parents cannot face their guilt and conflict with respect to a disturbed child, they seek someone to label the child. The label may provide them with a reason to treat the child differently and possibly exclude him. More caring parents don't want labels, they want explanations. Since explanations from professionals are hard to come by, they often have to settle for a label. It becomes apparent that almost everyone wants some kind of a diagnosis. With a diagnosis they can explain to themselves or to others why they are so unhappy or frightened.

Unfortunately, many child psychiatric or mental health centres provide diagnosis but few explanations and insufficient treatment. The net effect is that children, once labelled by a professional, are labelled by their family and eventually by themselves. They then tend to treat themselves and are treated by others as disabled. The net result is an increase in the number of children who are considered a liability by the community. When there is increasing demand to curtail the expenditure of funds in social agencies there is also a tendency to isolate those labelled children.

Professionals in the community and caring parents are often frustrated by having diagnostic labels given to children without any specific recommendations. When parents are given recommendations they may be unable to carry them out because they've never been taught how, or because they have conflicts which interfere with their understanding of the recommendation. In other instances recommendations don't work because they have never been tried on the child. Had they been tried it may have become apparent that a recommendation, although it might apply to other children with a similar diagnosis, does not work with this particular child.

Diagnoses in children are too often made from static tests given in an unusual environment. It is apparent that diagnostic tests and interviews in offices are not good indicators of the strengths or weaknesses the child usually exhibits at home or school. Even the best psychological tests say little about how children might improve under other conditions.

Programme

From the outset, The Family Restoration Programme has relied upon the rates of change in behaviour, attitude or dynamics to make diagnoses, treatment plans or recommendations. Although the usual tests from psychology, medicine, social work and occupational therapy are used, these are compared with or validated by rates of change. The greater credence is given to the rates of change. The shape of the curve representing the child's performance during a certain period and under controlled conditions of treatment is a good predictor of the child's future performance.

If the child has a learning disability, the rate of change in the growth of his vocabulary during inpatient treatment is a good predictor of how well he can learn if the environment approximates the same conditions. If the child is autistic, the increase in the amount of time he spends exploring is a good predictor of how well he will acquire new concepts at home if the parents use objects and techniques similar to those on the unit. If the child has a behaviour problem, the increase in compliance or in positive peer interactions are good predictors of the child's later behaviour. If the child is encopretic, the number of clean days and the size of the stools are good indicators of how long the child will stay clean once he leaves hospital.

Net Effect

All the staff are involved in measuring, therefore each staff member becomes aware of the elements of a child's behaviour that are important for accurate assessment. They become aware of their own skills and are able to indicate which type of problem they will work with best. Because all staff are involved in measuring they are all in a position to help assess the efficiency of a particular treatment technique or programme. Measuring rates of change in attitudes and behaviour provides corrective feedback to individual staff. Since staff tend to be influenced by halo or storm effects, accurate corrective feedback gives them opportunity to understand their own biases and blind spots.

The graphs that are used to illustrate the rate of change can also be used to convince parents they should give the techniques a good try. When confronted by sceptical professionals and colleagues outside the unit, staff members will demonstrate a technique and then illustrate its efficiency with accurate measures of change.

Although it is easier to measure behaviour only, attempts are made to define and measure attitude, conflict and emotion. We have found that it is possible to meaure a particular behaviour which is indicative of inner conflict. These behaviours are seen as sign behaviours which may accurately indicate the size of the problem in a particular area.

Appropriate Diagnosis

Problem

Too frequently, psychiatric patients have been admitted and then diagnosed. Unfortunately, the behaviour they exhibit within an institution may be more typical of that unusual setting than it is of their behaviour under their usual home conditions. The treatment may then depend upon the diagnosis engendered by the atypical behaviour in hospital. When the hospital behaviour is changed, treatment is considered to be successful, and the patient is discharged. Unfortunately, he is discharged into the community having changed few of the problems that he exhibited while in his usual home environment. In this way the patients become better adapted to living in the hospital situation than at home. Because the treatment is determined by the hospital environment, their behaviour is made more appropriate for that environment. In this way children are institutionalised.

Children in unusual environments often exhibit few of their usual strengths. A child may be very careful in cutting the lawn or caring for pets but doesn't have an opportunity to demonstrate these skills while in hospital. Because few strengths are seen, poor prognoses are made and low expectations are held by the staff. As a consequence, children are too often sent for further institutional care or for foster home placement. Children have an uncanny way of performing according to people's expectations and, if these are low, the child performs poorly.

With the trimming of medical budgets and the increasing cost of hospital care, it becomes important to evaluate the cost-effectiveness of treatment programmes. If the child is admitted and then diagnosed, he is taking up very expensive hospital space waiting for test results. While decisions are being made regarding his diagnosis and treatment, he may spend many weeks gradually regressing.

Programme

The Family Restoration Programme seeks to evaluate and diagnose a child prior to hospital admission. This evaluation will involve nurses, social workers and teachers observing the child functioning in his normal environment. While watching him in school and home, notations are made in such areas as his strengths and weaknesses, the conflicts he appears to have and the setting or reinforcing stimuli to which he seems to respond. Parents are asked to help in the pre-admission evaluation by completing questionnaires about themselves and their children. They are also given forms on which they can rate their child's temperament and a number of problem behaviours.

Because strengths as well as weaknesses are recorded, it is possible to see if the child loses some of his adaptive abilities once he is hospitalised. Having strengths in mind, the staff are in a position to reinforce growth and maturity which might otherwise remain unrecognised. While hospitalised, the child is given every opportunity to continue his participation in sports, Scouts or band.

Children are referred by a social worker, counsellor or agency concerned about a problem child, but ultimately the referral is passed through a physician. A screening committee looks at the available information, confers with anyone professionally involved with the family and makes a decision regarding whether he should be hospitalised and when. The admission date is influenced by the variety of children already on the unit. It has been found that having either too many depressed or hyperactive or behavioural problem children at one time creates a difficult environment. One object of the screening committee is to create an optimum environment by having the right mix of children. We make sure that there are not too many of any single diagnosis and that there are a sufficient number of children in the same age group so that every child has someone to relate to of approximately the same age and sex.

Once a decision is made to admit the child, a date for admission is fixed. For three weeks before the admission, the staff becomes involved in a detailed assessment of the child and his family. Standardised tests are used and compared with home and school evaluations. The primary care worker, intern, social worker and occupational therapist assess the child and family in their home and community. The teacher observes the child in his classroom and in the playground. Medical and psychological tests are done. The child is given an opportunity to see the unit and meet the other children. The parents are encouraged to begin attending parenting classes prior to the child's admission. By the time the child is to be admitted, the diagnostic evaluation is sufficiently complete to make possible a fairly comprehensive treatment plan.

Setting the date of the child's admission well in advance provides an opportunity for community professionals and the parents to make arrangements to be present at the admission conference. For parents who live far from the hospital, the admission date is set to coincide with times they are able to be away from home. They are encouraged to take at least two weeks of their annual vacation and live near the hospital. Sometimes the hospital can provide accommodation which is less expensive than the community hotels. At the Christchurch Unit, accommodation on the ward can be provided for one set of parents.

Net Effect

By assessing the children in their home environment, the parents develop a greater confidence in the staff and the assessment. 'Now you see him as we do.' 'Having been in our place during meal times, you can understand how irritated we become with his outrageous behaviour.'

Since more appropriate diagnoses are made when the assessment is done in the child's usual environment, the treatment can be more effective. The treatment plans include treating behaviours that may occur only in the child's home environment, whilst taking into account the child's strengths and weaknesses.

The child in the unusual environment of the hospital may not exhibit the maladaptive behaviour seen in his normal environment, so the unit is made to function as much like a normal home as possible. Children are expected to contribute to the ward maintenance by doing chores, making beds, setting tables, clearing up, doing some laundry and helping tidy the place. This may result in minor confrontations with the cleaning staff who insist that any cleaning is their job. When cleaning staff understand the reasons for this approach, they enjoy helping the children learn the importance of keeping house, resulting in some very therapeutic interchanges.

In the protective hospital environment, a young patient may quickly forget the harsh realities of school. For that reason our teachers are encouraged on some occasions to be more like their colleagues in the classroom from which the child came. Though our teachers have been specially selected because of their insight, understanding and empathy with children, in order to provide an opportunity for expression of school conflicts we sometimes ask them to be harsh and demanding. Children can then learn to cope and work even with a teacher who is under pressure or frustrated.

Continuing Community Involvement

Problem

It is important for community agencies and professionals to see The Child And Family Psychiatric Unit as a segment of continuing community care. Too often in their experience the child, having not made progress, is suddenly taken out of their care by the parents or a physician and placed in a hospital. This produces discontinuity in treatment and feelings of resentment by social workers, school counsellors, etc.

When the child is transferred from the care of one professional to another, information must also be transferred. Verbally transmitted information, although more accurate and complete means long conversations and expensive meetings. Written material obviously fails to provide all the nuances essential to a complete understanding of the child. It is virtually impossible for a community professional to provide the hospital-based professional with all the information they have gradually collected, without spending many hours talking together.

Children and families hate being passed from one professional to another. The family feels resentful having, say, to give a history all over again, especially when there are so many painful experiences. They begin to believe professionals are more interested in the information than they are in the people who endured the experience. The child begins to find it increasingly difficult to let people see into his life. He becomes increasingly distrustful and less able to provide the feeling aspects of the life history he gives.

The hard-won trust children have developed during outpatient therapy is usually broken when they are hospitalised. Having had bad relationships in the past they begin to suspect that professionals are just like everybody else. No sooner do you tell them about your real self than they leave you in the care of somebody else, thus reinforcing their belief that they are essentially bad or unlovable people. Children think people only need to find out how bad they are before they do not want to relate to them anymore. They may have started in treatment believing that professionals wanted to understand them in order to help them. By the time they get to hospital they may believe professionals are trying to learn only the bad things about them in order to reject them.

When community agencies become resentful about losing their charges to a hospital they tend to sabotage treatment plans. They may feel that they are only brought into the picture when somebody from the unit wants to discharge a difficult child back to them. Based on the assumption that institutions generally have a bad effect, particularly upon children, many social workers and counsellors are already suspicious. If they are not involved in decisions to hospitalise, treat and discharge, they resent being left with the responsibility of after care.

If the community does not appreciate a child and family psychiatric unit is there for their use, then the more effective the unit is, the more community resources feel envious or humiliated. They feel envious because the unit has such a rich complement of staff. The unit staff are a close-knit team and because they are able to focus their treatment they can be more effective. If the unit is effective when they are not, community professionals may feel humiliated. They wonder how the unit could achieve so much in such a short time when they have struggled with the child and his family for so many sessions.

Programme

When the community resource understands the hospital facility is there for their use and is part of ongoing treatment which they can help manage, they participate much more readily. They can understand that admitting the child is to accelerate treatment that is already in progress. Although sometimes that treatment is definitive, in many instances the child will be discharged back into their care. If so, they naturally want to have a major share in decisions regarding the child's hospital and follow-up treatment plans.

On the Royal Jubilee Hospital and Christchurch Hospital Units the family physician, paediatrician, social worker, minister or special counsellor, etc. are encouraged to continue their treatment of the child during his hospitalisation. They are urged to continue sessions with the child and family on a regular basis. Their time for seeing the family or children is scheduled into the programme and every effort is made to provide them with an office. If they can't visit the child he is given the opportunity to return to the doctor or social worker's office for continuing therapy.

When the admission date is set, the community professionals are sent an invitation to be present at the admission conference. At that conference they are asked what they consider to be the most important problems to tackle. When the key conflicts have been identified and when a list of problems and dynamics have been elucidated, the assembled family, child, professionals and unit staff are able to help decide who will deal with what part of the problem and what techniques will be used. At the admission conference all have an opportunity to help decide what measures and routines will apply to that child.

The primary care worker becomes the care manager with the responsibility of co-ordinating each therapist activity as it relates to his/her particular patient. By the end of the first day in hospital the primary worker can produce a weekly schedule for his/her child and the professionals. That timetable will indicate when community professionals will be on the ward and for which part of the treatment they are responsible.

The unit routine includes an hour and a half each week of clinical rounds. During that time the community professionals are asked to be present. Many counsellors and social workers have attended. They are there ostensibly to hear what is being taught to the families they care for. At the same time they may be picking up new techniques which they will use with other families they treat.

As those of the community agency become more confident in the usefulness of the unit, they become better able to assess their own ability to continue the outpatient treatment and more aware of when they should seek an admission. Feeling that they will not be humiliated by admitting a child, they are more ready to do so when they have come to the end of their resources. On the other hand, knowing that the intensive care resource is available to them when they need help, they will hang on to more difficult children and persist in treatment.

At the discharge conference, the same professionals and helping people are asked to be present to share results and make future plans. Verbally transmitted information is available in the appropriate amount to the concerned professional. A conference will usually begin with all of the staff present plus the child and his family. Generalisations about the child's problem and his success to date are provided for everyone. After that, various groups will split up with colleagues in order to share more useful and intimate details. The teacher will take the school teacher to his office, the social worker likewise. Because there are limits to what hospital records can be officially shared, information is made available on a verbal basis. The attending professionals generally take notes. They are encouraged to ask questions and to phone back on issues that need clarification.

A discharge summary is made available to the parents or foster parents and social workers when the state is the legal guardian. This carefully written document outlines the problems, the reasons for them, the techniques that have been tried, the success that has been gained, and detailed recommendations for further help. The child is also provided with a detailed set of recommendations on how to help his family and how to govern his own life. A report containing the results of tests and examinations, the problem and its background, the treatment, its results and the recommendations are sent to the general practitioner. The unit teacher provides a series of recommendations to his colleagues in the classroom. These are based on the diagnostic findings but more particularly on the results of various remedial techniques that have been tried with the child. Occasionally the child is recommended for another classroom, but in most instances the original classroom teacher is involved in planning the discharge programme. The occupational therapist, social worker and psychologist liaise with their colleagues and provide recommendations where required.

Net Effect

With this programme the community professionals have become increasingly involved. They begin to see the unit as their facility and therefore their support and co-operation are readily available. Because the facility is there for their use when they need it they have a lowered anxiety associated with dealing with problems in the community. Because they work harder at providing treatment within the community, there is a gradually decreasing demand for inpatient treatment for some kinds of problems.

Because the community agencies are given easy access to the children they are treating, there is a continual upgrading of community workers' skills. The unit staff and the community workers work side by side and there is a sharing of ideas and techniques, for their mutual growth. It becomes a type of patient care review that is well accepted. Community professionals are better able to acknowledge their failures and ask for help from the unit staff when they are working beside them.

Community agencies are asked to provide the information on which the screening committee will decide whether the child should be admitted. There have been occasions on which the information was incomplete or inaccurate and an unnecessary admission was made. However, it soon becomes clear which referring agents are accurate in their assessment of the child's need for admission. Once the screening committee becomes confident in the referring person's judgement it only requires a request with some basic information from that individual for the screening committee to agree to a child's admission. The agencies take the responsibility of making appropriate referrals very seriously.

Without attempting to do so, the unit eventually begins setting standards which are acknowledged by the whole community. When it becomes apparent that much more can be accomplished, community expectations of treatment increase. This may put greater pressure on hospitals and government to provide more of the same kind of treatment programmes.

Continuing Family Involvement

Problem

A psychiatrically ill child makes his parents feel very guilty. They cannot avoid realising that they are implicated by his illness. If he is depressed it is often because of losses they have created in his life. If he is anxious it may be because of uncertainties that they foist upon him. If he is phobic it may have something to do with the fears that they exhibit. If he feels hostile it may be because they use excessive punishment.

The psychiatrically ill child is often an embarrassment to his family. By exhibiting his symptoms in public he parades the inadequacies of his parents, drawing unwanted attention to all the family. In public he is an irritant. Trying to control his behaviour seems only to make it worse. If he behaves in a socially awkward way, correction only makes it more obvious that he is a real problem.

Psychiatrically ill children threaten parents' tenuous control. If parents have difficulty controlling their own anger, they try hard to control the child's expression of hostility. If they are anxious, parents are more anxious when the child expresses his fears. If parents are depressed, they try to keep their child from crying because his tears remind them of their own sadness.

Psychiatrically ill children are sometimes a stimulus which trigger marital fights and sometimes separations. The child becomes the point upon which they cannot agree about management. Parents may fight over how they should bring him up, how much allowance they should give him, how much time they should spend with him. Often this conflict is an expression of their own inability to determine the limits of their desires.

If the child improves in the programme it convinces the parents that they are the wrong people to care for him. They have always suspected the child may do better in another family. When he begins to feel better and to behave more appropriately, some parents are thoroughly convinced that it would be better to have the child placed in a foster home 'for his sake'.

When hospitalised, the parents feel considerable relief at the child's departure. The feeling of relief reinforces their belief that everyone would be better off without him at home. They then begin putting considerable pressure on the unit to find the child a foster home. In some child psychiatric units prolonged admissions occur because the parents are unwilling to accept the child back. The parents state or imply that unless the staff can prove the child will never be ill again, or embarrass them in any way, he should stay hospitalised or live somewhere else.

Because of the parents' guilty, embarrassed and irritated feelings, they don't want to remain associated with the child. When asked to participate in therapeutic programmes they often find excuses for not being there. If they come, they are often late and if they are not late they often take a passive, aggressive attitude. Sometimes treatment programmes increase the parents' guilt by emphasising their contribution to the child's illness. If so, the parents are more likely to stay away.

Parents are vaguely aware of the fact that through repetition-compulsion they often recreate in the child's life problems that they didn't solve in their own. In this way they force a child to experience many of the problems they couldn't deal with themselves. Aware of this tendency they more frequently prefer not to engage in any more interaction with the child than they have to. If staff can help them name the family games they have been playing, the parents gradually begin to see there is hope.

Parenting is diminishing in popularity. A cultural ethos which places emphasis on utility can easily demonstrate that children contribute very little to the economy and welfare of the community. They are mainly a drain on their parents' time and resources. The time they should be spending with their children they are convinced would be better spent enjoying themselves on a trip or playing golf. They soon believe that if it feels good why not do it. Too many believe a fling or swing would be good for them and thus good for their children. If it appears to hurt their children they can convince themselves that they didn't want the children anyway.

Programme

Families are asked to commit themselves to up to 12 hours a week. The elements of their involvment are:

(a) Learning to observe and evaluate their children more objectively.
(b) Participating in family training seminars and exercises.
(c) Involvement in marital, individual or group psychotherapy.
(d) Participating in a variety of new, recreational experiences.
(e) Learning and practising new communications and management skills.

When parents are reluctant to become involved they are asked if they would not basically much prefer that their children have a happier childhood than they had for themselves. We have seldom encountered any parent who didn't have some desire to have healthy loving children. Also there is an element of vicariously enjoying the child's enjoyment.

Families that live far away from the unit, i.e. 200–300 miles, are asked to take two weeks out of their holiday and spend that in a nearby motel. Although this means that for three weeks they are not very involved, it does mean that for two weeks we have their intensive participation. Some families will travel 400 miles twice a week to maintain their involvement. On only two or three occasions has the child been discharged because the parents would not participate. Those children were not discharged in anger but their parents were solemnly reminded that though they may not see the need for their involvement now, they probably will later. Children prematurely discharged are carefully watched by agencies in their community who have been alerted to the special problem.

One important element of the unit philosophy is that any question of placement must be decided prior to the child's admission. Although physicians and agencies often feel desperate about a child and his need for immediate treatment the unit resists pressure for an unplanned admission. If the agency is contemplating a post-discharge change of the child's living arrangements, they are asked to determine this before admission. This ensures that the child does not remain on the unit because no one can find him an appropriate placement. The unit social worker is thus free for more constructive activities. Although an agency may protest that the policy is inflexible, the majority of community agencies understand its necessity and make sure any question of placement is settled before making a referral.

At the weekly admission conference the designated patient and his family, the unit staff and professionals from appropriate community agencies, including the family's physician, are assembled to make specific plans for the child's admission. The family are asked what they believe are the most relevant and urgent family problems to tackle. Although they tend to concentrate on the behaviour problems as seen in the referred patient, they are soon steered to an understanding that any changes in the child to some extent, at least, depend on changes in the family. During admission conferences, key conflicts are isolated and the behaviours which reflect those key conflicts are isolated. Practical techniques will be applied to changing these behaviours. The families soon learn there can be major changes in a short time period when they apply their new insights and practical techniques.

At discharge conferences each Friday the family and community professionals are reminded of the key conflicts and goals that were determined at the admission conference. The staff then report on changes and the reasons for the changes in the children. Usually this is a very heart-warming experience for the child and his family. Many good things are said about them. If the family want to know details regarding the child's progress, the staff can produce graphs that show when changes occurred. Finally, the child, his family and whichever community professional will have a continuing interest in the family, are asked what more they would like to know.

The staff make every effort to include the parents in a greater understanding of themselves and their children. If they want to know the results of specific tests they are told these. Unless there is some reason to believe the parents will use specific scores to misunderstand the child or place unrealistic expectations upon him they are told the results of intelligence tests. We believe parents are in a better position to guide if they have the results of psychological tests, etc. Although IQ is a reasonably good predictor of a child's future school performance, there is no reason to believe that it is the only predictor. During the programme parents have been taught to develop realistic expectations based on an accurate assessment of themselves and their children. This sometimes involves coming to grips with the painful realisation of both their strengths and weaknesses. Too often parents avoid recognising their strengths in order not to exert their best efforts in parenting.

During the period of time they are involved with the ward programme, parents are taught how to observe their child. Too often parents make global assessments that depend upon a misrepresentation or some erroneous expectation, i.e. 'they are fighting all the time'. Standing behind a one-way screen and watching children together working at some task or playing a game, they are asked to count the number of occasions in which the child becomes combative. They are almost always surprised to learn that although they think the child is always fighting with his little brother they find he is aggressive only 10 per cent of the time.

Frequently groups of parents standing behind a one-way mirror commenting on their children will pick out strengths in the other parent's child, Jane. They are amazed to find other parents see good things in their Johnny when they can only see negative things. A particular parent may recognise that Jimmy, son of other parents standing beside him, is much nicer and more intelligent than Jimmy's parents think he is.

Watching children with their siblings has often given parents the opportunity to gain a considerably more accurate understanding of who initiates conflict. Whereas they thought that the older brother was being mean to the sister they soon realised that the little sister has often provoked him. The staff also use a portable video-camera to record children in other environments. Video tapes are played back to the parents who are asked to comment on what they observe and what they think is happening.

Parents are asked not only to count behaviours but are also asked to describe what they believe the child is saying and what feeling or conflict the child might be expressing. Often there are gross discrepancies between what the staff feel the child is trying to communicate and what the parents hear. This gives an opportunity for a lively discussion between staff and parents which is usually resolved by later asking the child what he was trying to communicate. Children on the unit are always notified when somebody is observing them. A tendency to become suspicious that someone is always behind the one-way mirror observing them is set to rest.

Family training consists of two three-quarter hour sessions each week for five weeks. These are held on Monday or Thursday evenings from 7.30 until 9 p.m. There is a coffee break between the two sessions. The first session is usually devoted to helping parents understand how children develop, think and feel. Although some parents have an accurate knowledge of how children develop they often cannot apply that knowledge to their particular child. The second session is devoted to helping parents learn how to handle a particular problem. In this session parents are taught communication and management skills. They are shown how to begin understanding the games their families play. They are taught how to relate to children at specific ages and how their aggressive or fearful messages affect children.

The families are assigned homework. This is designed to help families assess their functioning during the week. One parent will be asked to measure the ratio of praise to criticism of their spouse. Another parent may be asked to measure as accurately as possible the amount of time spent in one-to-one conversation with a particular child.

When the parents report back there is an opportunity to share with the staff their failures, frustrations and successes. This is an opportunity for them to abreact some of their own painful life experiences. Although there is no attempt to engage in group psychotherapy at training sessions parents are encouraged to talk about their own childhood. Soon parents realise they are not alone in having personal problems.

At the end of each session the parents whose children are about to be discharged are asked to report on their experiences. Almost invariably they have something good to report. It is a very important encouragement for the other parents who are just beginning the programme.

Although there is a sequence of seminars it isn't difficult for parents to begin in the middle of a sequence. They are told that the object of the family training is to make them better parents. There is no attempt on our part to remove the child from their care but rather we hope that they will be better able to parent their children wisely. We believe that if the parent enjoys being a parent the child will enjoy being a child. As children enjoy childhood so they grow up into happy adults and parents. It is our hope, therefore, that parents will learn techniques that will make it possible for them to enjoy parenting. If they enjoy being parents their children will also become good parents.

Families are also involved in considerable individual or family psychotherapy. Parents are told that they will have an opportunity to see staff alone if they so choose. After individual sessions, however, they are encouraged to share with the family all matters that do affect the family. Parents often have a fear that they will hurt a child by disclosing how they feel. At the same time children should be protected against the raw anger and hate that parents sometimes feel. In this case, parents are asked not to disclose these feelings until they have better control over them and have a better understanding of their children.

Family psychotherapy usually develops on both transactional and psychodynamic lines. The parents and children are asked to analyse and name the games that they have been playing. The staff have become adept at providing humorous names for rather disastrous situations. This helps them all to become more objective and optimistic in dealing with large problems.

Following the first two weekends that the child spends on the unit the family are engaged with the staff in developing guidelines and consequences. The children are encouraged to negotiate as well as they possibly can. In stating their case children are supported in attempting to put feeling or persuasion into their argument. They are encouraged to hope that a reasonable guideline can be put into practice. The parents are then given the opportunity to state their case pointing out to the child that while they sympathise with his point of view it is unreasonable because of time or financial constraints. Children are reminded that parents have needs of their own.

The children are first asked to state their position on both the guideline and the consequence. The parents are asked to give the child full opportunity to express his demands. Given an opportunity to suggest the consequences for some misdemeanour, it is often very surprising to find how severe children will be on themselves. This puts the parents in the position of being able to be less severe.

When two or three guidelines and consequences have been negotiated and written down, the parent is asked to try these on the first weekend home. They are given a form on which to report their successes and failures and comments. When the child returns to the unit, the parent can describe how well a particular guideline or consequence has worked. On the basis of the parent's and child's report the staff enable them to renegotiate some of the guidelines and consequences. By the time the final draft of recommendations are made, there should be a relatively complete set of guidelines and consequences available for the parents.

During follow-up, the staff are able to check with their patient and his parents on general progress and specifically on any difficulties with the recommendations. Frequently there is a honeymoon period of two weeks where everything seems to go well. Following this, some old problems may resurface. If so the staff can check with the parents to determine whether they have been following the recommendations. A careful review of the guidelines and consequences frequently shows that the parents have made some changes or have been unable to comply with the directions. Once again, the guidelines and conse-quences are renegotiated and everybody gives them another try.

Since discharge recommendations are carefully delineated and posted for everyone to see, the parents are reminded of their commitment and the child has no excuses for not knowing what is expected of him. If the recommended consequences are regularly applied the parents do not need to remind, threaten or coerce their children. The staff gain confidence in those guidelines that have been shown to work.

If certain recommendations don't work, staff work with the family to find the psychodynamic, transactional or behavioural reasons why they don't. They may discover that the parents have been unable to be consistent in some area. They may uncover old conflicts that make it impossible for the parents to change their attitude. This insight develops in the context of trying out well-proven techniques.

Net Effect

During the first week of the child's admission, the parents are asked to take a break away from their frequent involvement with their problem child. During this time they can begin new interactions with the other children, spend more time with each other as a couple, or go on a mini-honeymoon. This break gives them greater objectivity and renewed interest in tackling the problems of their hospitalised child.

During the time one child is hospitalised other family problems come to light. The problems of other children hidden by the over-whelming concern with the problems of the psychiatrically ill child become apparent. The other children become able to indicate they also need attention, or have difficulties that must be attended to.

Because the family training is designed to impart knowledge and useful information and to provide practical guidelines, parents attend regularly. They soon begin to realise that the information about human development applies also to them. They become interested in them-selves and soon begin attending sessions for their own benefit. In the discussion that follows the brief presentations, parents can share experi-ences from their own childhood.

Because the family knows exactly when the child is to return to them, the family system stays open to accept the child back. Since they are expected to pick up the child at specific times, they accom-modate to the coming and going of a child as if he is still part of their family system. Parents are asked to sign in and out to indicate when they are present. This information can be related to the eventual prog-nosis of the child. Often the number of visits by the family can be positively correlated with the amount of improvement seen in the hospitalised child.

The parents get a copy of the child's detailed weekly schedule so they know what treatment is going on and when. Family are always welcome but they must inform staff of their intentions. The staff will indicate whether the child is involved in a session that cannot be interrupted, or whether the activity is reasonable elective, or one in which the parents should participate.

Given an opportunity to observe their child, parents become more objective. They apply that increased objectivity to understanding themselves and their other children. The practical techniques of child guidance they learn are soon set to use with their other children. Although they may begin the programme determined to see the problem child adjusted to their family, they soon become aware that the programme is designed to help the whole family.

Child Involvement

Problem

Children anticipate hospitalisation with mixed feelings, predominantly fear. Psychiatrically disturbed children have often been dragged to visit many professional people; from these experiences they get the impression that adults are mainly interested in controlling their lives. Children who have had bad experiences with parents or foster parents, have learned not to trust adults. Though the staff on the ward are determined to help children unburden themselves and learn to take responsibility it is very difficult for children not to be defensive.

Many children are afraid to express their fears and longings. They may have been trying to hold the family together and this has meant that they cannot express their own feelings in case it would disrupt a precarious balance. They have a legitimate fear that if they are removed from the family to the hospital the family will be so relieved that they will not want their 'bad' child back.

Many children, aware that they need help, appreciate the determination of the staff to get on with the job, but when there is pressure to examine their thoughts, they wish to run away. They may fear that the staff will lock them up. Keys and some locked doors increase their distrust of staff on child psychiatric units.

Children soon become aware of the rules on a child psychistric unit. These rules often provoke an automatic anti-authoritarian response in children who have been struggling against coercive or manipulative parents. Staff may react by labelling a child as rebellious and see his greatest need as control. In child psychiatric units, the initial encounter with staff creates an impression which is difficult to remove. If staff are too involved with patients who have been on a unit for some time, children may feel they need to imitate the same type of behaviour to get attention.

Programme

The Family Restoration Programme has attempted to deal with these problems in getting children quickly involved in treatment by discussing the proposed hospitalisation with them after showing them around the unit and meeting the staff. Children are introduced to the concept of a time-limited programme from their first encounter. In most instances, children quickly realise this proposal is something from which they could benefit. There are children who appear to be definitely against admission. It isn't hard to discover there is an ambivalence which the family can resolve by being firm. If a family has difficulty in being sufficiently firm, the professional staff can add the weight of their opinion. In some instances the staff will visit the child in his home specifically to discuss the child's fears.

Even with the most difficult cases, it has never been necessary to involve the police or use any kind of certificate. Firmness on the part of the professional staff helps the parents be more definite, which in turn helps the child resolve his mixed feelings of wanting and not wanting hospital treatment.

Knowing that the period of time away from his family is time-limited the child has fewer fears that he will be extruded. He is given encouragement to explain to his friends, peers and neighbours where he is going. Many children are uneasy about doing this. The staff point out that he is not alone. Many other children in the community have had a similar experience.

In order to make sure that the hospitalised child does not lose his connections with community activities and friends, he is encouraged to continue with his Scouts, Cadets, choir, music lessons or sports. His peers are invited to spend time with him on the unit or join in swimming with staff and other patients. Friends soon realise that the special outings or trips make being on the unit a pleasurable experience. They like to be with their hospitalised friend during those times and feel no stigma joining in the unit activities.

During the admission conference the 'problem child' is given every opportunity to state what he wants changed. Sometimes the changes he wants most are in his siblings, or in the way his parents handle him. Most children recognise they must also change and are quite explicit. The child's self-proclaimed goals are carefully considered and given important weighting.

During the admission conference the child may be overwhelmed by the many reports, especially if they emphasise the negative aspects of his functioning and behaviour. It is important that whoever chairs the admission conference reminds family, community workers and ward staff to point out strengths as well as weaknesses. Most disturbed children hear very few reports of bad things that they haven't already heard. What they haven't heard is all the good things professionals may discover. Thus the admission conference is often a very positive experience for the child. The Family Restoration Programme emphasises a very careful introduction to the ward by the primary care worker. On the day of admission the child is shown about the whole ward, his bed is assigned, the key to his locker is given to him and his room mates are solemnly introduced. To ensure the initial experience is a good one, the ward should have a welcoming party. If the staff are able to, a small speech and song gives an air of joyful anticipation to the whole procedure. Part of the child's introduction is to be taught the guidelines and consequences which will govern his behaviour during his stay. These are carefully explained so that he clearly understands what happens if he contravenes or if he fulfils one of the guidelines. Since they are posted on a notice board, if the child forgets he can always refresh his memory by reading them again or by asking his worker.

The child is shown that there are no locks to the ward. However, the rules that govern the child wandering away are emphasised. Children are given time to leave the unit and be away on their own, but they must sign in and out. If they leave without approval then they are given a half hour in which to return. If they return during this period of time they are placed in pyjamas for a day. If they do not, their parents are notified. If their parents cannot locate them within an hour the police are notified. If they have to be returned, they must earn back their clothing over a three-day period.

A positive peer culture is encouraged by friendly competition and traditions. Because some children have been on the unit for up to four weeks, they tend to be more dominant. They may take the newcomer aside and try and frighten him with terrifying tales of huge needles. The staff keep an eye on how frightened a child may become but to some extent it is permitted because it is a type of initiation rite. In Kangaroo Kort the staff will go over the introduction of new people to explore all the feelings that are stirred up by newcomers to the ward.

The staff attempt to form a close relationship with their patient from the time the child is assigned to them. Since the primary worker is assigned before the child is admitted, that worker is able to see the child in his own home. During that home visit the child is asked to show the worker about and describe his home. From this the staff worker learns the child's perception of the spaces and events that are important to him. This provides the staff with an opportunity to help construct the child's ward space as much like his home as possible. The parents are encouraged to bring with the child all the teddy bears, pictures or models that are important to him.

Some depressed children begin their stay with a nurturing programme. The child is put to bed and tenderly cared for. Then he is gradually allowed to introduce himself into the ward routine. This regression in the service of the ego allows the staff an opportunity to get very close to the child. His primary worker spends much time reading to the child, talking to him about his past, tucking him into bed and bringing him food.

The child is reassured by the predictability of his environment on his first day in hospital. The staff encourage him to help put together his weekly schedule. Into that timetable are scheduled the routine events, getting up, breakfast, recreation, school, etc., and the particular occasions when he will be seeing various members of the staff. It is the primary workers' responsibility to ensure that the weekly schedule is filled in immediately after the admission conference. They must contact all the staff and family to co-ordinate therapy times and visits.

Although there is considerable anxiety relief in the predictability of the guidelines and consequences, there is also a definite flexibility. Each week children have a business meeting with the staff during which they can renegotiate certain guidelines and consequences. This process is important because it teaches them negotiating skills that they will eventually use in discussions with their parents. It helps children understand staff are not inflexible but will respond to reason and argument.

There are definite fun times during which the child is introduced to new activities. Because there are so many good things happening on the ward the child becomes increasingly attached to the ward.

During the first two weekends the child is on the unit, staff arrange recreational activities to include the whole family. Many parents learn for the first time how to play with their children during swimming or hiking, skating or bowling. The staff provide models which encourage parents to understand the rules of being a child with their children during certain times but also when to switch into parent or adult roles.

The unit has developed definite traditions. These traditions become focal points about which other activities revolve. The typical parties, routine and games are the things which children tend to remember when they leave. One very good tradition is a goodbye party the night before the child is discharged. The cake and games held in his honour are preceded by a session of strength bombardment. During this session staff and fellow patients are given the opportunity to tell the departing child all the strengths and changes they have noticed.

Net Effect

Judged on the criterion that runaways indicate an unsuccessful treatment programme, the Family Restoration Programme has been successful. Our patients seldom leave without permission and, even when they do, they are usually located nearby. The only time we lock the doors on Ward 24 is when everyone goes on an outing.

Because being in hospital has been a good experience for the children, they have no hesitation to come back. Our greater problem has been to keep away those children who might otherwise take up a lot of staff time. It is quite natural for the staff to want to see their old patients and find out how things are going. Follow-up is programmed to happen at home. Rules have been made to discourage children coming back to visit the unit until at least five weeks after their discharge.

The child's anxieties noticeably decrease within a few days of the hospitalisation. Very quickly the children fit into the routine and participate in structuring their own times. Because they are not struggling to control themselves in such an easily controlled environment, the child has freedom and energy to devote to the intrapsychic aspects of his problem.

Therapeutic Milieu

Problem

In many child psychiatric units the staff spend a great deal of time fighting to control the activities and the behaviours of children. Because so much energy and time goes into making the environment reasonably settled there is very little time or energy left for individual treatment. Consequently, children are poorly treated and staff are very frustrated. Because so much effort goes into controlling children, frequently the children respond by fighting the control. Not wanting to be part of the programme and watching the effort the staff put into control, convinces the children that the main exercise is a struggle for control.

If staff are unable, even for a short while, to control the environment, it stimulates within them considerable conflict. The aggression of children stimulates the aggression in staff. Staff have found that the best way to stop themselves from hitting provocative children, is to make sure the children are not allowed physically to attack staff. Unfortunately, if the staff do not have immediately available back-up resources, or techniques which can handle a child's assault on their person or feelings, people are injured.

If the staff are injured, they are frightened to become involved in treating children and thus a high rate of staff burn-out ensues. If the staff are frightened by their own feelings, they spend so much time struggling to control their responses, that they have little opportunity to express the happier emotional aspects of their personality.

In some child psychiatric settings, in an effort to control aggressive or behavioural or emotional responses, staff evoke a wide variety of contingencies. The children then become intent on determining whether these contingencies are consistent and firm. If they are not, the children become anxious and proceed to test the controls even further. As a consequence to this, the staff feel they must invoke more contingencies. The net effect is an invisible person. In this situation children are trying to find loopholes in the organisation and control system and the staff are spending an enormous amount of time plugging the small holes.

Whenever there are many contingencies, children elaborate a game in which they attempt to beat the system. Finding that they are often outfoxed by children with an intimate knowledge of how to frustrate adults, staff become more determined to control behaviour by invoking more contingencies. As a result, some child psychiatric units have an enormous number of contingencies.

Staff on some units have attempted to make children compliant by making sure that they enjoy their time on the unit. Much effort goes into entertaining the children, providing them with fun and games on the ward and taking them on outings. Unfortunately, that situation is so unlike the usual experience of many children, that anything they learn from the unit does not generalise into their home situation.

In some psychiatric settings staff are much more permissive than are the parents or schools. As a consequence parents become very suspicious of any change that they see in the child. They also know that once a child gets home they become increasingly strict to ensure that the necessary chores and routines are followed. Because the staff have made the children believe that many behaviours, formerly restricted, are permitted, they have an unrealistic expectation of their parents.

In some circumstances the ward routine has become too well ordered and too predictable. Again, the problem is that this is so unlike the home setting, the children's improvement cannot generalise to the home situation. Although children do benefit from the reassuring aspects of their predictable environment, they cannot expect it to be so when they return home. Thus it becomes necessary to allow a certain amount of unpredictability in order to see the anxieties children are attempting to deal with in their home environment.

Because of these difficulties it becomes necessary to provide a therapeutic milieu which is easily controlled, has predictable guidelines and consequences, is neither too much fun, too permissive nor too predictable. In a setting like that children will have time and energy available to work out their problems.

Programme

In the Family Restoration Programme it has been found important to establish a set of guidelines and consequences. These guidelines have been negotiated with the staff so that the staff feel comfortable with them. The guidelines regulate the usual activities of getting up, washing, teeth brushing, setting tables, manners at meals, going to school, outings and chores about the ward. The consequences are small but frequently applied. For example, periods of time-out averaging five minutes are more effective than long periods.

As much as possible, natural consequences are invoked. This gives the children a feeling of what might happen if they refuse to follow the guideline. If children are late in going to bed they feel tired in the morning. To reinforce that feeling, children who go to bed late are wakened that much earlier the next morning, i.e. 20 minutes late to bed, up 20 minutes earlier. If children are unmannerly at the table, they are asked to leave. If they do not want to work in school they are given additional chores about the unit.

Negotiation

The staff spend many hours negotiating and renegotiating those guidelines and consequences with which they have the greatest difficulty. There is always considerable feeling about aggression towards other children, breaking furniture or attacking staff. It has been found in these instances that it is essential to have an ultimate consequence. Time-out away from an activity is generally used, but if staff or children are attacked in an uncontrollable way, intramuscular chlorpromazine is used. Unfortunately, staff have very mixed feelings about such a procedure. It takes many hours of discussing their attitudes and emotional responses before such a procedure has general acceptance. If it is not generally accepted it tends to be undermined.

As much as the guidelines and consequences are negotiated among the staff, they are to a limited extent negotiated with the children. This gives the children an opportunity to learn the skills of expressing their feelings and opinions in the most persuasive way they can manage. Feeling that they have some part in determining the rules that govern their behaviour, the children find it easier to accept the guidelines. We have found that, given an opportunity to suggest consequences, children often suggest much harsher ones than the adults will. The children are provided a once-a-week management meeting during which issues of ward procedure are discussed. They are given the opportunity to express their opinions both on the guidelines and the consequences.

Chores

Children are expected to have an environment as much like their home as possible. Since many homes have chores and chores are useful, children from the Unit are expected to perform daily maintenance chores. In many instances this means a long discussion with the house cleaning staff who believe that it is their right and duty to perform all the maintenance chores. In some instances unions have objected. However, in most instances cleaning staff have become part of the therapeutic team and are quite happy to help apply consequences to children who do not do their chores around the ward. Chores include cleaning up, making beds, tidying up, setting table, washing dishes, etc. For these, children are confronted with consequences as natural as possible. Where natural consequences are not possible, the behaviour is regulated with tokens and back-up reinforcements.

The Role of the Parent and Teacher

As much as possible, the Family Restoration Programme seeks to make the unit adult like those the child encounters at home. Although it is not in the nature of the teacher to be harsh or to give homework, he is expected to do so because this is what children will find in their usual school. Although the child's primary worker will not be harsh or obstructive towards him, other members of the staff are encouraged to be somewhat inconsistent to simulate the child's usual adult environment.

Modelling

Children learn a good deal more from observing adult behaviours than from listening to adult instruction. The staff are encouraged to model interpersonal relationships and communication that will benefit the child. Expressions of affection are definitely allowed. Arguments in front of the children are allowed but must always end in an attempt to come to an agreement. The child must see that arguments do not result in disrupted interpersonal relationships.

Tradition

Many families anchor their 'programmes' through space and time with traditions. Traditions on the unit have had a great effect in providing morale for the child and for the staff. When the child first arrives he is taken through an elaborate ritualised routine of introduction. When he leaves he is given a farewell party, cake with candles and a session of strength bombardment. The children have initiated their own traditions which include not belonging to the group until you have had a needle for blood examination.

Stigma

To avoid stigmatising children, the unit functions within the community as much as possible. The child's friends and relatives are invited to participate in the ward programme. If the child is likely to be teased at school, he is given the skills with which to reply. Because his friends have seen him on the ward, he can always reply to their jeering comments that he was on a psychiatric ward with, 'I saw you there too.'

Net Effect

Children confronted with well-defined guidelines and consequences are in a position to determine their own legal boundaries. Coming up against regulations that are likely to be used at home, the child is able to begin reorienting himself to the programme that will be instituted in his home. When he comes up against rules, he finds that there are always consequences but these are not harsh. In that setting he learns how to take responsibility for his own actions.

Children will learn to negotiate. They begin to value a vote. In this way the concept of democracy is reinforced.

Because of the predictability on the unit, children are less anxious. They do not spend as much time trying to determine their environmental limitations and thus have more energy to devote to understanding their intrapsychic problems.

Because the staff are encouraged to be like other people in the environment, the child will invariably come up against problems in interpersonal relationships like those he encounters at school and home. He begins to realise that there are ways of coping with unpredictable adults and angry teachers.

The Best Utilisation of The Most Important Treatment Resource (Staff)

Problem One

Too often, those looking after psychiatrically disturbed children are doing so for mixed reasons. Part of it has to do with their desire to understand their own childhood conflicts, and part of it has to do with enhancing their identity by supporting their professional role.

In the professional games that people play, staff tend to ensure that they are what their professional identity indicates. They must find in children or their parents the problems that support their role as a helper.

To be a physician or a nurse, there must be sick people. Those who were primarily physician, nurse, counsellor, etc., will be looking for illness as maladaptive behaviour. When asked to describe a child, they will tend to emphasise his problems. If they asked one to talk about Johnny, they will say he is anxious, quarrelsome and obsessive, rather than that he has bright blue eyes and an impish way of teasing people.

Programme

The criteria for hiring staff should be:

(1) The best training.
(2) Good professional experience with good evidence of being effective therapists.
(3) The highest degree of maturity and ability to relate to children and families.
(4) The ability to tolerate ambiguity and to learn from experience.
(5) An identity that is independent of professional role.

When all other factors are equal, the job should go to those people who, when asked to describe themselves, would say, 'I am a painter' or 'I am a farmer'; i.e. those who have an identity distinct from their profession. Those people are more likely to be able to give up their professional role as a helper: because they don't have to be a helper, nurse, counsellor or psychiatrist, they won't have to find problems.

In hiring staff, we have placed emphasis on finding those people with a broad range of previous life experiences. Unfortunately, nurses have often come straight from high school into the nursing profession where they have remained ever since.

Using another category of workers variously described as child care workers, child and family workers, assistant child therapists, etc., it is possible to hire people with a much broader range of personal and professional experiences. We have found that a unit needs characteristics in staff that tend to represent all types of people in the community. For that reason we need older people, people who have been mechanics, teachers, housewives, etc. They bring individual skills and experiences which professional medical/psychiatric training cannot impart.

It is important to have an approximately equal ratio of male and female staff. This may have something to do with how the sexes get along best. We have found that there is less stress, competitiveness and role confusion where there is an equal proportion of adult males/females.

Since over half of the children admitted to most units are male, it is important to have male models. The difficulty is that advertising a preference for males is considered an intolerable, i.e. sexist, hiring practice. However, in most countries there is also some clause that allows sexual discrimination when hiring male and female clothes models. We have broadened that understanding to include modelling in a psychological sense. Although it has never been tested, there does not appear to be in the Human Rights Acts anything that precludes giving preference to one sex or the other, in order to obtain either a female or male psychological model.

Problem Two

In many psychiatric treatment facilities, staff have little idea of how best to utilise their time. Staff, the most expensive and the most useful treatment resource, are often badly under-utilised. Sometimes this is because the staff have not been given attainable goals with learnable, measurable, prescribable techniques. As a consequence, they operate with the vague impression that they must observe patients or talk to people and, though they know a great deal about illness, they have little idea of how to attain any treatment goal.

In many multidisciplinary units, professionals develop a hierarchy. Because nurses and child care staff have been left the primary responsibility of everything that nobody else deals with, they begin to feel that they are the people who are expected to do most of the work with the least guidance or knowhow. Although there are few overt criticisms of primary care staff, there are many implied ones. These lead to jealousies and rivalries. As a result, there is diminished effort, more frustration and hurt feelings. A great deal of energy burns up in solving identity conflicts.

When staff are unsure of what they are supposed to do, they hesitate. When they hesitate they tend to respond to crisis, thus inadvertently reinforcing the patient's most maladaptive behaviour. In this way, people who have an acute illness are made into chronic patients. Their condition worsens because staff inadvertently attend to their worst behaviour.

In some institutions, there is confusion about who is supposed to do what part of the treatment. When this happens, conferences have to take place during which staff try to sort out who is best capable of doing what. Every situation seems to be a new one. To determine who does what may take a great deal of time.

When there are so many problems and so many facets to these problems, there is always more to do than time and staff allow. Because of this, we believe that the burden of proof lies with those who state that others should not be involved in treatment. Our philosophy is that if somebody is volunteering, since there is so much more treatment to do than we can accomplish, it is our responsibility to accept or to demonstrate why they should not help. These helpers, volunteers and therapists are all readily accepted as part of the treatment team, unless we have evidence they are more a hindrance than a help. All of them take direction from the treatment team and regularly report back.

Programme

Our unit operates with the philosophy that staff may do what they can after they have done their chores. Chores are those duties that are basic requirements of a treatment programme. Who does what is determined by who is best qualified and who has had the most experience. Each professional on the ward will have clearly delineated chores. Among other duties, the social worker will do a family and community evaluation. The psychiatrist will do a physical and mental status examination. The nurse will check about immunisation and observe the child in his home. The psychologist will do routine psychological tests. The occupational therapist will do a routine sensory-motor investigation. Before staff are hired, they must understand these are their duties to be performed on every patient unless there is a good reason not to. When the chores are done and reports completed, all staff are given plenty of support and encouragement to become experienced and qualified in other areas of practice. Anybody may do family counselling if he/she has demonstrated good skills. Any staff member may engage on psychotherapy if he/she knows how. Competence in any skill is determined by two peers with acknowledged expertise. We have found with this philosophy, staff soon specialise. Some staff become very adept at dealing with battered children and their parents, others with autism.

When staff develop an area of interest and expertise, they are in a position to provide in-service training for other staff members.

To determine who can do what they are inclined to do, two peers or senior staff are asked to observe them in action. When any staff feel they are capable of doing assertion training, for example, they are asked to perform this in front of those who are acknowledged experts. Once approval is given, the staff member is publicly acknowledged as having gained new skill expertise also. Once skill expertise has been clearly delineated, it is possible to draw up a staff skill inventory (see Chapter 7). When patients are admitted and treatment plans made, a look at the skills inventory will determine who should do what with which patient.

Net Effect

With this philosophy, staff have found great freedom to develop skills in the areas where they have a natural inclination or curiosity. Because there is more to do than anybody can accomplish in one period of hospitalisation, there is never competition for pieces of a child that people feel they should treat. Consequently, there is a good feeling, with staff readily consulting their peers who are acknowledged experts in particular techniques. There is little fear of exhibiting one's ignorance.

Treatment Methods

Problem

For too many years many difficulties with psychiatric treatment have arisen because primary care staff have not known what to do with their time. In the treatment of psychiatric patients, heavy reliance has been placed on the use of drugs, talking to patients and, more recently, operant conditioning. When drugs are used staff are asked to monitor the patient's progress. This usually means asking patients if they are still delusional or noting whether they are hallucinating. This attention tends to reinforce maladaptive behaviour. Where the emphasis has been on talk, staff who have not been trained to do psychotherapy tend to get into conversations which often lead nowhere.

More recently operant conditioning has become popular. Primary care staff have been glad to have some technique that gives them specific directions. Unfortunately, with very little experience they often do operant conditioning poorly. Or they find that operant conditioning may change certain behaviours but hardly touches the core conflicts.

Many primary care staff are humiliated by continually having to ask, 'What do I do now doctor?', The physician often responds with, 'I want you to observe the patient' or 'I want you to talk to them' or 'I want you to do some recreational or occupational activity'. If the primary care staff press for more direction the physician often becomes angry stating, 'I can't tell you exactly what to say.' In a lot of these exchanges both the physician and the primary care staff feel a sense of futility.

In attempting to promote good treatment much time has been taken up developing a therapeutic programme followed by tentative forays with one technique or other. When the staff don't see an immediate effect they tend to neglect the patient or to demand further direction. This usually involves another conference, more wasted time and not infrequently more uncertain directions. Physicians and primary care staff have yearned for the opportunity to know exactly what to do and what results to look for.

Programme

The Family Restoration Programme has concentrated on describable, prescribable, measurable techniques. Because they are describable it is possible to have a high rate of agreement between therapists. Because they are prescribable it is possible for staff to know when to use which technique for how long. Because these techniques are measurable it is possible to determine whether the desired effect is taking place.

When these delineated techniques are used, the child's week can be organised around so many sessions of various techniques. As a result the child's primary therapist can organise a weekly timetable for each child. Sessions with various staff members, beginning after breakfast and going on throughout the day, are pencilled in. The tentative time-table is carefully gone over with the child and family who may indicate the need for certain changes. As a result there is a high utilisation of staff skill and their valuable time.

The techniques in this book are not all new but we have attempted to describe them in such a way that others could learn almost all they need to know from the description. Obviously it is not possible to rely entirely upon any book. Using the description as a guide will help staff members orient themselves. Once a technique has been tried a few times many staff become innovative and develop their own style.

At admission conference we find it is possible to isolate key con-flicts. Then behavioural problems or dynamic difficulties are enume-rated and described. To each a technique is prescribed. Staff estimate how much time will be required for each of these techniques. Staff who are particularly good at those techniques are assigned. Thus by the end of the first day of admission it is possible for the primary care staff to put together a fairly comprehensive weekly timetable for the hospi-talised child.

The weekly timetable will include the usual group activities, the school programme and in addition times that are set aside for specific therapeutic tasks. Since the primary care staff are responsible for organising the timetable they must contact other professional staff and family members. They co-ordinate times for each activity including school, recreation, individual psychotherapy and each treatment technique.

Net Effect

These techniques can be learned without too much difficulty by most staff who gain a reasonable level of confidence in most of them. Because some techniques take more experience and training, staff have always something more to add to their expertise.

Having techniques which can be defined gives the staff a clear idea of what works with which child and what doesn't. Because what is expected is clearly specified the staff work hard. Because they are aware of what they are personally accomplishing staff on our unit have always been known as people who work hard, and who have a high level of personal satisfaction.

Because the techniques are measurable it is possible to know almost immediately when something is not working. This makes it possible to change the programme with little time wasted.

The staff become aware that there is no limit to what they can learn. Once they have grounding in basic techniques they attempt to learn the more difficult ones such as interpretive play therapy. If staff leave, it is possible to write recommendations about their work which specify what techniques they are good at.

Staff Burn-out/Job Satisfaction

Problem

In most child psychiatric units, there are special stresses which result in high levels of fatigue, absence and individual sickness. Too often staff feel they are working hard but with little tangible evidence of this effort. At the end of a shift they feel exhausted and go home wondering what they have accomplished.

All staff who work with psychiatrically disturbed children are subject to special stresses.

1. Self-restraint. Frequently, child psychiatric staff must look into the sad eyes of emotionally starved children. With the effects of that appeal burning in their hearts, they must restrain their strong desire to rescue and nurture and must give the parents the first opportunity to respond. Not infrequently many staff would like to take a child home for proper care. When they see an abused child they become enraged at the parent. Yet they cannot express that rage and still gain the parent's co-operation. When they see a neglected child they yearn to provide the affection he doesn't get; but if they do that, they may alienate the parents.

2. Optimism and Real Expectation. In most areas of medicine a grossly deformed or diseased child creates in staff an appropriately low expectation that he will recover. In psychiatry, the most severely disturbed children often show little easily observable evidence of the extent of their disorder. Childhood autism is probably the most difficult of all psychiatric conditions to treat, yet autistic children appear fair, bright-eyed, and well formed. Because there is little evidence of severe disease, the staff tend to have unrealistically high expectations. When their attempt at treatment quickly fails, it is easy to become extremely frustrated. Their expectations are met with few successes, and it is hard to see why.

In the homes of many disturbed children, there are feelings of anger or despair. The community is also angered with the child's bad behaviour and the family's apparent refusal to change. On the one hand, everyone is clamouring for an immediate change, on the other, no one expects much good to result from hospitalisation. The staff must deal with a large measure of family and community ambivalence regarding outcome.

To get a therapeutic process started, ward staff must inject considerable optimism into the depressing system. Attempting to make everybody wait while they have a chance to begin changing the situation, the staff have to hold back a tide of accumulated angry or sad feelings. They need time to help the child and his family to try once again. They have to engender hope and struggle to maintain their own realistic expectations.

3. Strong Emotions. Child psychiatric ward staff continually ride an emotional elevator. While they empathise with the child's sadness, they are sad; with his anger, they are angry; with his frustration, they are feeling frustrated; with his despair, they tend to want to give up. All day long their emotions are dragged up and down. But for the child's sake, they must control the expression of their own ambivalent feelings.

Few children can cope with raw adult emotions, and psychiatrically disturbed children have experienced too much turmoil already. They need to be able to express their strongest feelings and feel their staff members can handle it without losing control. Having to control the hormonal and psychological changes engendered by a child's strong emotions, it is small wonder that at the end of the day, staff can feel drained.

4. Surrogate Scapegoat. There is an ancient tendency to use children as scapegoats. Thus, when a primary worker stands up for his patient, he is likely to have dumped on him all the hostility that has gathered about the child. Not infrequently ward staff encounter an enraged parent who demands the child change right away, a teacher who threatens to dismiss the child tomorrow, or a probation officer who intends to put the child in jail if he ever steps out of line again. The moment a primary care worker defends or protects a child, he becomes the object of much displaced hostility.

5. Feeling of Responsibility. Every child should have a good life experience and a bright future. No child should be dragged through the crisis of parental turmoil. Believing this and sensing the child's helpless confusion, the primary staff cannot help feeling a personal responsibility.

Because the child hurts so obviously, the staff share his feelings of helplessness. Commonly, there is a strong desire to take the child away from the parents and place him in a kind, nurturing environment where he can be properly cared for and protected. Not infrequently, staff members become angry at a neglecting parent. They would happily take the child into their own home for proper love and affection but acknowledge that their duty is to encourage the parent to take responsibility.

6. Effort-Outcome Ratio. Unlike other areas of medicine, it is not possible for primary care staff to medicate the patient and go home feeling confident that the child will soon be well. Primary child psychiatric workers know that they cannot rely on a biochemical or a technical procedure. They know that the degree to which a child improves is more directly related to the amount of effort they put in. They must then face the uncomfortable realisation that they are seldom able to give enough to a family. Somehow they must accept the fact that some families continue to suffer because they did not have enough staff time.

7. Gratitude. In many areas of medicine, parents express considerable gratitude to the staff who care for their children. In psychiatry, there are so many mixed emotions of guilt, abhorrence, shame and pity, that it is hard for the parents or the community to express their feelings of appreciation. Compared to nurses on paediatric units, it is seldom that primary care workers on psychiatric units receive a gift.

8. Job Satisfaction. Many staff have been medically trained to stick with patients until they are well, dead or gone away. They find it hard to stop treating a family that made minimal gains even though the child is symptomatically better. It would be much more satisfying to see the patient cured.

In psychiatry, we hope that the family will become more mature than they were before one member became symptomatically unwell. It may be an impossibly high expectation but, unless the family members have more insight, better communication and improved management skills, staff know the problems will soon recur.

9. Appeal. When a child screams in distress, the staff are reminded of their own psychic pain. When a family wanders in confusion, staff members will recall the times of futility in their own families. The child's fears and sorrows reawaken old fears and losses which must be either repressed or worked on.

Because it may take time to deal with the child's distress, there are long periods when staff feel helpless. That sense of helplessness reminds them of similar feelings from childhood.

10. 'Push me pull you'. At the same time that the child appeals for help with his eyes, facial expressions or behaviour, his verbal message tells the staff to leave him alone. The staff caught by this ambivalence must work to determine to which message they should respond. Should they leave the child to his privacy but also his distress, or should they push through his defences and rescue him from his difficulties?

11. Misinterpreting Motives. A disturbed child may easily misinterpret the staff's earnest desire to help. The child may think, 'This adult is just like all the rest who try to control me.' The adults in the family may interpret the staff's attempts to mean, 'You are just another one of those people who are trying to take my child away from me' or 'You say that just to make me feel guilty.' It is easy to be frequently misunderstood.

12. Self-consciousness. There is good evidence that thinking about one's self tends to raise levels of anxiety, blood pressure and heart rate. Yet, in psychiatry it is important to examine yourself in order to know whether the patient is responding to some characteristic in you or some personality feature they are projecting onto you. Primary staff who, of necessity, must think about themselves have to endure the stresses of being increasingly self-conscious.

13. The Complexity of the Problem. The human mind is the last frontier. The work involved when one mind tries to understand another mind is hard. When the child's mind interacts with the minds of parents and community, it becomes a very complex puzzle. Trying to understand all the possible combinations at all the levels of meaning is something like three-dimensional chess played over extended time. There are few more complex problems in all the world than trying to understand the interaction of one mind with another. Because the child's mind is often much more closed to an understanding, the staff must infer deep complexities from very little information.

14. The Borders of Science. Since each child's mind is unique, each child's problem is new and different. There are few family difficulties that are exactly like any other they have ever seen before or read about in a textbook. Previous experiences will help guide the staff, but each experience is sufficiently unique that each family problem is like starting from scratch. The lack of familiarity creates uncertainty which must be constructively handled.

15. Can't Turn Off. Outside of working hours, staff often think about not only the child and his problem but the turmoil engendered within themselves. They go home with a mixture of conflicts in their minds. When they should be relaxing, they continue to work on their patient's problems or their own conflicts. Much of that work is material which is not to be shared with friends or spouse.

16. Fountain of Hope. Faced with a disintegrating classroom, home and interpersonal system, the child's psychiatric staff ask everyone to hang on with, 'Give us a chance to clarify the situation and possibly rectify it.' Staff must convince the family to be patient and have a reasonably hopeful expectation. To convince teacher, counsellor and coach that it is worth another try, staff must pour in considerable optimism that the child will change, that the parents will become more understanding, that the system can adjust and that, in the long run, everybody will benefit. After the parents have tried 'for years' and agencies have 'attempted everything', it takes a large reserve of hope to counter the growing scepticism towards the child. It is tempting to join the cynical with, 'Yes he is a sociopath' and difficult continually to dredge up more hope.

17. Psychic Energy. There is a sense in which supporting patients means supplying them with the energy, determination or desire to keep working on the problem. This energy drain, plus the need to be constantly alert to the nuances of communication, plus working hard to solve complicated personal and interpersonal dilemmas, can make anyone feel flat by the end of the day. It is not unnatural for staff to search for someone or something to give them a boost.

18. Misunderstood. While many of their colleagues are rushing around a hospital doing desperate deeds to save lives, the primary workers in the psychiatric unit are seen to be doing little more than sitting and playing with children. When they talk with their colleagues, they may be teased or derided. When asked to explain what they do all day, they find it very difficult to put into words just exactly what it is.

It is hard to explain to colleagues why they feel so stressed when there is so little apparent activity. Being misunderstood tends to annoy and frustrate, but to express that annoyance seems inappropriate.

19. Hellos and Goodbyes. To be therapeutic, the staff must have a personal involvement with their patients. Personal attachment to disturbed children can grow very quickly. The child is desperately reaching out and the staff are eager to help. When it comes time to say goodbye, primary care staff must go through all the pain of a personal loss. If they cannot anticipate when the child is about to leave, hospital staff are confronted with an abrupt loss. The hurt and anger they feel is seldom dealt with. Yet they are expected to make another attachment to a new patient the next day, just as easily as the last.

20. Suspended Decisions and Judgements. In psychiatry, it is difficult to reach a quick conclusion about a family problem. It is more important to watch carefully the development of the interactions between child, family and staff. Some people who become primary care workers have previously been given major responsibilities as nurses, teachers, etc., where they have been expected to make quick decisions. In child psychiatry, it is necessary for them to suspend judgement and delay decisions. This change of pace may result in a feeling of wanting somebody else to make the quick decision so that they can get on with it.

21. Identity. Few people go into child psychiatry without an established identity in some other profession. When they go into child psychiatry, they must then struggle to change a fairly secure identity. Unfortunately, the child psychiatric primary worker is not a work identity that is well recognised in the community. It is certainly not an identity that is easily picked up second-hand. Each identity must be worked out personally.

Programme

In order to deal with all these problems which may result in burn-out, the Family Restoration Programme has emphasised the need for job satisfaction. The staff attain this through careful follow-up and feedback. Feedback is provided by measures applied to each technique before, during and at five weeks' follow-up.

It is a good feeling to visit a child at home or school and notice that changes in the family are being sustained. Since there is built-in feedback, there is less need for individual direction. Thus, those who are responsible for the administration of the unit have greater opportunity to become clinically involved themselves.

Even with good results and good feedback, staff lapse in their zeal and enthusiasm. On these occasions it is important to get them together for a variety of group activities, parties or a session on personal positive feedback. During strength bombardment, staff are singled out, and their strengths described. They can usually take one or two comments of correction. It is a very warm and enjoyable experience from which staff leave determined to give it another good try.

Staff will work hard at what they enjoy. They will enjoy what they do well. They do a good job when they have been trained and when they have feedback which shows how effectively they are working. Children tend to imitate adult behaviour when adults are enjoying themselves. When the staff are enjoying their work, children are more likely to imitate their good interpersonal relating.

Strong emotions engendered within staff simulate the production of catecholamines. Staff will find it relaxing to join in some kind of vigorous sport. It has been the tradition of The Family Restoration Unit to have a weekly game of floor hockey. It is a primitive sport with few rules and much exercise but, when words cannot release tensions, body contact can.

Although it has always been a practice not to socialise only with those with whom you work, the staff have found it most enjoyable to have parties highlighting certain occasions. It has been the tradition to have a party welcome someone. (There is less emphasis on partying for those who leave.) Sometimes it is a party centred around a swimming pool when all staff, their spouses and children, can find enjoyment in the same activities.

In order to keep the staff from a disrupted personal life, and patients from disrupted therapeutic relationships, the programme has concentrated on regular shifts. This has been made possible by having only four out of the ten children on the Unit during the weekend. The majority of staff not only have regular shifts but regular weekends off. To provide continuity it is very helpful to have a regular night nurse. This nurse has often been someone who is taking courses at university and enjoys the opportunity to study when it is quiet.

Net Effect

Good therapeutic results have always been the best motivator to keep staff treating difficult problems. They are pleased that the Family Restoration Unit has been effective. Staff keep struggling with impossible problems partly because they know that there are increasing numbers of grateful families and grateful children. Some staff have been around long enough to meet the children of children once treated on our child psychiatric unit. To see the much improved way in which treated children handle their children is a joy.

High levels of hopefulness are necessary to keep staff optimistic about the continual stream of deeply disturbed children from chaotic families they must treat. That hopefulness springs from mutual encouragement, personal strengths and spiritual resources in individual staff members.

Since staff are accurately aware of their patient's progress, they are accurately aware of each other's successes and failures. When they become aware that some children have not progressed as well as their colleague had hoped, they are quick to encourage that staff member with reassurance and support. A close camaraderie develops in which there is opportunity to express a wide variety of hopes and frustrations.

By learning useful techniques, staff build up an inventory of skills. Should they need to move or change jobs, these skills are useful in a wide variety of settings. With the inventory of skills that have been checked on by review committee, a referee has no difficulty writing in a letter of recommendation, an accurate assessment of a primary worker's experiences and abilities.

Compared with other psychiatric or medical units there has been very little turnover of primary care staff on The Family Restoration Unit. It appears that the staff enjoy their job and feel they are making a significant contribution. Generally they have good health with few sick days. This means that there is little disruption to the child's therapeutic programme.

The good reputation of the unit makes it easier to hire good staff.

Generalisation

Problem

Many child psychiatric units demonstrate good success in changing the child's behaviour and attitude while he is in hospital, but these beneficial changes do not generalise into the community environment. The child may do well for a short period immediately upon discharge and then problems tend to recur, resulting in a high readmission rate.

The parents are painfully aware of the fact that staff often do not see the child as he behaves in his usual environment. They complain 'You staff think that he is such a good kid but that's only because you give him so much attention and so many enjoyable outings.' 'If you saw him at home you would see quite a different child.' Most frequently this complaint is quite genuine.

Programme

The Family Restoration Programme has attempted to deal with the problem of generalisation by making the unit as much like home as possible. The decor and furnishings are home-like and each child is expected to care for his own hygiene, do various chores and attend school on a regular basis.

The staff are chosen to represent the kinds of people who live in the child's real world. There are old and young staff, fat ones and skinny ones. A handicapped staff member would be a real asset. Staff represent a variety of attitudes towards children. If we cannot get staff who are reasonably representative of the population, we ask them to role-play certain characteristics that children are likely to encounter in the real world. The staff do not wear uniforms. This allows them greater opportunity to adopt different roles and greater flexibility to express their individual interests and personality characteristics.

During the five weeks of hospital admission, children are sent home for two trial weekends. For these weekends tentative recommendations of guidelines and measures are drawn up. Parents reporting back after the weekend can do so on the basis of specific recommendations given by the staff. The parents can report that the child's compliance rate was only 50 per cent, for example.

The Family Restoration Programme emphasises the necessity of observing the child in his natural environment and of making a diagnosis before admission. The programme is designed to deal with the problems that take place in the school, in the home and on the playgrounds.

Our programme emphasises teaching management skills, teaching parents and teaching family communication aids. Parents are given instruction and practice in using techniques that the staff have found useful in helping their child. In learning to negotiate guidelines and consequences the parents learn a management skill that they can apply with all members of the family.

The programme provides the parents with a detailed prescription to follow on discharge. This prescription is usually a reminder of those things that the parents have already tried and found useful. A number of the issues that are covered are fairly common to all families, e.g. parents need to be reminded to spend time with their children individually. Too frequently families feel they must always go out as a family. This does not give parents an opportunity to see how their children behave when they don't have to compete for attention.

The child is given a brief set of recommendations of his own, e.g. 'Don't forget when the kids tease you, you must look them straight in the eye and stand up for yourself, without getting too mad or walking away.'

On discharge the family physician is sent a report which includes a summary of the problem, diagnostic findings, and the recommendations given to the parents and children. The unit teacher sends a summary of his findings and recommendations to the child's regular teacher.

The five-week follow-up period provides staff an opportunity to contact children in home and school. They try not to respond to emergencies but to make pre-arranged visits. As already mentioned, it has been our experience that there is a two-week honeymoon period, after which a problem may briefly reappear. It is vital at that time that parents don't react with old ways of responding. Often the staff can check up on the way the parents have been dealing with small difficulties, make a slight programme change and see the improvement continue.

Net Effect

As a result of the programme's follow-up parents do not feel abandoned. They know, however, that treatment will only last a total of ten weeks so that they must utilise all the time available to gain the greatest amount for themselves and for the child. Because of the five-week follow-up the staff are better able fully to say goodbye to the child and the parents. During follow-up parents relinquish their dependency on the staff and begin to actualise their own strengths. Results indicate that change in the child and family during admission generalise well into the home and school.

Making Parents Successful at Parenting

We assume that if parents could see themselves as successful parents, they would feel warmer towards their children and spend more time at being parents. With proper methods of communication and management, parents who humiliate, criticise or batter could find that they would no longer need to abuse their children. When there is no longer continuing hostility between child and parent, the child feels more inclined to please his parent, who in turn responds with greater warmth.

We found that 85 per cent of those parents who have had children on the unit, attend family training willingly and quite regularly. Even parents who came from as far as communities on the north end of the island, 100 miles away, would attend quite regularly. There have been fewer fathers than mothers attending, but the rate of fathers was still high. Some parents attended the parent training many weeks after their children were discharged. Because the parent training proved to be such a useful activity, we considered requiring that parents attend twice a week.

We combined seminar presentations with discussions of specific family problems. Presentations were enlivened with role-playing, video tapes and staff dramatisations. The one and a half hour session was split between two staff; the first half devoted to a better understanding of children and the other three-quarters of an hour to practical solutions to frequent problems. Parents were given homework and asked to report their detailed observations, successes and failures. At the end of the five weeks for each parent, they were provided with group acclaim and invited to attend a five weeks' post-graduate seminar.

During the follow-up, parents would attend a 5-week, 1-hour session during which time, further topics pertinent to their struggles were discussed. However, more time was spent in giving the parents an opportunity to air their difficulties, which, when shared with the other parents, often resulted in practical solutions.

Seminar Topics

1. Why Did it Happen to Me? An outline of the constitutional, psychodynamic, transactional, existential and behavioural aspects which pertain to the origins of the problem in a family.

2. How Large is the Problem? An emphasis on objective measures of the child's behaviour, realistic expectations of what their child can and cannot do and hope, which is neither too great nor too small.

3. A Behavioural Explanation of Problems. The parents are taught to define punishment and reinforcement, given an explanation of mutual reinforcement, child and mother, with examples including temper tantrums, thumb sucking, bed wetting, lying, stealing, etc.

4. Techniques of Modifying Behaviour. This includes primary and secondary reinforcement, primary and secondary punishment, shaping, time-out, response cause and reinforcing incompatible responses.

5. Guidelines in Confidence and Consequences. The parents are taught to start with the behaviour that is most likely to change their given examples of negotiating and a demonstration of how it is done.

6. Three Parts of a Person. This is an outline of transactionalism. The parents are given an opportunity to try and name the games in their home.

7. The Child's Perspective. The parents are reminded that the child is a small person and sees things very differently than they do. They are given an understanding of children's developmental stages and emotional responses.

8. How the Problem Gets Larger. This seminar outlines principles of reinforcing maladaptive behaviour, from small beginnings to large problems such as prolonged temper tantrums.

9. Expressing Our Feelings. Parents are taught the origin of feelings, how children manage them, the benefits and disadvantages of expressing or withholding feelings.

10. Techniques of Changing Behaviour. The parents are given a variety of ways of tackling problem behaviours in their children.

11. Praise, Criticism and Correction. Parents are taught to distinguish between them, then asked to go home and measure the amount of praise and criticism they use on each other and their children.

12. Putting it into Practice. Parents are given a review of the practical techniques that are used, then some helpful hints on how to handle problems.

13. Developing Family Strengths. Parents are asked to enumerate the strong points of the family and rate the weaknesses.

Parents are required to commit themselves to up to 12 hours per week in therapy with their children. Although this is not always possible, they are expected to spend at least one and a half hours in training seminars, 1 hour in conjoint counselling or psychotherapy and 3 hours a week working with nurses learning observational management and communication skills.

Staff

As previously discussed, the unit's philosophy is that a person may also do what they are able to do, not only what they have been trained to do. It is unnecessary to place restrictions on therapeutic endeavours restraining one profession to one kind of activity because there are so many activities that need to be done for each family. The emphasis rather, is on using each individual where they are most effective with their particular skills. Many staff have individual talents and these are highlighted. Some staff are good at behaviour modification techniques such as assertion training; others are good at individual psychotherapy. Because there is no end point to how skilled an individual can become, continuing emphasis has been placed on staff training.

In addition to flexibility, we believe that each staff member should have a distinctive role and professional identity. We found that where roles and identities are confused, professionals have a tendency to promote the existence of their profession by finding patients that need their skills. The more secure an individual is in his identity, the less he needs to find patients to support his professional role.

The philosophy in hiring staff has always been that where two individuals have similar qualifications and skills, preference will be given to that staff member who has an identity distinct from his profession. The nurse who also sees herself as an artist will be given preference to a nurse who has no other major interest.

Therapists' abilities increase by developing their interest and experience in specific skills. Each staff member is required to fill out a skill inventory on which are listed 60 or more hospital skills that they may be proficient in. They list both those in which they feel competent, and those in which they would like to learn more. If they exhibit competence in a specific skill, they are reviewed by a peer group who have proven ability on that skill. Once they have been checked out, there is no restriction placed on their functioning in that area.

Part of the good morale stems from the fact that there have been controlled admissions with pre-planning of the programme in which each staff member can participate. Staff who are available are acquainted with the children and given some opportunity to determine whether that child in that family, are people they feel they can work with. There is a certain amount of mutual selecting between staff and patients. Staff are pleased to be able to follow children into the community and learn what becomes of them.

Since all staff have a tendency to become very attached to children and want to remain attached, we are quite firm about the limit on hospitalisation. When a child, parents or staff want to maintain that attachment, they are reminded of the rules that state a child must be discharged whether he is apparently well or ill. When staff plead that the child is just getting better or about to make a major change, they are assured that responsibility is in the hands of the child's physician but that they will be able to continue treating the child during the follow-up.

Some staff find it much easier to communicate with older children. For this reason, staff are allowed to select the age group with which they wish to work. There is sufficient flexibility, however, that staff may change to work with younger children if they wish.

Ward Co-ordinator

The ward co-ordinator, a child psychiatrist, provides overall direction and accepts responsibility for the family unit programme. Child psychiatrists, adult psychiatrists and general practitioners may admit to the programme as long as they will accept the responsibility of detailing the child's individual programme, meeting with the nursing staff to discuss direction and accept the unit's overall programme. They adhere to the philosophy that:

(1) The child should be returned to his home environment, school and family.
(2) The ten-week termination of treatment.
(3) Continuous care by staff before, during and after admission.
(4) Pre-admission, diagnosis and planning.
(5) Predetermined placement following admission.
(6) Utilisation of staff which is not limited to their professions but is determined by their skills.

The ward co-ordinator (or other senior staff) chairs admission and discharge conferences. He conducts follow-up reviews, teaches the staff, leads family training seminars and liaises with a variety of professions in the community. With the screening committee he is responsible for the appropriate mix and match of the patients. With a management committee he co-ordinates unit activities.

The ward co-ordinator is part of a team in Victoria that travels throughout the adjacent countryside in order to follow up children who have been treated on the unit. This trip takes place three times a year and involves a child psychiatrist, social worker, nurse, teacher and, alternatively, the occupational therapist or psychologist. This provides an opportunity to maintain contact with community agencies and to discuss children who might be referred for admission.

The Primary Therapists and Child Care Workers

Primary therapists are responsible for a pre-admission home visit to collect essential baseline assessment data of psychological and physical needs. Data collected include a record of immunisation, current medications, physical impairments, bowel and bladder patterns or problems, dental care and sleep patterns. A physical assessment data form is completed with the parents' assistance. The child is interviewed in his own home and preferably in his own room. Information on how he thinks and feels about his family, his interaction with peers and his functioning in the community is obtained. The information is shared with a team at the pre-admission planning conference. This facilitates realistic goal-setting and provides well-structured treatment plans.

During hospitalisation, primary workers assist children and young adolescents in interacting in more appropriate ways with their peers, siblings, parents and teachers. They provide corrective feedback, cue children when to respond, and engage in individual psychotherapy. Primary workers may use all the techniques outlined in this book once they have demonstrated they have the skill.

Primary workers function in the classroom as ego auxiliaries. They provide children and adolescents with a sounding board and will demonstrate mediational modification. To do this, they sit beside the child and attempt to see the school situation from the child's perspective. They are discouraged from teaching the child.

Primary workers teach parents during the seminars but more particularly in individual sessions. They help them provide limits in consistency in a way that is acceptable to all members of the family. Parents learn to negotiate with others for desired behaviours and reinforce the positive changes that occur.

In preparation for discharge, primary workers write prescriptions for the parents and adolescents for future care and self-control. For the two weekends of home leave, the child and parents are given trial recommendations. On the child's arrival back at the unit, the recommendations are gone over with the parents and staff members. Prior to the next weekend visit, appropriate changes are made. By the time the child is discharged, there is a comprehensive record, written by the nurse, of observations and recommendations which have already been tried. These recommendations are sufficiently specific that on follow-up home visits, nurses can request from the child or parents detailed information on how things have gone.

A discharge summary is sent to the referring physician with a copy to the consultant. The discharge summary includes the identified conflicts, goals and nursing intervention. The nurses in their summary indicate the progress made during hospitalisation. A separate summary is provided to parents and another one for the older children and adolescents.

Experience indicates that approximately two weeks after discharge a crisis is very likely to occur. It is important that the nursing staff be available to make a home visit and intervene where necessary. Prescribed treatment ensures consistency and assists the family towards a more comfortable and secure way of handling problems.

For children who live outside the city, the telephone number of the staff is provided, with instructions that the child may call at any time the staff are on duty. More frequently the staff call parents and child at pre-arranged times. It is important that even though the staff cannot see the child, they are able to talk together by telephone.

Staff Duties

Every staff member is carefully selected for their maturity, training and attitudes to families. Each person is given a carefully described job description which becomes his chores, those duties which must be finished before he or she starts other treatment. Usually the chores take up 40–50 per cent of the time. The rest is spent doing various treatments.

3 INDIVIDUAL TECHNIQUES

Introduction

For those who are about to learn and use these techniques we would like to emphasise that all of them are dynamic and developing. It is up to you to take the basic idea and adapt it to your abilities and your situation. As you do so, if you describe your modifications you will build up your own bank of techniques to use in treating children.

The ideas were developed and described by the authors but much credit must be given to the staff on the Child and Family Psychiatric Units of Victoria, Hong Kong and Christchurch, Rick Hana, Philip Williamson and Jan Brooker to name a few, who have contributed to and modified various techniques. The names of each technique have grown with popular usage. The children often have their own terms and those are indicated in inverted commas. The abbreviations, in brackets, are used in the skill inventory and in charting. Our manual of techniques sits on the ward with blank pages attached where staff can make notations to indicate what they believe is working well and what should be changed.

In all the techniques the importance of making measures before, during and after, in order to determine whether they are really working, is stressed. The data you collect will also provide a baseline to determine whether any modifications work better for you.

The techniques have been rated according to difficulty into three categories. As you become more experienced you will want to learn and develop the more difficult techniques. However, remember that all of these techniques can be learned by reasonably intelligent, frontline staff regardless of their background training.

Treatment Techniques — Explanation of Assignment and Levels

Treatment techniques have been evaluated and divided into three categories on the basis of: their risk to the patient, the skill and training necessary for the staff performing the technique.

Technique — First Level (Low Risk)

These techniques are considered low risk techniques and could be

74

administered by all regular and relief staff after reading the appropriate instructions. Even if the techniques were administered incompetently or incompletely, risk or damage to the child's physical or psychological health would be low.

Compliance Training	Play Therapy — Observation
Delayed Gratification	Self-esteem
Locked Box	Teaching Machine Instruction

Technique — Second Level (Moderate Risk)

These techniques require some specific supervised instruction in addition to the write-up. The majority of the front-line staff and some regular relief staff are proficient in the use of these techniques.

Abreaction	Listen to Your Body
Amorphous Blob	Mediational Modification
Assertiveness Training	Nurturing Child
Body Impulse Directing	Play Therapy — Corrective
Body Painting	Pushing Red and Green Buttons
Child Free Play Acting	Relaxation Techniques
Conflict Displacement	Saying Goodbye
Corrective Feedback	Self-control
Delayed Impulse Response	Sex Education
Ego Auxiliary	Shaping
Feelings Rehearsal	Sphincter Control
Individuation	Therapeutic Wrestling
	Time-out

Technique — Third Level (High Risk)

Unless properly administered, these techniques involve potential risk to the child. These techniques should be performed with supervision. This category also includes techniques that require a very high level of expertise, regardless of risk potential.

Aversive Conditioning	Parent–Child Contract
Biofeedback Training	Play Therapy — Interpretative
Brief Insight-oriented Psycho- therapy	Psychological Testing Interpre- tation
Empathy Training	Rage Restraining
Giving Medication	Rebonding for Battered Children
Grief Facilitation	Secret Disclosure

Hypnotic Therapy
Name Change
Operant Conditioning of
  Children

Systematic Desensitisation of
  Phobic Children

Brief Description of Individual and Group Techniques (Chapters 3 and 4)

Abreaction — 'Let it all hang out'
Reviewing traumatic experiences in such a way as to diffuse the emotional charge associated with the experience.

Amorphous Blob — 'Who am I?'
A paper and pencil exercise of discovering one's inner self and improving one's self-image.

Anatomy and Physiology Teaching (A & P Teaching) — 'Teach me Doc'
A rationale and guide to anatomy and physiology teaching to children.

Assertiveness Training — 'I'm not afraid of the big bad wolf'
A procedure to teach and train children to respect their own and others' rights.

Aversive Conditioning — 'Getting rid of bad habits'
The use of unpleasant stimuli to distinguish maladaptive behaviour.

Biofeedback Training — 'Bells and buzzers'
The use of mechanical monitoring of body responses in order to train the child in self-control.

Brief Insight-oriented Psychotherapy — 'I can figure it out'
A process to assess children and their families to gain insight into their behaviour and thereby increase their motivation and their power to change.

Body Impulse Directing — 'Know your body'
A process of education, experience and self-discovery which alters misconceptions of one's body.

Body Painting – 'Colour me carefully'
A process of concertising the body boundaries and emphasising body parts and properties.

Child Free Play Acting – 'Let's dress up'
An activity which involves all the children on the ward in a play based on a well-known fairy story, during which they identify with the conflicts in the play and learn to understand more of their own conflicts.

Compliance Training – 'I'll do what you say'
A technique which assists a child in carrying out adult requests.

Conflict Displacement – 'Oh, no you don't'
A process of education, experience and practice which assists children and their families to disagree and rebel about issues which are not life-threatening.

Corrective Feedback – 'This is what you are'
A process of making objective assessments of a person and sharing that information in order to correct previous misconceptions.

Delayed Gratification – 'You gotta be patient'
A technique which trains children to wait to have their needs or desires met.

Delayed Impulse Response – 'Keep your cool'
A series of sessions using role-model, role-playing, mediational modification and practice that lead an impulsive child to gain self-control and become more objective in situations of stress.

Ego Auxiliary – 'Be my friend'
A process of identification with the child in order to support him through a situation of conflict to more adaptable behaviour.

Empathy Training – 'I know how she feels'
The way children can be taught how to recognise the feelings of others from their facial expressions and non-verbal communication.

Family Counselling – 'Help for parents'
Use of family dynamics and support to effect change in behaviour.

Feelings Rehearsal – *'Say it with feeling'*
A step-by-step educative, demonstrative process of teaching children about their emotional life.

Giving Medication – *'It doesn't have to hurt'*
A description, rationale, precautions and guidelines for using medication with emotionally ill children.

Grief Facilitation – *'It's time to say goodbye'*
A step-by-step system of guiding individuals through the grieving process.

Home Maintenance Skills – *'Chores'*
A procedure for education and attitude change in home care.

Hypnotic Therapy – *'Let's relax'*
An aid to eliminate resistance that exists from habit or to change underlying belief systems.

Individuation – *'I'm myself'*
A series of prescribed verbal and non-verbal exercises which enable a child to separate from the parent and vice versa.

Kangaroo Kort – *'What is right and what is wrong'*
A psychodrama group that evokes conflictual feelings and assists children in learning more adaptive responses.

Limit Challenge – *'Reach for the stars'*
A series of experiences where the child is asked to extend and exceed his physical limitations.

Listen to Your Body – *'My body tells me what it needs'*
A procedure to sensitise children to their own inner sensations with a view to self-control of urges.

Locked Box – *'It's in the bank'*
A programme which teaches by experience, possession, value and ownership.

Mediational Modification – *'Going gopher'*
A step-by-step process of cognitive restructuring.

Messy Play – 'Being messy is fun'
A process to desensitise children with a strong aversion to dirt and to disinhibit unnecessary repression.

Name Change – 'I like my new name'
A practical procedure of name change to assist in development of more positive self-esteem.

Negotiating Guidelines and Consequences – 'Bargaining rules and pay-offs'
Teaching by example and practice the process of compromise and consensus in helping families formulate house rules.

Nurturing Child – 'Really being looked after'
A period of regression for the purpose of nurture, care, relationship building and history reconstruction.

Operant Conditioning of Children – 'Learning good habits'
A brief description of the way children's behaviour can be modified by carefully applying the correct consequences.

Parent-Child Contract – 'You signed it Dad'
A procedure to assist parents in making a firm commitment to each other and to a child, and also to assist the child in trusting that commitment.

Play Therapy – Corrective – 'Play my game'
The formal use of play to structure more adaptive responses to conflict situations.

Play Therapy – Interpretative – 'What can your play tell me?'
The use of play as a psychotherapeutic tool.

Play Therapy – Observation – 'Can I watch?'
The rationale and guidelines for observing children's play.

Psychological Testing Interpretation – 'Mind testing'
An explanation of the administration and interpretation of psychological tests.

Pushing Red and Green Buttons — 'Pleased and mad parents'
A technique which helps children identify their parents' temperamental characteristics and those triggers which stimulate pleased or angry responses in their parents.

Rage Restraining — 'Lion taming'
A procedure to remove an aggressive child from the environment against his will or physically to restrain him when he is out of control.

Rebonding for Battered Children — 'It will be better this time'
A method of systematically desensitising the parent and child and reintroducing them in a positive controlled manner.

Recreational Introduction — 'It's a beautiful world'
A step-by-step procedure of introducing a child and/or parent to the activities available in the community.

Relaxation Techniques — 'It's good to relax'
A procedure to teach relaxation to people with special adaptations for young children.

Role-playing — 'Play a part'
A step-by-step method of using role-play to teach empathy and understanding of new behaviour patterns.

Saying Goodbye — 'So long, it's been good to know you'
A process of guiding a child through the ambivalent feelings of saying goodbye to important relationships.

Secret Disclosures — 'I have a right to know'
A guideline to use with a family who need to reveal a family secret.

Self-control — 'Flying level and steady'
A combination of techniques designed to assist the child to know when and how to let their feelings go and learn confidence in their own judgement.

Self-esteem — 'I'm okay'
A procedure of modelling, monitoring and goal setting which improves one's self-perception.

Sensitivity Exercise — 'Getting to know you'
A series of games that develop self- and other awareness, so designed and scheduled that they support the intra- and interpersonal process of the treatment programme.

Sex Education — 'The birds and the bees'
A guideline for teaching children about their developing sexuality.

Shaping — 'New ways of behaving'
A process of developing, reinforcing and establishing new behaviours.

Social Skills Training — 'The right way to treat people'
A series of procedures involving feeling release, modelling, analysis, re-enactment and practice to improve interactional and social skills.

Sphincter Control — 'I can hang on or let go'
A series of exercises and techniques designed to give the child greater control over his spinchter.

Strength Bombardment — 'You're pretty good'
A process of flooding in order to establish a healthier self-concept.

Systematic Desensitisation — 'I'm not frightened anymore'
A step-by-step procedure using relaxation, visualisation and practical retraining in order to assist children in overcoming their phobias.

Teaching Machine Instruction — 'Computer teacher'
A method of using a machine to overcome learning difficulties and to reinforce work habits and general knowledge.

Teaching Parents Skills — 'How to be better parents'
A guideline to assist staff in helping parents learn healthier relationship skills with their children.

Therapeutic Wrestling — 'The bigger they are the harder they fall'
An experience of controlled wrestling in order to abreact previous situations of abuse.

Time-out — 'Penalty box'
A rationale for isolation as a method of distinguishing behaviour.

Tradition Engendering — 'Remember when . . .'
A process of education and selection of family traditions and celebrations.

Ward Control — 'Let's vote'
A rationale and guidelines for maintaining a therapeutic milieu on the ward.

Compliance Training (CT) — 'Yes sir, no sir'
Technique — First Level

Rationale

Usually when children are easy to manage they are more liked by their parents. When there is less hassle, parents are more likely to spend time with their children, enjoy parenting more, see themselves as better parents and praise rather than criticise each other and their children. Consequently, children have an improved self-image.

Non-compliance may increase when parents inadvertently reinforce disobedience by speaking again to a child after requesting a certain behaviour. Over-controlling parents tend to have negative stubborn children. Parents increase a child's resistance or stubbornness when they attempt to force a child to obey them in an area where the child should have autonomy. Non-compliance increases where parents do not let natural consequences govern the child's own decision-making.

Applications

Any child who disobeys inappropriately or unnecessarily can benefit. Do not use this technique with children who are over-compliant, e.g. obsessive, compulsive, anorexic or school phobic. By learning gentle techniques of control, parents who abuse their children are in a better position to control their own aggression.

Measures

Calculate the percentage of compliance, i.e. obedience divided by the total number of requests X 100. There should be at least five requests per shift and more requests in particular situations.

Procedure

1. Make baseline measures using at least five requests/shift. Note the conflicts, the setting stimuli, antecedents, reinforcements and games played.

2. Explain the procedure to parents and children after negotiating reasonable goals.

3. Demonstrate using another child who has already made some progress.

4. Make a hierarchy of requests with increasing probability of compliance. Begin by making requests in areas where the child is most likely to comply. Make each request once only. Don't ask if they want to do something. Many parents do, but become annoyed if the child quite rightly states 'no', he doesn't want to do it. Say, 'Johnny I want you to . . .'

5. If the child begins to respond within five seconds of the request, it is recorded as a compliance. Make requests increasingly difficult. Then make requests involving two activities. Use continuous and, if possible, natural reinforcements. The child must reach for his reinforcement.

6. The child should succeed at 70–80 per cent before you proceed to more difficult tasks.

7. Once a sufficiently high rate of compliance is achieved, place the child on a ratio reinforcement schedule and substitute natural reinforcers for the artificial.

8. Negotiate guidelines and consequences with the family in all the usual areas of hassle.

9. Make sure the parents have learned the techniques before the child is discharged.

10. During follow-up, check to see if they are falling back into old patterns.

Untoward Effects

If the shaping is not done properly, increased rebellion or resistance will occur. Be careful not to reinforce inadvertently non-complying patients who are not your direct responsibility.

Charting Requirements

A hierarchy of requests should be included in the 24-Hour Progress Notes. Compliance measure on graph.

Delayed Gratification (DG) — 'Waiting it out'
Technique — First Level

Rationale

Demanding children irritate their parents, who in turn become increasingly angry and frustrating to their children. Parents may become abusive in spite of themselves. When angry, some parents become increasingly uncertain and inconsistent. This produces uncertainty in the child which makes him more demanding. Demanding children may make parents feel trapped and thus more desperate in their determination to spend time outside of the home in activities without their children. Demanding behaviour is often reinforced on a variable ratio schedule by parents who give in to the demand.

When children learn to delay gratification, it provides them with a greater sense of integrity and security. Parents are grateful for the greater peace and quiet, 'maybe those kids aren't so bad after all'.

Application

Impatient, immature and anxious children usually benefit.

Measures

1. The interval required to wait.
2. The percentage of successes. At least two tests of this kind should be given per shift.

Procedures

1. Obtain a baseline. Try measuring it with parents present and preferably in the child's home.
2. Explain the object and procedure to the child and parents. Alert fellow staff to when you are carrying out the technique.
3. Negotiate, e.g. 'How long do you think you can wait?' Begin at an interval below which a child thinks he can wait.
4. Intervals should be increased as tolerated. The interval should depend on the age of the child, e.g. 2 X the child's age. A three-minute wait is a good starting point. Once the child has successfully waited at each level three consecutive times, then increase the time interval by intervals of two minutes.
5. The first request of the child is deemed to be the most important. If the child seeks to engage in an alternative activity and requests this of the staff, the staff must use their own judgement whether it is a legitimate request for an alternative activity while the child waits, or whether it is another demand that should also be put on delayed gratification.
6. If the child becomes very frustrated give him one or two additional explanations. Reassure him that the staff are not being inconsistent or inconsiderate.

7. If he succeeds in waiting he gets what he was promised. If he asks again he gets nothing but an explanation of why he failed.

8. The parents must take over doing the delayed gratification of their children before discharge.

9. On reaching your goal, make sure the behaviour is set by using a variable ratio reinforcement schedule.

Untoward Effects

Children may become increasingly irritable and whiny. It is possible they will further distract adults. If so, the therapist must explain what is happening and demonstrate how consistency in other areas of the child's interaction with them pays off.

Charting Requirements

Measures and observations.

Empathy Training (ET)
Technique — Third Level

Rationale

Children are born self-centred, not necessarily selfish. They become selfish if they have never had an opportunity to care for others. They learn to empathise with the needs and feelings of others by watching their parents. Children are by nature careful to observe their parents' responses, mainly because they depend upon their parents. They cannot afford to offend or overwhelm them because they dare not break up their own support system.

If parents do not show emotions or if they show too much emotion or confusing emotions the child cannot learn to read his parents. If the child has sensory perception problems, is partly blind, deaf or developmentally delayed, the child may not learn as readily. In these instances it is important that children learn to read other people and understand from their gestures, facial expressions and emotional tone what that person is feeling. We have found that once children learn to understand the emotions of others they become much more careful of how they interact with them.

Staff can model a great deal of empathy during their normal interaction with children. The child may soon pick up from staff, who make it very clear that they are not only concerned but actively trying to understand the other person's responses.

Some children can be overwhelmed with too much emotional

feedback from their parents. Because children are sensitive to emotional feedback from the adults upon whom they depend they may feel immobilised if the parents show too much fear, anger or sorrow. Thus, it is important for the parents to let children know how they feel, within the bounds of their child's capability of dealing with those feelings. Since the child will attempt to meet his parents' needs, parents should not overpower their children with needs they cannot meet. If the child can do nothing about the parents' needs, then to let him know about them does the child a disservice. He will spend many hours worrying about what he could or should do to help his parents.

Some parents rely on creating an atmosphere of secrecy and ambiguity to control their children. They may feel that to be well understood by their children detracts from their power.

Application

This procedure is very useful with children having conduct disorders or children who have been so emotionally traumatised that they do not want to or are unable to empathise with people.

Procedure

1. Obtain a baseline of the child by watching his response to his parents interacting for a few minutes. Ask him to guess at their feelings, record the mistakes, particularly in which emotional area.

2. Explain to the parents and the child that you are able to teach them how to understand and read the feelings in other people. Obtain their consent.

3. Demonstrate using another child who has gone through the procedure or another staff member.

4. Using pictures showing the emotional expression of a variety of people, ask the child to describe what that person may be feeling. Gently correct any mistakes. Teach the child the correct words to describe emotions and when to apply adjectives — very, quite, etc.

5. Use your facial expressions and ask him to guess at what you are feeling. Give corrective feedback.

6. Use gestures in addition to your facial expressions. Teach the child what questions he might use to clarify any ambiguities.

7. Show the child how words and non-verbal expressions of feelings may be incongruous. Get him to guess at what feelings you are expressing when your words say one thing and your facial expressions or gestures say another. Ask him if this occurs in his own life at home.

8. Using a mirror ask the child to look at his own expressions. You

should guess at what he is feeling. He must be encouraged to be honest but he can try to fool you.

9. In a crowd of people you can stand quietly aside and ask the child to guess at the feelings of the people going by.

10. Using one parent, see if the child can now read his parent correctly. Teach the child empathetic statements — 'Mum you really look very sad.' Encourage his parent to respond to correct analyses and empathetic statements with appropriate approval.

11. Teach the child how to read his parents' feelings while they are interacting. Get them to stop in mid-transaction and ask the child to guess at their feelings, give empathetic statements and then determine how correct he was.

12. Teach the child how to empathise with his peers and at home with his parents. Make sure during follow-up that he continues to work on empathising.

Untoward Effects

Children may become too worried about how mothers are feeling and become stilted or stifled in their own responses. Make sure that the whole procedure is kept sufficiently light-hearted. Encourage the child to feel confident in making a few mistakes or even ignoring some emotional expressions.

Charting Requirements

Note the number of sessions required to teach a reasonable degree of empathy with the child and the emotions that they cover. Be sure to describe how their parents respond to the procedure.

Locked Box (LB) — 'My stuff in my box'
Technique — First Level

Rationale

Some children steal because they have no sense of property, i.e. 'mine' and 'not mine'. This may occur because the child has had little privacy of person or security of possessions. This procedure is to help them become more aware of the sense of ownership and security of property. A loss from their own locked box can be used to help understand that the victim is suffering loss and hurt.

Taking things from the locked box of the one who steals can be used as an aversive stimulus. It can be used to encourage restitution, teaching a stealing child the value of repayment in order to deal with the guilt and to re-establish a broken relationship between thief and victim. The child can be encouraged to negotiate what is reasonable punishment. By checking the locked box, staff can monitor the amount and frequency of theft.

Application

Thieves, deprived children can benefit.

Measures

1. Observe how the child receives the locked box from his parents and what he puts into it.

2. Record how often valuables are put in or taken out.

Procedure

1. Establish a baseline on the child's stealing.

2. Explain to both parents and child, that the object is not to punish but to help break a bad habit.

3. Demonstrate by using another child's locked box.

4. A parent should buy or build a box and provide a lock and keys. Fishing tackle and tool boxes with hasps are ideal. One key is kept by staff and placed, with the child's knowledge, in a very secure place.

5. As a child places his valuables in the locked box, give him the opportunity to comment on the importance of each and why.

6. Check the locked box randomly. If you find something in it which isn't his, first give him the opportunity to explain how it got there. Be neither excessively gullible nor suspicious.

7. If he steals, ask him to repay voluntarily. The victim is asked what he would choose from the child's locked box. If the victim is vindictive in what he chooses, participate in negotiation. Staff should remember that victims may contribute to the crime.

8. Before discharge make sure the parents can handle this technique calmly.

9. On follow-up, check to see if it is still working.

Untoward Effects

A child may become increasingly secretive.

Charting Requirements

Measures and chart incidents of stealing.

Play Therapy — Observation (PTO) (Play time)
Technique — First Level

Rationale

When children play freely, they express their thinking, including their conflicts, fears and anxieties. They also reveal their ego strengths, imagination and intelligence. By observing and recording a child's play, you can learn a great deal about the thought life they could never put into words. To play freely, children need plenty of time, the right materials and a feeling that they are not too vulnerable.

Measures

Record a narrative description of play. Observe for repetitive patterns, areas of intense emotions, description of interpersonal relationships, spontaneity and any verbalisation. Special observation may be requested for each child.

Application

All children under 12.

Procedure

Use sand, water, clay, paints, string, cloth, blocks and bendable human figures. Avoid mechanical, one-purpose toys. Allow the child to play freely, alone or with another child. Do not interact with him or try to direct him. Let him know it's OK to do almost anything but break toys, harm himself or you.

Untoward Effects

Some children don't like people to know their inner thoughts. To be watched may be frightening.

Charting Requirements

Record narrative document. Graph if special observations are not to be counted.

Self-esteem (SE) — 'Walking tall'
Technique — First Level

Rationale

An unrealistically negative and critical perception of self is an integral part of the depressive syndrome. In some depressed children, low self-esteem seems to have an inertia of its own. The depressed child will tend to reject any information inconsistent with his negative self-image. Thus, realistic self-perception may have to be taught explicitly. Children tend to believe statements made of them by the adults important to them. Often children simplify a negative or critical statement an adult makes of them, then they address themselves. They may identify with their aggressor and become angry at themselves. To impart self-esteem, the child must be able to separate his internal, correcting feedback from statements of him by adults. Usually children are accurately aware of their capabilities but aren't given the opportunity to evaluate and listen to themselves.

Application

Depressed, anorexic or obsessive-compulsive patients can benefit most.

Measures

Note the number of positive self-statements within a given setting and a given time period.

Procedures

1. Obtain a baseline before the child is admitted.
2. Explain to child and family the importance of self-esteem and how to achieve it.
3. Demonstrate to the family the way you have encouraged another family to enhance each other's self-esteem.
4. Model self-praise. By hearing a significant adult or adults praise himself, the child will be more prone to do the same. This self-praise can help enhance self-esteem.
   (i) When modelling self-praise, begin by complimenting yourself for your personal accomplishments, e.g. 'I think I did a good job on that.'
   (ii) Later in the programme, focus on more global personal qualities, 'I guess I'm not so bad after all, in fact, I think I'm all right.'
5. Accurate self-monitoring. Children need to evaluate their behaviour realistically. The feelings a child has about himself are largely derived from his attitudes towards his own behaviour. If a depressed child perceives his accomplishments as failures, self-praise is inappropriate. Although an unrealistically negative evaluation of behaviour produces low self-esteem, a realistically negative evaluation may provide a basis for behaviour change. For instance, reflect on the difference

between a child who considers 79 per cent a failure and one who considers 49 per cent a failure.

6. Encourage the child to monitor success rather than failure experiences. The teacher who grades papers by marking the number right, rather than the usual practice of citing the number wrong, understands this fine point. While half a glass of milk is both half-empty and half-full, you should encourage the child to see it as half-full.

7. Evaluate the child's performance against his own baseline rather than against the norms of his age-mates. Accentuate the positive.

8. Realistic goal-setting. Research shows that people with low self-esteem tend to set their goals unrealistically high or unrealistically low. Either creates a no-win situation. The former produces frequent failure, the latter produces accomplishments that are so Mickey Mouse that they do not count as successes. Learning and behaviour change are achieved in small increments. Goal-setting should reflect this. Teach the child to think in terms of step-goals as well as a bigger end-goal. Short-range, attainable goals increase the opportunity for self-reinforcement and self-praise.

9. Self-praise. Self-esteem is ultimately internal. The child must become his own evaluator and reinforcer. Traditionally, positive self-communication (or 'blowing one's own horn') has been thought of as impolite.

   (i)   Elicit self-praise with questions like: 'Do you think you did a good job on that one?'

   (ii) If the child uses self-praise, confirm it by praising him yourself: 'Yeah, I think you did a good job too.'

10. Teach the child to praise others. Praising others and self-praise are positively correlated. Apparently, praising is still a skill which can be applied to anyone, including oneself. Moreover, praise of others tends to bring praise in return. People reciprocate, stroke-wise.

11. Model the reception of praise from others. Teach the child that it is all right to accept compliments matter-of-factly, without either becoming embarrassed or letting it go to your head. Teach him to say thank you or to correct a mis-impression.

12. Show the family how to enhance each other's self-esteem.

13. During follow-up, do some more appropriate modelling.

Untoward Effects

Children may become boastful or arrogant until they learn to self-monitor accurately and appropriately.

Charting Requirements

Graph the number of positive self-statements. Chart positive areas that a child is able to see in himself so others may reinforce these. Chart levels of achievement and encourage progress.

Teaching Machine Instruction (TMI) — 'Computer teacher' Technique — First Level

Rationale

The natural curiosity of many children is killed by teachers too eager to teach and examine. The most important skills and concepts are learned without formal instruction. Teachers and classrooms gain aversive qualities from long associations with restriction and anxiety. Teaching machines give feedback without derogatory connotations. Children are very interested in machines that teach and very pleased to find they can learn without the usual amount of frustration. Teaching machines can give children a head start on their school mates in areas of rote learning (e.g. times tables) and problem-solving. The main object is to improve the child's motivation to learn.

Instruction is maximally effective if it is programmed so that:

(1) It holds the child's interest (important with distractable children).
(2) It requires attention to a small amount of information at a time (shaping).
(3) The student must make a response to each segment of information before him.
(4) There is immediate feedback of results.
(5) Material reinforcement (tokens, Smarties) are provided intermittently.
(6) The child competes against his own baseline, rather than against his classmates'.
(7) Sequences are so gradual that learning is almost errorless.
(8) The response button and critical stimulus are very close.

Application

All children struggling with school.

Measures

Elapsed time, number of errors, reinforcement ratio, etc. Use the record form provided for this purpose.

Procedures

1. Obtain a baseline for each skill.
2. Give a careful explanation of the benefits and hazards of teaching machines.
3. Other children using teaching machines can demonstrate the enjoyment of learning on teaching machines.
4. Check with the teacher about what programs are most suitable.
5. Carefully explain the machine's operation.
6. Check out the child's ability to change programs, etc.
7. Stay nearby so the child can appeal for help or ask you about difficult problems.
8. Encourage him to share his frustrations and excitement.
9. Provide an opportunity to let your patient demonstrate his new skills to his regular classroom teacher.
10. To the extent it is feasible, arrange continued access to teaching machines after discharge.

Untoward Effects

Mechanical breakdowns, paper tearing, bugs (errors) in the programs. 'Ripoffs' of candy and tokens. Inflation: children generally should not work at programmes below their grade level, or earn reinforcements too easily.

Charting Requirements

Measures only necessary.

Abreaction (A) – 'Let it all hang out'
Technique – Second Level

Rationale

The brain appears to be programmed to relive traumatic experiences until the emotions lose their impact. Highly-charged memories appear to become less influential in the child's thought and behaviour after both dreaming and abreaction. As emotional tensions diminish, the body tension is lowered. If the charge is lowered soon after a traumatic incident, there is less likelihood of a continuing painful memory. Children who survive a close miss or the death of someone near or dear to them, will have many conflicts to resolve.

Abreaction provides the child with an opportunity to gain greater objectivity about a painful event, some understanding about his own ambivalence and some insight into his own reactions. Once the psychic pain subsides, it is easier to work with other techniques.

Application

All children who have either personally or vicariously experienced an event that deeply disturbed them, e.g. rape, car accident, parents fighting, marital separation, frightening movies, etc., could benefit from abreaction. Chronically anxious children are particularly helped.

Measures

Pulse and pupil dilation are measured while the child is recalling a specific event. Record verbatim statements of the child's emotional reaction and his growing insight.

Procedure

1. Record the baseline, i.e. the child's reaction to a memory before any therapy.
2. Give the child an explanation of the procedure and a brief demonstration.
3. Reassure the child you will not make him re-experience painful events too quickly. To help evoke the memory with greater clarity, some of the objects or pictures associated with the event, should be handy.
4. Request the child to 'Tell me as much as you can.'
5. Focus on the circumstances surrounding the traumatic event.
6. Describe the details of the event (colour, size, speed, etc.).
7. Discuss some of the things that were said at the time.
8. Help the child describe his own emotional reactions to the trauma.
9. Encourage him to discuss feelings of responsibility and ambivilence.
10. Don't forget, it's very difficult to be a survivor.

Untoward Effects

There is a possibility that abreaction could precipitate a psychosis by overwhelming a child's fragile ego. More likely there may be an increase in anxiety, resulting in nightmares, night terrors, inability to assimilate traumatic experiences.

Charting Requirements

Measures and verbatim statements are necessary.

Amorphous Blob (AB) – 'Who am I inside'
(The Shape of the Child's Inner Self)
Technique – Second Level

Rationale

Many children are unaware of their inner selves or have distorted perceptions of their ego. The amorphous blob technique is an attempt to help them describe those less easily defined components of themselves. Specifically, the amorphous blob technique will:

(1) Monitor changes in the child's self-concept.
(2) Clarify changes in self-image.
(3) Determine those components of the child's self he will accept and those he wants to reject.
(4) Allow the child to compare his self-awareness with his family's and friends' view of him.

Application

All children without insight and/or shaky self-concepts, particularly depressed children, can profit.

Measures

Obtain a drawing plus a self-description, which should be recorded verbatim, at least once per week.

Procedure

1. Don't forget to obtain a baseline, give a careful explanation and demonstrate what you are going to do.

2. Ask the child to try and draw a picture of his ego. 'Show me what the person inside looks like even if it looks like a blob.' If he has trouble doing this, a staff member draws a blob on a piece of paper, leaving room inside and outside for comments. The patient is told at this point, he may be as amorphous as the blob – that we know very little about him and that's what 'amorphous' means.

3. 'In order to understand what's part of you (inside the blob) and what is not (outside the blob), we're going to write things that are you, good and bad, inside. Things that aren't you, but that you would like to have as part of you – outside the blob; and things that people say about you that aren't true, also go outside the blob.'

4. Items to consider with patients fall under the following categories: likes and dislikes, temper, hopes, ideals, friendliness, trust,

April 13   JACKIE   (first)

HOW OTHERS SEE ME:

— others think I am really good at making jokes sometimes.
— easy to talk to — good listener.
— good friend.
— brat, lazy.

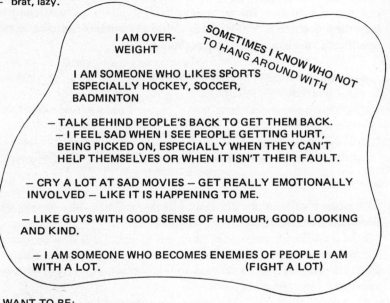

I AM OVER-
WEIGHT

SOMETIMES I KNOW WHO NOT
TO HANG AROUND WITH

I AM SOMEONE WHO LIKES SPORTS
ESPECIALLY HOCKEY, SOCCER,
BADMINTON

— TALK BEHIND PEOPLE'S BACK TO GET THEM BACK.
— I FEEL SAD WHEN I SEE PEOPLE GETTING HURT,
BEING PICKED ON, ESPECIALLY WHEN THEY CAN'T
HELP THEMSELVES OR WHEN IT ISN'T THEIR FAULT.

— CRY A LOT AT SAD MOVIES — GET REALLY EMOTIONALLY
INVOLVED — LIKE IT IS HAPPENING TO ME.

— LIKE GUYS WITH GOOD SENSE OF HUMOUR, GOOD LOOKING
AND KIND.

— I AM SOMEONE WHO BECOMES ENEMIES OF PEOPLE I AM
WITH A LOT.   (FIGHT A LOT)

I WANT TO BE:

— THINNER
— HAVE MORE FRIENDS
— BE ABLE TO STAND UP FOR MYSELF WITH OTHERS
— NOT FEEL GUILTY WHEN MY FRIENDS ARE MAD AT ME
— TO BE ABLE TO WORK OUT DISAGREEMENTS, BEFORE THEY BUILD
UP.

suspicions, temperament, career goals, emotional characteristics, and problems cited at admission conference, etc.

5. The first blob is done during the patient's first week, preferably on the first or second day of admission.

6. In the second and third blob, the child should be encouraged to work the shape into a more recognisable human form. Children who are poor artists and who will accept it, should be offered assistance.

7. The first blob can then be looked at and comments transferred to where they belong at this point. Hopefully, good, desirable characteristics

April 20   JACKIE   (Second)

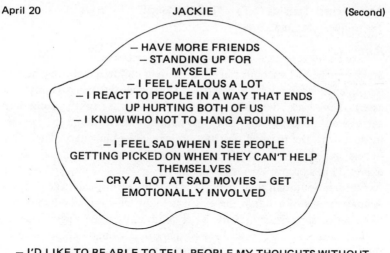

– HAVE MORE FRIENDS
– STANDING UP FOR
  MYSELF
– I FEEL JEALOUS A LOT
– I REACT TO PEOPLE IN A WAY THAT ENDS
  UP HURTING BOTH OF US
– I KNOW WHO NOT TO HANG AROUND WITH

– I FEEL SAD WHEN I SEE PEOPLE
GETTING PICKED ON WHEN THEY CAN'T HELP
  THEMSELVES
– CRY A LOT AT SAD MOVIES – GET
  EMOTIONALLY INVOLVED

– I'D LIKE TO BE ABLE TO TELL PEOPLE MY THOUGHTS WITHOUT
HURTING THEM

will move into the blob. Undesirable characteristics inside the blob which are no longer applicable, will disappear. It may be necessary or helpful to remind the patient that this is movement into or out of themselves. Work on items that haven't been moved should be encouraged and aided with new programmes. Always encourage an honest appraisal.

8. Another method of doing the second blob is to work with current information from the child rather than with reference to the first blob. Difference in methods would depend upon particular patients and their programmes.

9. During the patient's fifth and final week, he is asked to draw another picture of his ego. This is compared with previous ones. Encourage the child to draw and understand a sharper definition of his inner self, good and bad. Help him to see the differences in how he sees himself and how others see him.

Untoward Effects

The child might become embarrassed by revealing himself too suddenly. He may not be able to represent himself correctly and get discouraged.

Charting Requirements

File drawings and verbatim comments in front of chart. Document any untoward effects or resistance in the 24-Hour Progress Notes.

Assertiveness Training (AT) – 'Talking tough' Technique – Second Level

Rationale

Some parents feel uncomfortable about their children maturing, becoming independent and more assertive. Consequently, when children do assert themselves, they are 'put down': somtimes subtly, sometimes aggressively. Because the child is naturally determined to become independent, the parents' obstruction may make him angry. The object of his anger may be displaced to a sibling or authority figure or expressed in a passive–aggressive manner.

Children imitating their parents may learn to put each other down. Among groups of children there is usually at least one child who does not comfortably assert himself. That child tends to be singled out and be put down by other members in the group. Some children react to this with explosive aggression. Because they explode so predictably and so dramatically, the group likes to provoke them into rage and then enjoys watching them. It is very much like setting off firecrackers. Other children, feeling anger but not knowing how to express it, withdraw and become passive in their aggression, e.g. refusing to do their homework or chores. Others become aggressive towards themselves, shy, depressed or suicidal.

Children should be taught to assert themselves appropriately and comfortably, or to stand up for themselves, but not by putting others down. 'I make no demand on others except they recognise that here I stand.'

Children tend to discriminate derogatorily against one another and they do so on the most observable characteristic. If it is race, then they are called 'wop'; if intelligence, 'retard', etc. Knowing the child and his background gives the staff an insight into what is likely to be used to put this particular child down.

Application

Children who have difficulty with explosive anger, passive–aggressive behaviour, or are depressed because of internalised aggression, need assertiveness training. Anorexic, encopretic, enuretic, anxiously over-pleasing, obsessive-compulsive, battered, obese, physically or intellectually handicapped, school failures and phobic children usually benefit from assertiveness training.

Measures

1. The frequency per shift of explosions or tailturning, wimpy behaviour, assuming that he is exposed to a certain amount of nasty teasing by his peers.

2. Appropriate assertive statements in the face of staff or peer provocation.

3. Empathy, the percentage of times a child correctly identifies the feelings of another person.

Procedure

1. Obtain a baseline at home or school and for the first two days on the treatment unit.

2. Explain to the child and his family the procedure you are about to use. Get the parents' agreement and consent to the words that the child will eventually be taught to use in his assertive responses. This is very important because otherwise you may be teaching the child to use expressions the parents find offensive.

3. On one or two occasions demonstrate, using another staff member or child.

4. Obtain a hierarchy of words and situations to which the child responds with high levels of anxiety, e.g. called 'retard' or told to do his reading out loud in class.

5. Teach the child ways of interpreting social situations correctly, e.g. watching facial expressions, gestures and listening to the conversation, so that they can properly understand what is appropriate assertion. It is important for the child who cannot interpret social situations correctly to learn only those assertive responses that are unlikely to get him into trouble when used indiscriminately.

6. Teach the child to empathise, e.g. get the child to watch people and guess their feelings. Then check with those watched what their feelings actually were.

7. Teach the child self-affirming statements e.g. 'I am not a retard, I'm pretty smart.' Only when these are ineffective should you teach him expressions that may put his antagonist down.

8. Teach the child to respond to the provocation with equal intensity, no more or less. This will eventually make his antagonist either start laughing, begin to respect the child or at least go away in disgust. It will prevent escalation evoked by an automatic sadistic or hostile response.

9. Model gentle, assertive responses to small provocations and continue escalating until they include a wide variety of difficult put-downs

and social situations. These should include the whole hierarchy of mean things, being told to get lost, and being told to do things they cannot perform easily.

Untoward Effects

If this is done too hurriedly it may make the child increasingly sensitive to certain situations or words, less able to assert himself, or may give him the use of words or assertive responses that will get him into further trouble.

Charting Requirements

Anecdotal description of behaviour and emotions, counts and graphs.

Body Impulse Directing (BID) — 'I don't have to fight myself'

Rationale

All humans are constructed with finely-tuned feedback mechanisms which maintain fine homeostatic balances. This applies not only to body chemistry and temperature, but also to the control of sleep, eating, rest, sensory input, posture, etc. Unfortunately, some of these feedback mechanisms can be confused by:

(1) Override: parents telling children what and when they should eat, sleep, defecate, etc. Since the child needs to believe his parents, he tends to doubt himself.
(2) Conflict: when a child grows up feeling he must struggle to control himself, an acute control conflict may centre in one particular area, such as eating.
(3) Titillation: subtle effective advertising aimed at increasing the person's desire for food, drink, etc. may confuse basic human mechanisms which indicate a need has already been well filled.

As a result of confusing physical and emotional inputs, persons may no longer trust their body. They must then rely upon artificial measures to tell them what is going on inside. Unfortunately, if they are habituated or emotionally conflicted they begin to cheat and then to rationalise. 'I need it, just one more, I won't have another one for a week.' Unfortunately, this is usually followed by failure which increases a feeling of shame or guilt. Their feeling of conflicted dis-ease is eased by a repeated ingestion of the unwanted chemical. For a short period following the eating or drinking or smoking, there is a warm feeling of relaxation which reinforces the relapse. It is quickly replaced by remorse which increases the conflict.

For many foreign chemicals the human organism has no sensory mechanism to determine its level in the body and no mechanism in the mind to indicate what the level should be. When there is no built-in corrective feedback and powerful rewarding sensations, the human organism has great difficulty controlling itself.

This technique first seeks to provide conflict-free feedback to the mind. It has been noticed that once this happens, the mind will tend to assert more control and the 'bad habit' tends to stabilise. Once this occurs, it is important to provide some objective. We have noted that, given an easily achievable goal without any sense of reward other than a hope of achieving it, the body takes automatic aim. This automatic aiming happens more rapidly when the mind receives corrective feedback fairly frequently. The objective measures should be recorded and plotted. To increase the effect of automatic aiming control, the individual should also record and plot his desires for the forbidden behaviour.

Application

This procedure is useful for children struggling with obesity, anorexia or other areas where automatic control has been confused. It also used in any situation, child or adult, where foreign chemicals, caffeine, nicotine, etc. have established a difficult habit. This technique should be used together with Limit Challenge, Conflict Displacement and Listen to Your Body.

Measures

The staff should record the child's attitude towards the problem and themselves, usually once a week. Also make weekly honesty spot-checks in a random manner and explain that this is because the staff distrust only some of the individual's behaviours.

Procedures

1. Obtain baseline measures prior to the child's admission.

2. Explain the procedure to the parents and child. Check to see if other members of the family would like to work on a similar issue.

3. Demonstrate how it works with another child or adult with whom the procedure has already has some success.

4. Help the child become more objective with himself and his problems. Encourage him to have a more clinical detachment towards the problem. Tell him of other instances in children you may have known.

Introduce A & P Teaching at this juncture.

5. During the latter half of the first week of admission, encourage the child to count the number of times he engages in his 'bad habit' and the number of times he desires to do so. Start him reporting the occasions to the staff, e.g. 'I am starting to feel very hungry.'

6. Teach your patient to record his temperature and his unwanted behaviour for short and then increasingly longer periods of the day. These should be recorded in two columns, not necessarily side by side.

7. Teach the child to graph the number of behaviours. Use plenty of colour and small illustrations on the graph.

8. Once graphing is well established, draw a line which averages the number of behaviours. Teach him routinely to connect the average points.

9. When the daily fluctuations diminish, draw a red line 2 per cent above the average and a green line approximately 2 per cent below the average line. 'Above' or 'below' will change depending on the direction you want the behaviour to go. Calculate the percentage as the portion of the total change that is wished by the individual.

10. When the average moves in the direction of the green line, draw another green line 5 per cent in the direction to be moved and make the previous green line the black one and the black one the red one.

11. Move in increasing increments in the direction desired. If the behaviour does not automatically move in the desired direction, start the child on some incentive. It is essential that there be no hassle. If the child does not automatically and regularly record and graph his behaviour, it may be necessary to use Shaping until it becomes an automatic response. The whole procedure should be light-hearted.

Untoward Effects

If the child fails to move automatically in the right direction he may get discouraged. If so, stop for a period while other techniques are beginning to take effect then start again. Operant Conditioning can be used as a back-up. Make sure that psychotherapy regarding conflicts is going well.

Charting Requirements

Keep a copy of the graphs on the child's chart.

Body Painting (BP) – 'I'm turning green'
Technique – Second Level

Rationale

Some children are not well aware of their skin's capacity to protect and insulate them. To allow them to paint it, reassures them that they are intact and resistant, at least to paint. Those children who have obsessional defences against dirt can gradually learn that discoloration of their skin can be dealt with easily. Psychotic children can be helped to define ego boundaries by understanding the outer limits of their bodies. Body painting is used to facilitate A & P Teaching. When the child's face is painted he can pretend to be any character he likes.

Applications

Obsessive-compulsive patients, anorexic, psychotic or borderline patients with poor ego boundaries, inhibited or depressed patients with excessively controlled anger, can all benefit.

Measures

Sketch the patient's own painting, with the extent of body covered and colours used. Note his responses, particularly any fantasy associated with a particular design. Indicate which parts he is most reluctant to have painted.

Procedure

1. Explain the procedure to the child and his family. Be sure to understand the origins of their anxieties.

2. Each child requires baseline observations of his initial reaction to paint or discoloration.

3. Staff can demonstrate by painting their own hands or those of another co-operative child. Then view the paint in the mirror and exclaim over the brightness of the design and the effects on the expression given.

4. The therapist should first paint himself and then a small portion of the child. Gently encourage the child to paint himself. Gradually enlarge the area and include a wider variety of colours.

5. Use Indian or Maori markings on his face to demonstrate the impact of non-verbal expressions. Use vivid colours and expressions that he might not usually exhibit. Encourage him to paint a clown's face then play the part of the clown he has painted.

Untoward Effects

An angry child might take the opportunity to cover the therapist with more markings or mess than the therapist would want.

Charting Requirements

Measures plus narrative charting of verbal and non-verbal reactions.

Child Free Play Acting (FPA) – 'Theatre time'
Technique – Second Level

Rationale

Children feel very vulnerable and try to protect themselves with privacy. To portray themselves they need an additional protective coating – a mask, costume, stage props – which will allow the child to display more easily what is on his mind. Children are ambivalent about being known. They want to be understood but are afraid of rejection or criticism. They feel freer to show other aspects of their character while portraying play characters.

Children need a structure within which to act out. The basic story of a play provides guidance, but lack of script allows latitude for individual expression. Children need corrective feedback. The audience reaction (generally applauding) gives permission and encouragement to be free with expression of feelings. Some booing might not harm but it must be done with good humour.

Children learn through participation. An academic understanding comes through experiencing the subject being taught. Children learn English and history by enacting its dramatisation. The well-known, enduring and endearing children's stories portray common human conflicts in stylised, acceptable fashion. A child learns to understand more of his own conflicts by enacting the conflicts of the story, e.g. Jack and the Beanstalk – male child destroys bad (giant) father who went up to heaven (died or went to live with another woman).

The children use dress-up clothes, painted faces, and the 'bare bones' of a fairy story to produce a play which is videotaped. The emphasis is on what each child brings to the play. The choice of character, clothes and how they paint their face is their own. The fairy story provides a structure and style but there is freedom to pursue one's own imagination.

Application

This should involve all the children on the unit, including psychotic or disabled children. They should all get something out of it.

Measures

Make observations of the child's involvement and which play he becomes most caught up in.

Procedure

Phases.

   (a) Introduction of play and theme.
   (b) Choosing characters — 'Who am I really?'
   (c) Dressing up — 'I would like to appear to be . . .'
   (d) Getting started — 'I'm scared, but here goes'.
   (e) Acting it out.
   (f) Closure.
   (g) To see myself as I might also be. Replay.

1. Baseline. Before the child is admitted, invite him to watch a play and note his reaction.

2. Explain to parents and children, the basics of the procedure and why it is so important. Parents may feel the child does enough acting up without your encouraging him to be more outlandish. Remind them of their own enjoyment of becoming involved in drama.

3. Watching a play with his parents before admission assures the child it is permissible and safe.

4. Prior to choosing a story for the day's play, a choice of activities to explore expression of feelings and movements, and a chance to experiment with the dress-up clothes is done, usually in the form of games. These warm-up activities include games such as Chinese Whisper, Queen Dido is Dead, the song 'Soldier, Soldier' with dress-up activities, miming and using facial masks.

5. Discuss play to be done, placing the limit that a well-known story (not from television) be chosen. Reach a choice acceptable to the whole group. If it is a story as well known as 'Cinderella', the children take turns to re-tell the story in sequence. If not, the story is read aloud.

6. Make a list of characters on the blackboard. Each child chooses who he wants to be. This is surprisingly straightforward, each child having some feeling, from hearing the story, about who he would like to portray.

7. Sometimes at this point, the group works in pairs to paint large pictures about the story, which are pinned up as backdrops. If a child particularly requests a prop he considers necessary for the character, this time is used to make it.

8. Each child chooses clothes he feels are appropriate for the character. The emphasis is on the children choosing what they feel is right for the character. If the adults make choices for them, it is imposing on them our ideas and limiting the child's chance for free expression of himself. Make sure there is a wide range of clothes available — dresses, trousers, blouses, shirts, wigs, shoes, bags, hats, lengths of material, coats, belts, tights and waistcoats.

9. The face painting, too, is an expression of the child. It is important that each child paints his own face, because only he knows what he really wants to show. Make the suggestion that it does not have to show the character, e.g. it does not have to look like a cat for the part of Puss-in-Boots. Each child paints his own face to create a mask from behind which the child can begin to show tentative aspects of his own character.

10. After the children are in their dress-up clothes and painted faces, you may sit in a circle and talk through the story as a reminder. This depends very much on the particular mix of children in the group. It can raise the anxiety level of 'will I do it right?' or 'will I forget my words?' The desired aim is to take it as it happens. Occasionally it is necessary to clarify the beginning, otherwise make no other suggestions or instructions and no suggestion of props, where the children situate themselves while waiting, what to say or what direction the play will take.

11. One child introduces the play and the characters to the camera and the audience. As the play progresses the camera catches as much of the performance as possible, including any of the working-out or discussions, the stops and starts, the blank looks and the arguments of out-of-character characters. The ending is at a point of the group's choosing. It sometimes continues on past the story-book version of the story and sometimes barely makes it to that point.

12. After the clothes have been put back into the dress-up box, and the masks have been washed off, the children watch the video, during which many comments are made. Gently encourage the children to understand why a particular character was important to them.

13. The children sit together and discuss their own part, how they felt playing the part and watching it. Staff can help children identify the human dilemmas and suggest how it might turn out differently.

Suggested Fairy Stories.
1. Sleeping Beauty — the girl is awakened by the kiss of an unknown lover.

2. Hansel and Gretel — caring parents who abandon their children. The wicked witch (social worker) tries to entice them into her house where they will be devoured.

3. Cinderella — the child no one wants until someone discovers her real worth.

4. The Wolf and the Seven Little Kids — the difficulty for children of separated parents both wanting the children.

5. Goldilocks and the Three Bears — the danger of poking into someone else's business.

6. Snow White and the Seven Dwarfs — the unappreciated child is cared for by imaginary playmates.

7. Rumpelstiltskin — the father keeps his daughter locked up for himself.

8. Jack and the Beanstalk — the father who deserts or dies.

9. The Elves and the Shoemakers — the importance of children to a parent's happiness.

10. Little Red Riding Hood — don't talk to strangers.

11. The Three Little Pigs — how to outwit a hostile environment.

Untoward Effects

Much of the impact is lost if the children don't have an opportunity to discuss their perceptions and feelings. Sometimes children get too excited and need to be taken outside for a few moments.

Charting Requirements

Record the child's part and responses with a very brief description of the play.

Conflict Displacement (CD) — 'Why should I?'
Technique — Second Level

Rationale

Conflict often arises in areas where the child is legitimately striving for autonomy but where the parents feel they should have control. In these areas the child is usually able to win but the parent may exert such pressure, the child never learns easy self-control. Sharp conflict occurs because the child is not prepared to give up and the parents are determined to be in charge. The child can show the parents that they cannot control something that is legitimately an area of his autonomy but the parents become increasingly angry and punitive. Children may win the battle with their parents but never really trust themselves thereafter.

Parents may battle for control because they don't trust the child in areas such as eating, sleeping, bowel or bladder control, learning or talking. They don't trust the child possibly because they don't trust themselves. They may have severe conflicts of self-control which stemmed from pressure that was placed upon them by their parents.

When the parents recognise they are losing, they get angry at the child because it shakes their own self-control. The anger the child receives makes it hard for him to learn easy control of his own functions. The child expresses his reciprocal anger towards the parent by unconsciously withholding or letting go when it is socially inappropriate. To parents of encopretic children this is like being 'shit on'. They sense the child's hostility all too easily.

The object of this technique is to shift an intense conflict between parent and child, into an area where there are fewer emotions, where it does not matter from the parents' view if the child wins, and from the child's view, where it is not important to have self-control. As the battle for control in an unimportant area intensifies, the child's ability to assume self-control in the previously problem area improves.

Application

Conflict displacement works well with anorexia nervosa, encopresis, enuresis, obesity, insomnia, learning inhibition, school phobia and elective mutism.

Measures

There should be a subjective measure of the intensity of the conflict and an objective count of the frequency with which these conflicts are expressed. Measure both of these on the conflict that is being given up and the new conflict that is being fostered.

Procedure

1. Baseline should be measured prior to the child's admission and in his own environment on both old and new conflicts.

2. The child should be told that you want to help him gain self-control. For that reason you are suggesting he fight for control in an area that is less important to both him and his parents. The parents should be reminded that they cannot win in this area of a child's autonomous control where they have been fighting. They should examine some of the problems surrounding their own mistrust in these areas.

3. Demonstrate using another staff member. The staff or a willing patient can role-play the situation in which they are being forced by

parents to do something that is obviously in the child's area of self-control, such as going to sleep. A third staff member may step in and suggest they should fight about something else since it is obvious that neither of them will win. The model can then demonstrate to the child how one can go about asserting oneself and maintain self-control. You should verbally mediate your legitimate objections to another person's attempt to control you. Model how you feel you would like to respond in anger, how your body seems to take over and do or say for you what you cannot put into words, and how, rather than expressing it indirectly, you feel so much better expressing it directly.

4. The provoking staff member should suggest something that is far out, e.g. 'I think it would be good for you as a fourteen year old, to go to bed at seven o'clock.' When the child is able to begin asserting himself against such a ridiculous idea you can then modify the directive to something more reasonable.

5. You should become increasingly insistent, monitoring the child's response. This technique should be paired with Assertiveness Training.

6. Encourage the child to express all the old frustrations that come to the surface when they struggle with over-controlling parents.

Untoward Effects

The child may be made more passive–aggressive if the staff are too forceful. If the child is not given sufficient opportunity to express his conflicts he may become withdrawn.

Charting Requirements

Chart subjective measures of intensity. Graph the frequency with which conflict is expressed. Statements of verbal mediation should be charted. Note the degree of aggression expected before negotiations and chart on a 24-Hour Progress Note.

Corrective Feedback (CF) – 'How am I doing now?'
Technique – Second Level

Rationale

There are times when families, and/or communities, project onto a child characteristics that are not true of him. Sometimes these projections are so strong that they become part of the individual's self-concept. Corrective feedback may change the opinion of the individual, family and the community about that individual. Then they are able to see the individual in relation to his strengths and abilities.

Although children generally accept what important adults say about them, you cannot expect them suddenly to change their self-concept just because you tell them they are not like that. On the other hand, most children are intuitively in touch with a fairly accurate picture of themselves and they sense the discrepancy. To correct a false impression can produce a marked change because it resonates with their true self-image.

Most people can organise their lives more appropriately when they are accurately informed about themselves. Most parents are better able to guide their children when they have realistic expectations of them. Although people may abuse vital information about themselves, the large majority become more responsible. If expectations are too high parents will be disappointed in a child. Their negative feedback will give a child a poor self-image or a feeling that he can't win, so why try. As his performance drops, the negative comments about him increase and thus a destructive cycle ensues.

If expectations of a child are too low he may be allowed to coast along and never realise his full potential. It should be possible for the child to meet parental expectations most of the time, but they should sometimes give him the impression he could do better. A child who usually pleases his parents usually tries harder.

Application

Children who have been given negative labels, or possibly positive labels that are unrealistic to their natural abilities, e.g. 'dummy', 'bad girl', 'irresponsible', 'brain', 'artistic', benefit most. These are usually depressed, obsessive or phobic children.

Measures

Do a weekly Amorphous Blob with the child. For the family and community: note changes in how they treat the child and how they describe him.

Procedure

1. Obtain a baseline of the stated behaviour. Give sensory-motor assessments, IQ test, aptitude tests, a personality rating scale, etc. Use Limit Challenge to define the child's abilities and attitudes towards himself. Collect as much supporting data as you can to establish the fact that the child is not as he is seen.

2. Explain to the child, family and community workers (at different times) in as much detail as possible, the results of your baseline and

tests. Allow them as many questions and objections as possible and answer these with a careful description of the results from your tests.

3. Give the child and family opportunity to explain fully why they have a particular view of him, before trying to correct this misperception. It is also important that the same people hear the same or similar information from a variety of different sources; e.g. if a community and/or family have felt that a child was very bright and was not performing at school because of poor attitude or not working, they should be told the facts. If your academic and IQ testing show that his IQ is below average and that he is performing at the level he should be, then the family and the community will need to hear this information from the doctor, the psychologist, the teacher and the primary worker, each one speaking from a different viewpoint but all giving the same information.

4. When family and community workers have agreed on a new perception of the child, tell them all once again in the child's presence. Encourage him to say 'Yes, that's right.'

Untoward Effects

The family and/or community may reject the feedback and become more set in their 'image' of the child.

Charting Requirements

Baseline and all test information. Narrative reporting on information given to parents and their acceptance of information.

Delayed Impulse Response (DIR) — 'Counting down' Technique — Second Level

Rationale

Hyperactive, impulsive and aggressive children are continually getting themselves into trouble because they cannot delay their response to some kind of provocation. Consequently, they are more frequently punished. The punishment, which is usually physical, makes them more aggressive. The build-up of unexpressed, aggressive feelings tends to make them even more irritable and impulsive and less able to restrain their anger. Some aggressive children cannot seem to ignore any provocation and will fight at the drop of a hat.

Parental reminders to ignore the provocateur, given at the moment they feel most angry, will make them angry at both the provocateur and the restraining parent. Sometimes reminders to ignore teasing inadvertently reinforce the impulsive activity.

Impulsive children often cannot finish required routines such as schoolwork. They are scolded for not getting on with it. The continuous stream of irritating injunctions to keep on working is aversive conditioning which can eventually turn a child completely off his schoolwork.

For constitutionally hyperactive children, the impulsiveness may be an adaptive mechanism which, in the past would have allowed them to develop into excellent hunters and warriors. But in today's sedentary, confining society, impulsiveness is maladaptive and unappreciated.

Application

Constitutional and chemically hyperactive children, aggressive children and temperamentally reactive children, can learn to delay impulsive responses.

Measures

Record the types of stimulation to which a child responds most strongly. Measure the number of seconds in the delay of response to provocative stimuli.

Procedure

1. Baseline: measure the interval between stimulus and response to a variety of stimuli and in different settings.

2. Explanation: Parents and children need to be reassured that impulsiveness *per se* is not necessarily bad, but it should be controlled. The child's improved self-control will benefit him greatly.

3. Demonstration: Use another child or staff member to show how it works. Both the stimuli and the response, with reinforcement in delaying a response, should be demonstrated. Demonstrate various tactics a child might use in delaying a response, e.g. counting, self-explanation, distraction, etc.

4. Use mediational modification, e.g. 'Boy, would I like to hit him right now, but I don't think I should because I will only get into trouble, and I might hit him too hard. So I will count to ten, then I will let him know exactly how I feel.'

5. Without any provocation, use as many practice sessions as necessary to establish the mediational process.

6. The child should be first encouraged to count to two and then progressively lengthen the interval up to at least ten. He should be reinforced for successes. Progress gradually, depending upon at least 80 per

cent success rate.

7. Encourage the child to voice his emotional reactions to increasingly irritating or distracting stimulation.

8. There should be a gradual increase in the intensity of the distracting stimulus, from whispers to loud crashes, while the child is trying to concentrate on some schoolwork.

9. Include the parents in the training sessions when the child is successfully restraining his reaction to a variety of irritants. Give them an opportunity to demonstrate their skill in helping the child with this technique.

10. The responsibility of demonstrating and practising should be handed to the parents before the child is discharged.

11. During follow-up, do some more practising.

Untoward Effects

If you proceed too rapidly, a child might become frustrated and give up. Children with cerebral irritability will respond less well to this technique, but it can be tried.

Charting Requirements

Graph the delay in responding. Chart the mediational statements used and the intensity of responses. Chart parents' demonstrated ability to carry out this technique.

Ego Auxiliary (EA) – 'My buddy'
Technique – Second Level

Rationale

In the stressful situations of family, teacher or peer group activity, emotionally disturbed children may not be able to use all their capabilities. When he can't cope, a child becomes progressively more anxious, uses maladaptive defence mechanisms and gets angry at himself for being so stupid.

What these children need is someone to support or direct their ego as if from inside. This can enable them to react to the stress more rationally and capably. Since it is impossible to get inside another child, the ego auxiliary gets as close alongside as possible.

The ego auxiliary provides the child with:

(1) A variable barrier to external stimuli so that stress is filtered and integrated before reaching the child.

(2) Strength to support his ego so he can better handle his anxieties and use his best potential.

(3) An opportunity to experience vicariously how someone close to him can function under the same stress by choosing alternative defences and adaptive behaviour and by appropriately expressing feelings of distress.

(4) Mediational modelling of adaptive thinking through a problem.

(5) Coping strategies.

Application

Any child who decompensates when dealing with teacher, peer or family stress, and who has a sufficiently strong ego.

Measures

1. Note heart rate or pupil dilation after exposure to stress.

2. Record the percentage of successes in dealing with the key stressful situations.

Procedure

1. Baseline: Obtain measures of anxiety felt by the child in a variety of common stressful situations to which he has shown maladaptive responses.

2. Explain to the parents and the child the object of this technique and how you are about to proceed. Parents and teachers are able to give the most comprehensive list of situations in which the child tends to decompensate.

3. Demonstrate using another child.

4. Establish a hierarchy of stressful situations. Start with the least stressful and work in the least stressful manner.

5. Identify the teacher or staff members or children who will be the provokers. Indicate to them when they should apply stress, e.g. ask the teacher to give the child five arithmetic problems in rapid succession. These problems should be well within the child's capabilities.

6. The ego auxiliary needs to sit beside the child, trying hard to experience the situation just as the child would.

7. Don't give more support or help than the child needs. Give him opportunity to try and handle a demanding situation on his own.

8. If he appears to be too angry, frightened or frustrated to think of any way to cope with the stress, first try just putting your arm around him and giving encouragement, e.g. 'I think you can do it.'

9. If that doesn't work apply the same stress and briefly observe the

child struggling. When it becomes obvious that he cannot handle it, the ego auxiliary proceeds to function as part of the child's ego.

(a) Empathise with the child in his struggle, e.g. 'Boy, this sure is hard.'

(b) Interpret the stress and label the most probable feelings, e.g. 'When he gives me so much work at once, I get confused and angry.'

(c) Wait to see if the child copes. Then point out the good parts of that attempt.

10. If the child cannot cope given this amount of help both child and auxiliary should leave the room and rehearse the child's response.

(a) Encourage him by helping him realise his assets and abilities.

(b) Suggest ways of applying these abilities.

(c) Give him another try. If he copes, describe to him the essential elements of his success.

11. If he still cannot deal with the stress, leave the scene of the stress together.

(a) Model alternative ways of dealing with the stress. Use mediational modification to establish different cognitive functioning.

(b) Provide in detail the full development of thought process necessary to cope with the stress. This includes interrupting the stress, considering the alternatives, defining the best behaviour and carrying out the appropriate behaviour.

(c) Rehearse the thoughts and coping behaviour till the child has got it down pat.

(d) Expose the child to the same amount of stress.

12. If he still cannot cope, model the strategy and the necessary behaviours and keep practising. Don't diminish the demand unless nothing else works.

13. Once the child is coping, encourage him to rehearse in the real situation and a variety of increasingly stressful ones.

14. This procedure should be repeated until the child can handle any similar spontaneously developed situations on the ward.

15. Test his ability to handle similar demands at home and school.

16. Gradually withdraw your support.

Untoward Effects

If the child cannot deal with stress appropriately and if he decompensates too often, he may become more anxious and less capable of dealing with demands.

Charting Requirements

Measures, chart various stages of treatment reached, note reactions, changes and the future focus in order to provide continuity.

Feelings Rehearsal (FR) — 'Say it with feeling'
Technique — Second Level

Rationale

Many children do not have the concepts or words to express properly their feelings. In fumbling for the right expression they become increasingly anxious, frustrated and very often misunderstood by adults, e.g. Mother: 'Johnny, what's the matter with you?' Johnny: 'I feel . . . I feel . . . I don't know.' Mother: 'Well, when you know what you are feeling, let me know. Until then, stop looking so glum.' Johnny: 'Okay, Mum.'

Children who cannot talk out their feelings are sometimes driven to act them out, often in inappropriate ways. Acting out evokes in adults repressive exhortations, making the children even less capable of explaining themselves and their feelings.

Feelings expression is inadvertently repressed in many ways. In some instances parents repress in children emotions and thoughts that the parents cannot deal with in themselves. Parents may say: 'Dry your eyes, Johnny' because they cannot deal with their own sadness. Parents in poor control of their anger try to control the child's angry expressions so that they themselves will not be provoked to anger. Unfortunately, this may result in a vicious cycle of repressed, inhibited and sometimes explosive anger.

To label a child's feelings and give him an appropriate word for it helps the child gain:

(a) Insight.
(b) Better ability in providing parents corrective feedback on their management skills.
(c) A release of feelings associated with conflict and anxiety.
(d) Ability to identify in himself those uncomfortable feelings that he can usually only express with naughty behaviour.

To teach the child the appropriate expression of strong feelings will:

(1) Give him guidance on how and when.
(2) Improve his social interactions.

Application

All children with poor facility for emotive words, or those who are particularly depressed, psychosomatic, anorexic or stutterers.

Measures

Each week a typical session should be documented in a 24-Hour Progress Note. Record the number of reinforcements that are used to encourage the feelings rehearsal. Measure the accuracy of each imitation session and how it changes from session to session. Record the percentage of times the child expresses appropriately or inappropriately a major affect during a given period of normal peer or adult interactions.

Procedure

1. Establish a baseline on the child's ability to express emotion-laden words and concepts.

2. Explain to the child and his parents the necessity in interpersonal relations of expressing oneself clearly and why it is important in maintaining health.

3. Demonstrate what you hope to achieve to the child using other children who have had the experience, or use a staff worker. The child should be given ample opportunity to express his anxieties about expressing feelings, e.g. 'My father would never let me get away with it.' The therapist, in dealing with the child's resistance, should point out the various benefits and get the parents to indicate approval.

4. Make a hierarchy of all the child's emotional expressions, indicating the most easily and the least easily expressed.

5. Use the 'moods and emotions' pictures. This can give the child an idea of how he can read moods and emotions in others. Encourage him to indicate how accurately he can identify them.

6. Have the child portray moods and emotions as he sees them. This can be done in front of a mirror. The child's response may be, 'Do I really look like that?' or if this is too threatening, have the child draw people portraying moods and emotions.

7. If the child has difficulty identifying what he is feeling when you see a specific affect, label it for him. This technique can be used in conjunction with 'empathy training'. It is helpful to have the child look again in the mirror. 'See how you look when you are angry-happy-sad, etc.'

Take the feelings that the child has difficulty in dealing with. Discuss how he is presently expressing them. Then, suggest alternative ways which would be more appropriate.

8. Help the child relax. Then model the expression of the feeling, giving him plenty of opportunity to imitate and rehearse it.

9. In a situation where a child is having difficulty dealing with what he is feeling, take him aside and run through a role-play of how better to deal with what he is feeling. Then encourage him to go back into the everyday situation. Hopefully, after doing this once or twice, cueing him will be necessary only when he is really stuck.

10. Reinforce the child with praise or physical contact for each everyday occasion in which he speaks out with a feeling appropriately and adequately.

Untoward Effects

If the therapist tries to force the procedure, it could backfire making the child clam up and become more resistant. Determine the parents' ability to tolerate the child's expression of any particular emotion. If they have difficulty dealing with a similar emotion, they should be helped in a session of their own. Children should be taught to express feelings only in a manner acceptable and tolerated by their families. Otherwise family stability may be shaken.

Charting Requirements

Measures, rating scales.

Individuation (CI) — 'I am me'
Technique — Second Level

Rationale

In the child's early life, parents and children are symbiotically attached to each other. As normal development occurs the child gradually begins to recognise himself as a separate entity and has enough of his parents inside him to feel secure as the attachment gradually weakens. Some insecure or ambivalent parents unconsciously foster symbiotic attachments. The result is a very high level of anxiety in children as they try to detach.

Symbiotically attached children cannot distinguish their own individual desires, wants and needs. They often confuse their perceptions with those of their parents. They also believe that without them, their parents would suffer, especially if while they try to individuate they fantasise aggression against their parents. In feeling anger towards his parents, the child may wish they were ill or dead. The child must then stay close to the parent to make sure that the wish does not come true.

If the child cannot perceive his own desires, he is less likely to be able to distinguish the legitimate needs of other people.

Pathologically attached children do occasionally attempt to individuate and separate, but they may be overwhelmed with anxiety. That anxiety is only relieved when they reattach themselves. The anxiety relief reinforces their clinging to parents. The staff must deal with this anxiety by supporting both the child and his parents as they separate. As a child gains insight and maturity, so he will gradually loosen the attachment. Gradual detachment will allow the child to reattach in the future as an individual. The process of letting go is facilitated by systematic desensitisation and training in assertion.

Application

Agoraphobic, asthmatic, battered, scapegoated, disabled, handicapped, symbiotically psychotic, schoolphobic and anorexic children can be helped. Individuation is also useful where there is intense sibling rivalry.

Measures

1. The level of anxiety as a function of distance from the parent.
2. Personality rating scales, particularly on temperament.

Procedure

1. Baseline: Observe parent and child together. Measure anxiety and distance apart. Get both parents and child to assess each other and themselves on the temperament scale. Stay around to interpret to the parents any questions they don't understand. Put the questions into language the child can understand.

2. Explanation: Make sure parents and children understand that the object is to help them have a better relationship, one which is based on a more complete and separate identity. It is not designed to make them dislike each other.

3. Demonstrate using another staff member or child who has already been through the procedure.

4. Help the child describe the parent and the parent describe the child and themselves, without the other present.

5. Bring the parent and child together, help them comment on each other's characteristics. Give the parent then the child an opportunity to describe each other while the other listens. Then they must speak directly at each other without interruption. At first empathise observable details then describe personality characteristics.

6. Provide corrective feedback to the child's self-statements and

descriptions of the parent. Note agreed similarities and differences and write a list of each.

7. They should engage in an exercise of mutual clinging and, while doing this, say how much they enjoy each other's company. Then they should start pushing away while verbally asserting how they need to be separate.

8. Teach the child assertive responses to the parent's cautionary remarks, e.g. 'Be careful', with 'I'll be all right', 'I am quite capable of looking after myself'.

9. Engage the parent and child in a joint project and gradually get them working on separate parts.

10. Help them draw a diploid amorphous blob, i.e. an amorphous blob made of both of them and then an amorphous blob which is separate.

11. In the presence of each other, they should talk about individual interests, past events and future hopes for their individual, personal development.

12. Re-do the scale on temperamental characteristics.

Untoward Effects

Very anxious symbiotically attached children might become psychotic if the process is too abrupt. If the process is shortened and not completed the symbiosis might be intensified.

Charting Requirements

Measures, temperament rating scale both before and after technique. Narrative description of untoward reaction.

Example of Individuation Form

Direction.
Make a tick on the line at that point you feel most truly represents your child. Give your best guess if you are unsure.

1. Activity. Likes to be on the move, busy, moving, playing, drawing, etc.
Always) . . . .(Never

2. Compliance. Happily does whatever he/she is requested.
Always) . . . .(Never

---

3. Regular. Naptime, waking, sleeping, defecating, breathing are all regular and predictable.
Always)........................(Never

4. Quiet. Peaceful and happy to be alone.
Always)........................(Never

5. Perceptive. Understands what is happening in people and events.
Always)........................(Never

6. Approach to New Experiences, Food, People, etc. Goes right up to new people without hesitation.
Always)........................(Never

7. Inquisitive. Likes to investigate new things and places.
Always)........................(Never

8. Adaptive. Adjusts easily to any new environment.
Always)........................(Never

9. High Threshold. Does not startle easily or react to sudden new sights or sounds.
Always)........................(Never

10. Positive Mood. Happy and agreeable whatever happens.
Always)........................(Never

11. Playful. Enjoys playing with friends.
Always)........................(Never

12. Clean. Prefers to be neat and tidy.
Always)........................(Never

13. Intense Responder. Gets very emotional or easily excited when upset.
Always)........................(Never

14. Self-initiating. Starts activity for himself with work or play.
Always)........................(Never

---

15. Intrusive. Butts into others' activities or conversation.
Always). . . . .(Never

16. Distractable. Frequently changes activity with very little distraction.
Always). . . . .(Never

17. Persistent. Sticks with activity even if frustrated.
Always). . . . .(Never

18. Content. Happily accepts whatever he/she is given.
Always). . . . .(Never

19. Courage. Will face danger and difficulty without fear.
Always). . . . .(Never

20. Self-esteem. Thinks he/she is the best at job or school.
Always). . . . .(Never

21. Sadness. Never finds enjoyment or pleasure in life.
Always). . . . .(Never

22. Anger. Flies off in a rage for no reason at all.
Always). . . . .(Never

23. Ambition. Would like to be at the top in everything.
Always). . . . .(Never

24. Concern. Puts other people's needs ahead of his own.
Always). . . . .(Never

Listen to Your Body (LYB) — 'What does my body say?' Technique — Second Level

Rationale

Children lose the ability to sense their body's corrective feedback. This corrective feedback provides the basis for automatic control over a large number of physiological and emotional functions:

(a) Sleep
(b) Hunger
(c) Social contact
(d) Elimination
(e) Exploring
(f) Washing
(g) Clothing
(h) Tidying up
(i) Obeying parents
(j) The discharge of emotions

Parents who are afraid of their own lack of control tend to regulate children excessively. In some cultures parents are socially encouraged to regulate children's functions. The child naturally wants to control his own body functions but he also wants to please his parents and 'go' when they say he should. If he is inclined to listen and respond to his own inner sensations, he will have to disregard his parents. The parents may be able to exercise sufficient control through punishment or guilt that the child stops responding to his inner sensations. Once established, the conflict doesn't easily fade. The child gradually loses sensitivity to his body's corrective feedback, though his inner sensations never die out completely.

In order to please his parents, he must keep ignoring or repressing those quiet but persistent messages from his body senses. This effort makes him tired and irritable. Put another way, he must keep reinforcing the prohibitive parent inside of him. When he becomes older, or when his parents are absent, he must substitute his repressed, natural feedback with artificial monitors, such as weight scales. Thus, to control his eating and to replace his lost awareness of when he is hungry or full, he weighs himself and counts calories. This artificial control breaks down when he gets tired or discouraged. The times when he loses control results in excesses, which make him afraid of his emotional expression. It also inhibits his curiosity about his body.

To restore the child to an easily balanced self-regulation, the child's inner sensations must be awakened. He must re-learn how to receive and understand his inner sensations. When he can listen to his inner sensations, he can then learn to respond with self-control. It is important to reassure the parents that the child is basically able to control himself. Remembering their own childhood will help them see that their impositions only confuse him.

Application

Children with problems of self-control (enuresis, encopresis, etc.), children who are overly controlled (anorexics, obsessives), children who are excessively aggressive or have learning inhibitions are also helped by this technique.

Measures

Take measures of body tension and areas of self-control, i.e. weight, enuresis, etc.

Procedure

1. Baseline: Obtain measures prior to the child's admission.

2. Explanation: Provide the parents with a complete explanation of how the problem came into being and what procedures are being used to rectify it. Allay their anxieties about losing control of their children and reinforce any desire they may have to help the child gain self-control. The parents may need psychotherapy directed at their own problems of self-control.

3. Demonstration: Use another child on which this technique has been used or a staff member to demonstrate how they can learn to identify and respond to inner impulses.

4. Describe body mechanisms, emphasising homeostasis. The child may also be included in A & P Teaching with emphasis on the particular area of concern.

5. Appoint another staff member as temporary controller. This staff member will remind the child that he must do what he normally has been told to do by his parents. 'It's time you . . . you had better go.' The controller will take over the functioning of the parent and gradually and systematically relinquish during the early part of the child's hospitalisation.

6. Using modelling, teach the child to report when he thinks he is feeling a sensation. Start with non-conflicting areas. If there are areas of more than one conflict, start with the one that is least involved. 'Tell me when you think you are tired, hungry, needing to go to the bathroom, etc.' If necessary, use reinforcement.

7. Do 10-minute checks. 'Are you feeling tired, hungry, etc.?' 'Okay, it's no problem, I was wondering if you were listening to your body.' The child should be able to report yes, no or maybe. Gradually lengthen the interval between checks by 10 minutes.

8. Note the discrepancies between when the controller is requesting the child to do what he must and the child's own desire. Discuss the

implications.

9. Involve the child in psychotherapy specifically designed to deal with the problems of control, particularly fears of loss of control, his or his parents'. Discuss the graph that is used to indicate the number of times the child is reporting a sensation.

10. When the child is reporting regularly and reasonably on his impulses, get together with the controller and negotiate a transfer of control. After this the child will be allowed to do whatever he feels like, eating, sleeping, etc., whenever he feels so inclined, and to the extent that he wishes to do it.

11. If the child experiences a rebound phenomenon, that is an excessive indulgence in his impulses, allow this to occur unless the child or the parents become excessively anxious.

12. Negotiate with the parents and the child a generous upper and lower limitation to the expression of the child's impulse to eat and sleep, etc.

13. Before discharge, hand over control entirely to the child and watch the parents' reaction. Reassure them if they wish to reimpose their control over the child.

14. Check the child on home visits to see how well he is functioning in terms of listening to his own body and self-control.

Untoward Effects

If this technique is not done with sufficient care, it is easy for the child to force the parents or the staff member to exercise control and no progress is made.

Charting Requirements

Measures only necessary.

Mediational Modification (MM) – 'Going gopher'
Technique – Second Level

Rationale

Mediational modification, also known as cognitive restructuring, is a technique to modify the thought process of a child. It has become increasingly apparent to clinicians and researchers that thinking patterns must change before behaviour does. The process requires role-playing, imitation, practice and reinforcing successively more adaptive responses.

Many disturbed children get into trouble because they tend to act without thinking or they react too quickly. Mediational modification attempts to provide thought processes which will mediate between the stimulus and the response so that the behaviour is more adaptive. Constructive thought processes are taught by staff who model adaptive responses to a provocative stimulus. Since the child cannot see the adult's thought process, the adult must verbally express them and do it in such a way that the child sees how one thought logically follows another. Closer approximations by the child to the adult model's way of thinking through the problem, are reinforced.

Application

Anxious, impulsive, irritable, hyperactive, aggressive children and those with social or antisocial behaviour disorders, may benefit.

Measures

1. Note changes in the rate of target behaviour, e.g. temper tantrum, shouting, fighting or running away.

2. Record the strength and the duration of the provoking stimulus and the delay in responding appropriately.

Procedures

1. Baseline: Measure using varying intensity of provocation, the child's usual response prior to modification.

2. The child and parents should be given a full explanation of what the procedure is and what the objectives are. The parents must commit themselves to learning the procedure so that upon discharge they can continue to reinforce the child's more adaptive cognitive style.

3. Using either a staff member or another child, the technique in its usual form should be demonstrated.

4. Set up a situation which requires the child, a reactive model, a rational model and a provocateur. The provocation should be enough to produce anxiety but not overwhelming anxiety. If the child becomes too anxious he can watch a few times from behind a one-way glass with a staff member commenting. Make a complete list of situations, to which the child responds with undue haste or with self-defeating behaviour.

5. The provocateur should make demanding or irritating statements that would normally excite the patient's usual maladaptive response. To this the reactive model will respond modelling the child's usual behaviour plus the kinds of thoughts that would be going through the child's mind.

6. The rational model will then begin by empathising with the child's emotional response, thinking through the implications and suggesting alternatives. The reactive and rational models will respond back and forth to each other in such a way that the reactive model eventually begins incorporating the thoughts from the rational model.

7. Over a period of time, the reactive model begins using the suggestions in his own thinking that have been made by the rational model. The staff portraying the rational model gradually fades from the scene.

8. The remaining staff carries both the reactive and rational model and begins coaching the child to express some of the same words that he was using to typify his thought processes.

9. Gradually the child is encouraged to perform both the reactive and the rational components of the model's behaviour. When he does so, he is reinforced with praise or primary reinforcement.

10. The provocateur increases the intensity of the provocation. The child is encouraged to respond, speaking his thought processes and eventually providing a rational adaptive response.

11. Once the child is comfortable in doing this, the parents should witness the whole process so that they understand and will give him the opportunity to think through his responses before they demand an immediate reaction.

12. The child should be taught to keep his thought process silent but should have some prearranged signal, e.g. tapping his finger, to indicate he is working on the problem and needs a little time.

13. Make sure the parents understand this technique well enough so that they can encourage him at home.

14. On follow-up give a few tests to see if the child can still handle the most provoking situations. If he can't, give him some more coaching.

Untoward Effects

If this procedure is rushed or not sufficiently well taught, the child becomes more inhibited and his behaviour more maladaptive. Children who have difficulty in discriminating social situations should be taught empathy first.

Charting Requirements

Graph the changes in the target behaviour and the increase in intensity in the stimulus. Chart any approximations that are to be reinforced and what reinforcement was used. Responses incorporating both the reactive and rational models should be charted as well as clear documentation of each stage of the process.

Nurturing Child (NC) — 'Really looked after'
Technique — Second Level

Rationale

Deprived children are suspicious of any new relationship. From their experience, they expect to be disappointed by those who offer to help. They often set themselves up for repeated rejection by asking the wrong people. Yet children with incomplete parenting persistently keep hoping for parental recognition and nurture. The persistence of hope is often directly proportional to the number of rejections. This forlorn hope continues into adulthood. The unresolved conflict is expressed by the deprived child, when grown up, repeatedly getting into disappointing relationships.

The purpose of nurturing is to:

(1) Teach the child he can trust the staff who offer to help him.
(2) Overcome resistance to a therapeutic staff/patient.
(3) Provide rest during which neurophysiological functions stabilise and dreams allow abreaction.
(4) Strengthen the ego for psychotherapy.
(5) Allow regression during which a child finds it safe to allow nurturing at many levels.
(6) Demonstrate to parents and child that needs can be satisfied.

Application

1. Deprived (angry and sad) children.
2. Traumatised children.
3. Detached children who have not mourned previous losses.

Measures

1. The amount of time asleep.
2. The amount of time spent with staff.
3. Verbatim comments on the experience.
4. Activities engaged in during the nurturing programme.

Procedure

1. Baseline: Obtain estimates of how well the child is nurtured at home.

2. Explanation: Tell the child: 'I think you really need a rest.' 'Even though you may not feel tired or sick, your body is tired from trying to overcome problems and difficulties.' 'I want to get to know you.'

'There won't be an operation.' 'You will be up in three days.' 'We two staff will look after you and try to give you whatever you need.'

3. Day 1: Provide continuous bed rest, meals, pillow fluffing, stories and sometimes special food. Obtain a careful history and give considerable empathy for the expression of feelings.

4. Day 2: Allow the child to get up and explore the ward. Allow one or two visits. Review the history and in light of that provide the child with hope. Engage in abreaction of traumatic situations. Do some teaching of mental mechanisms and relaxation.

5. Day 3: Allow the child up for meals. Review his history and make appropriate interpretations. If identification is being used in a programme, start with such statements as 'You and I are struggling with weight', or 'You and this other child seem to have the same problem.' Empathise the ability to overcome difficulties even though there have been some hang-ups. At the end of day 3, explore with the child his reactions to nurturing, his previous disappointments, how he feels about being looked after and whether he thinks he will be looked after in the future.

6. Day 4: Spend time with the child and parents discussing their needs for nurture. Demonstrate to the parents how the child responds to nurturing. Give them encouragement to take over the nurturing.

7. Day 5: The child should be up and dressed, fully involved in the ward programme. At night and meal times the parents should continue nurturing him. Often deprived parents find it hard to nurture. Even when they are shown how, they may feel jealous of the child getting something they never had as children and are unlikely to have as adults. During the time the child is being nurtured they should have intensive psychotherapy aimed at resolving their nurturing conflicts. Badly deprived parents can be nurtured at the same time as their child is being put to bed.

Medications such as Diazepam and Amitriptyline can be used to enhance relaxation. A physical must be done first. Blood pressures and pulse must be recorded frequently at the beginning.

Untoward Effects

Some children fight against nurturing because they fear regression and losing control.

Charting Requirements

Measures and document any resistance and how it is handled.

Operant Conditioning of Children (OCC)
Technique — Third Level

Rationale

If a good deal of human behaviour is determined by the environment, we now know many of the rules that describe how this happens. If the human organism finds that the change in the performance of a certain activity in its internal or external environment is to its advantage, it will tend to do it again, i.e. if it is given something that it finds rewarding it will engage in the activity more frequently. The activity is thus reinforced by gaining a rewarding stimulus. If it finds that as a consequence of a certain activity it encounters a stimulus that makes life somewhat more unpleasant, it will feel punished and the activity will diminish in frequency and intensity.

It is important to note the organism really rewards or punishes itself. This puts the emphasis less on the determining nature of the environment and more on the self-determining nature of choices people make. The organism may not consciously figure it out, but biologically it is adapting quickly to environments that will make life more pleasant and profitable.

People can change each other's behaviour. The person who has the best advantage in changing another person is the one who is more aware of what is happening. Usually the parent or staff can reward or punish the child's behaviour to make it happen more or less frequently. But the child will reflexly reward or punish the adult's behaviour by complying with what is desired of him by the adult. This makes it important to understand the mechanisms that govern adult or staff behaviour. If to enhance their self-image they depend too heavily on the child's compliant behaviour, the child will soon learn to govern the adults' behaviour by complying or not complying.

In many cases parents and children, or staff and children, are mutually conditioning each other's behaviour. At the same time the parent reinforces crying behaviour by picking up and comforting the child while it is crying, the child is reinforcing the parent for picking it up, by no longer crying. Parents become very tense when their children cry and very relaxed when they stop. The relaxation that follows the child's cessation of crying is strong reinforcement for the picking-up behaviour of the parent. In this way parents condition children to maladaptive crying behaviour and children condition their parents into habitual picking-up behaviour, if they are not careful.

Operant conditioning can be used in many other techniques. We prefer not to manipulate a child but to teach him how to control his own behaviour. We want to teach the child to use operant conditioning on his own behaviour when he finds he can't make his decisions stick.

We prefer to use natural rather than artificial reinforcers. When there are no immediately available natural reinforcers, however, we proffer a 'smorgasbord' of artificial reinforcers to find which the child prefers. Although some autistic children appear to have no reinforcers, it's possible to find something that reinforces almost every behaviour.

In using operant conditioning it is particularly important that we obtain the parents' consent. The principles of operant conditioning are used with Negotiating Guidelines and Consequences, and Shaping.

Application

Whenever it is possible, we try to teach parents and children to control their behaviour with an understanding of how and why it occurs. In situations where they are no longer able to control themselves and with their permission, we use operant conditioning to help them overcome previously conditioned maladaptive behaviours. Operant conditioning can be used with almost every technique whenever staff are stuck. Autistic children, oppositional behaviour, non-compliance, encopresis, taking medication, concentrating on schoolwork and wheezing less frequently are a few of the areas where operant conditioning can be used.

Procedure

1. Carefully define the target behaviour so that everyone monitoring it will agree when it occurs and when it does not.

2. Obtain baseline measures of the target behaviour, preferably before the child's admission but, if not, in the first two or three days of his admission.

3. Give a careful explanation to the parents about the procedure upon which you are about to embark. Make sure you obtain an informed consent.

4. Demonstrate the procedure to the parents using some other child.

5. Find out the most useful reinforcers. This is best achieved by finding out what activities or goodies the child finds most rewarding or what is most likely to make rapid change in the child's behaviour.

6. In giving the reinforcement, it is essential to give it immediately upon the completion of the required behaviour. The reinforcer is more potent if the child must exert himself, i.e. stretch out his hand, to get

the reinforcer.

7. Since most primary reinforcers cannot be given to the child within the 0.5 sec. immediacy requirement, it is useful to pair it with a secondary reinforcer, e.g. 'good boy', until the 'good boy' takes on the reinforcing properties of the primary reinforcer or acts as a signal to indicate that a primary reinforcer is about to be given.

8. With oppositional children there is an advantage to being very subtle about reinforcing. Autistic children sometime are so resistant to change, they do not like to be seen complying. Therefore, one must deliver the reinforcer in a very indirect, no fuss way.

9. Reinforce the desired behaviour at baseline rates until it is happening more frequently. Increase your expectation whereby you reinforce more selectively desired behaviour at higher rates. Refer to the Shaping technique.

10. Reinforcing is generally most powerful if there is a state of relative deprivation. For this reason, if you are using social contact you should not be spending too much time with the child in other pleasurable ways. Once the desired behaviour is happening frequently change to a ratio or interval schedule to make the behaviour well entrenched.

11. When the behaviour is well established switch to a more mutual reinforcer.

12. Teach the parents the method you have used and hand over the control to them.

13. Once the parents are well in control of that behaviour, teach the child how to do it for himself.

Untoward Effects

The child may become too worried about approval or disapproval. Operant conditioning should be used in combination with insight psychotherapy to facilitate the child's greater freedom and awareness.

Charting Requirements

Note the defined behaviours. Include the graphs of rates of change, indicating when reinforcers or ratios have been altered.

Play Therapy — Corrective (PTC) — 'Play time'
Technique — Second Level

Rationale

Children experiment with different roles within their play. They learn new concepts, knowledge, facts and connections through play. It is possible in a structured setting to measure their ability to learn.

Children who are either resistant to new relationships, stuck in patterns of interaction, frightened to learn new patterns or have developed a negative attitude towards exploring, benefit from corrective play.

Application

Depressed, deprived, retarded children who have been scapegoated or abused and need to learn new interactional patterns start slowly but learn quickly. Children with previous school difficulties and those who are obsessive may benefit.

Measures

Measure the behaviour within the play, the skill or knowledge that is being learned.

Procedure

1. Obtain a baseline while watching from a distance.
2. Explain the rules that almost anything goes provided he doesn't hurt anyone or break property.
3. Demonstate by letting another child play with the same material.
4. Select one behavioural skill, concept or piece of knowledge to be learned.
5. Model the behaviour that is required to learn this new skill.
6. Divide the learning into small steps. Set up tools, toys or situations in the playroom.
7. Interact with the child in a supportive manner, encouraging development along each step.

Untoward Effects

An increasingly anxious or restricted child may result from the lack of structure.

Charting Requirements

Chart steps and record narrative report on responses and reactions of child.

**Pushing Red and Green Buttons (PRGB) — 'Stop and go'
Technique — Second Level**

Rationale

Although children wish to believe that their parents can meet all of
their needs, supply them with a secure and predictable environment and
protect them from the parents' own inner confusion and distress,
children become all too soon aware of the fact that their parents are
vulnerable, have foibles and are inconsistent. Not only are they unpredictable, but frequently the parents are as child-like in some areas as
the children themselves. Though they may try to avoid the realisation,
children discover their parents are very human with very human needs
and insecurities. When the children see their parents' needs, it stirs their
desire to nurture and protect their own parents and to blame themselves. Some of this tendency is useful in stimulating the growth of the
parent-like characteristics of the child but if they are exposed to it too
often, children become too anxious to function as a child who explores
the world and enjoys life.

Children need to learn to understand their parents so that they can
react to their parents' unpredictable behaviour. We find it necessary to
tell children that their parents are scapegoating them, or their parents
have such deeply-rooted problems they cannot respond to their needs.
This is not intended to demean the parents but to give the child an
increased ability to use his own resources to find what he needs. The
child can then respond rationally. He will know how to please his
parents and if he displeases them, he will know why.

Children learning how to push their parents' red and green buttons
correctly are first encouraged to identify temperamental characteristics.
They learn to recognise the triggers that stimulate irrational responses
in their parents. These triggers are 'red buttons'. The conditions which
will stimulate spontaneous approval in the parent are known as
'green buttons'.

Application

Almost all children can benefit from understanding the red and green
buttons in their parents. This technique should not be taught to manipulative or antisocial children, nor is it of great value to psychotic
children.

Measures

1. The number of times the parents become irrationally enraged.

2. The number of times they express pleasure at their child.

Procedure

1. Obtain a baseline on the above measures, preferably before the child is admitted.

2. Explain to the child and his parents the procedure of this technique and why it should be used. Parents who are frightened of being controlled by their children will need to understand that if they wish they can learn the red and green buttons in their children.

3. Demonstate how the technique works by using another child who has been well taught and that child's parent. If no other child is at that stage, role-play with some of the staff members.

4. Provide an opportunity for the child to observe his parents interacting with other parents or with his siblings. Ask the child to describe the parents as best he can and see if he can pick out what triggers various responses in the parents.

5. Using the temperamental characteristics form, help the child understand his parents' temperamental features and how they may differ from his own. Briefly describe the parents' major conflicts and point out to the child what environmental situations or behaviour of his own may trigger an enraged or pleasurable response.

6. Select six buttons, three red and three green, and rank order them in terms of intensity. A bright red button would be something that is sure to make the parent very angry, a medium, less so and a dull one, hardly angry at all. A bright green button is sure to get a pleasurable response from the parent, a medium and dull green button, less so.

7. Modelling a parent, encourage the child to push your buttons, beginning with a dull red and a bright green button. Rehearse it often enough so the child can do it without thinking too long.

8. Having identified a bright green and a dull red parental button ask another staff member to role-play the part of a parent and see if the child can turn the buttons on. The staff should react as naturally as possible.

9. Having primed the parents as to what may happen, get the child to try pushing one of his parent's bright green, then dull red buttons. Make sure the parent is visibly pleased or displeased.

10. Try the same with a medium green and a medium red button, making sure the child has plenty of time to rehearse it before trying it out on his parents. The parents on this occasion should not be primed.

11. Using the same technique try a bright red and a dull green button on parents who have not been tipped off.

12. Once these have been well established, tell the child to use them whenever he wishes. Continue to watch the child recording how often he pushes a button and how well he achieves the desired results.

13. Involve the child and parent in other activities, having indicated to the child that he should not press any red buttons at all. Measure the number of occasions the child does or misses opportunities to push buttons.

14. Tell your patient to try pushing the right buttons while on weekend passes.

15. During follow-up, check his button-pushing for accuracy and desired effects. Provide the child with corrective feedback and reinforce him for successes.

Untoward Effects

Staff and parents may worry that the child will become manipulative both with parents and other adults. We have found this seldom occurs and if it does it is usually because the parents are not meeting the child's needs in other ways.

Charting Requirements

Chart measures and anecdotal explanations of successes and failures.

Relaxation Techniques (RT)
Technique — Second Level

Rationale

When children are anxious and tense, they cannot be really perceptive of themselves, others or the environment. Anxiety makes it difficult to learn, gain insight or change behaviour patterns.

Various relaxation techniques have a number of features in common. These include muscle relaxation, self-discipline, focusing attention to the exclusion of other stimuli, suggestion and putting oneself into a better perspective.

The purpose of teaching children these techniques is to help them learn that they can govern their automatic and effective responses, even when situations about them are very anxiety provoking.

Children are better able to make use of a variety of therapy sessions if they are first relaxed.

Application

All children can benefit, especially anxious and phobic children.

Measures

Objective — pulse, respiration.
Subjective — body posture, facial expression.

Procedure

1. Baseline: Obtain measures in a variety of anxiety stimulating situations.
2. Explain to the parents and child, making sure you respond to all their anxieties about who is in control. Demonstrate the basic procedure with a co-operating child.
3. Carefully explain the technique to the children as one of helping learn to control his reactions. Considerable emphasis must be made on the fact that he is learning to control himself and that nobody is taking over control from him. Emphasise the many advantages: learning how to concentrate, doing better in school, feeling more relaxed.
4. Teach the child systematically to relax his muscles. This involves deep-breathing exercises. Make suggestions of how to begin to feel relaxed. If biofeedback equipment is available, hook him up and show him how he is controlling his own responses.
5. Give the child control over his own relaxation. Encourage him to do it on a regular basis. Reinforce him on those occasions when he is able to conduct the whole exercise for the appointed periods of time. Emphasise self-induced muscle relaxation.
6. The child first induces muscle relaxation you then teach him to concentrate by saying over and over to himself a magic word. The child is given a specific nonsense double-syllable word which becomes his magic word. He says this to himself, to focus his attention.
7. Once the child is relaxed introduce anxiety provoking stimuli (APS). Begin introducing the stimuli at the bottom of the hierarchy of APS. The therapist, in describing these stimuli, watches carefully to ensure that the child is still in control of his relaxation. If he loses control, the APS is discontinued until he once again regains control, and it is then gradually reintroduced.

Untoward Effects

If the APS is introduced before the child has good control of basic relaxation techniques, or if he loses control too frequently, there could be an increase in his anxiety which might cause him to feel more hopeless about himself.

Charting Requirements

Graph pulse and respiration. Chart number of relaxation sessions and duration. Chart magic word used. Chart hierarchy of anxiety producing stimuli in 24-Hour Progress Note and record which one being worked on and response.

Saying Goodbye (SG) — 'It's been good to know you'
Technique — Second Level

Rationale

Most disturbed children have had many goodbyes, most of which have been incompletely resolved. These unresolved conflicts are carried into their adolescent lives, making them vulnerable to hurts from friends and relatives and frightened of making attachments.

Children do become attached to staff, often much more than the staff realise. This is not surprising. Being on the Family Unit is usually a bright, warm experience in the child's life. The child is naturally drawn to any staff member who understands him well and is so attentive to his needs. The growing attachment to staff evokes fears in the child, which may be expressed in anger or withdrawal. It is therapeutic for the child to re-experience another hello and goodbye with a fuller understanding and resolution. Before the child is able to re-establish himself thoroughly in the family, it is important for him to say goodbye to the staff. Thus the staff also must learn how to say hello and goodbye.

It appears children can maintain only a few very important relationships at a time. They mature best when they have only one set of parents. There comes a time when they must say goodbye to a separated father or mother, especially when the parent they live with has remarried. If they don't say goodbye, they keep yearning for the return of the absent parent and may try to manoeuvre their return by splitting up the new marriage.

Application

All children can benefit to some extent, particularly traumatised, depressed, deprived and withdrawn children.

Measures

Record verbatim statements of sadness and anger regarding the relationship and your own emotions and intuitions.

Procedure

1. Record in detail the child's history of attachments and loss. Remind the child that his hospitalisation is only for five weeks (eventually he will have to say goodbye) but do not bring it up too frequently because it will interfere with attachments.

2. It's vital to explain very carefully to parents why it is so important for a child to finish his goodbyes.

3. The child should witness goodbyes being said by the staff to other children.

4. Beginning in the fourth week, the staff should make a conscious attempt to start disengaging: 'Next week you will be leaving and we will have to say goodbye.' Make sure you recognise and deal with all of the child's ambivalent feelings.

5. On the last Friday, hold a goodbye party during which Strength Bombardment and a special meal is used to celebrate the occasion. Children fear that things at home have not changed or that they will have been forgotten. Remind them you will continue to have contact for a period of five weeks' follow-up.

6. While saying goodbye on Saturday, review the mixed feelings of sadness and anger, e.g. 'Saying goodbye hurts and hurts make you angry. I am sure you must be angry that you are just getting to know me and I am now saying goodbye'; 'This has happened to you before'; 'I can imagine how hurt and angry you are.'

7. In situations where children have unresolved losses of parents, etc. they should be reminded of those occasions and given an opportunity to compare the effects upon them.

8. When getting a child to say goodbye to a separated parent, get that parent to initiate the process by saying goodbye to the child. Eventually the child and parent should be able to look each other in the eye and say a mutual goodbye.

9. If the parent is absent encourage the child to phone. Inform the parent you are on an extension phone and encourage both parties to make their goodbyes very explicit.

10. If the lost parent is dead or too far away, get the child to write a letter. Make sure the child is definite. The letter can be taken to the cemetery and laid on the grave.

11. Help the parents to say their goodbyes where appropriate.

12. On follow-up, check to ensure the mourning and reattachment process is still in progress.

Untoward Effects

An unresolved hurt associated with the child's hospitalisation and attachment to a staff member could add to his list of incomplete goodbyes.

Charting Requirements

Measures only.

Self-control (SC) – 'Flying level and steady' Technique – Second Level

Rationale

Good self-control is possessed by those who can restrain impulses, but on other occasions can let go their inhibitions – whoop, weep or laugh uncontrollably. Some children are unnaturally inhibited, partly because of parental disapproval and partly because of a bad experience when they did express their feelings. Other children are so impulsive they cannot restrain themselves when the need arises. They may lack maturity or they may have been reinforced by parents who inadvertently attend to their impulsive reactions. Sometimes impulsiveness is modelled, sometimes it is a result of brain dysfunction. Children need control but blanket-type inhibition tends to hinder a child's ability to question and explore the unknown.

The object of this technique is to teach children:

(1) When and how to let go of their feelings.
(2) To learn confidence in their own quick judgements and reactions.

Application

Inhibited, doubting, obsessive, autistic children should learn to express their feelings and trust their own reactions. Impulsive, hyperactive children should learn how to restrain their responses and question their first responses.

Measures

1. The number of appropriate responses in any given day.
2. The number of self-initiated questions.
3. The amount of exploring.
4. The child's creativity as shown in pictures that are drawn three times a week at a standard time under standard conditions.

Procedure

1. Baseline: Measure 1-4 for three days without intervening. Time the interval between the irritation and the response.

2. Explain the procedure in detail to the child and his family. Any questions raised need to be given consideration and anxieties reassured.

3. Demonstrate the technique using another impulsive child who has almost finished the programme. If no child volunteers, one of the staff may role-play a situation, i.e. someone provoking by teasing or hitting.

4. Obtain a self-statement of how the child gets into trouble and why it happens. Give an opportunity to inhibited children to describe how they would like to react and what stops them.

5. Combine Self-control with Delayed Gratification, Mediational Modification and Social Skills Training. Stimulate impulses under pre-set conditions. Carefully measure the time interval between the provocation and the impulse. Graph these. Eventually teach the child to measure that interval himself.

6. Give impulsive children a specific method by which they may inhibit their impulsive reaction, e.g. counting to 10, turning in circles four times, muttering aloud for 30 seconds.

7. Rehearse these procedures until they come naturally and easily.

8. Allow the child to engage in the usual ward activities. Give corrective feedback on his success and failure.

9. Reinforce inhibited children for questions. Help them develop new ideas and shown how scientific methodology can be used to advantage in exploring the world around them.

10. Teach children how to be determined by:
   (i) limiting the challenge;
   (ii) having been given an opportunity to face a challenge, ask them how long they would persist at it if they were frustrated on more than one occasion.

11. Provide inhibited children a variety of new situations, puzzles and problems to see how well they respond.

12. Show the parents how to estimate the child's self-control and not to push it too far with either frustration or excitement.

13. In follow-up, check to make sure the child is maintaining self-control with friends and family.

Untoward Effects

If the programme is done too quickly, inhibited children may become increasingly inhibited because of failure. Some frightened parents may become concerned that their quiet, compliant children become too aggressive or demanding.

Charting Requirements

Chart measures and graphs of time intervals between provocation and impulse.

Sex Education (SE) — 'Birds and bees' Technique — Second Level

Rationale

Learning about sex should be part of normal development and, there-fore, part of general health education for both children and adolescents. The emphasis should not be on physiology and contraception but on relationships and respect.

Feelings, attitudes and facts about human sexuality are often an area of misconception. The resulting conflicts and stresses are frequently cited as problem areas by the children's parents. Before doing any sex education, staff must obtain the parents' informed consent.

Reviewing these feelings, attitudes and facts with an objective adult assists the children in developing their understanding and moral code. Pre-marital promiscuity correlates with extra-marital promiscuity, so there is a pragmatic reason for virginity. Children also need to learn how to say no and how to sublimate their sex drives.

Increasing awareness of their sexuality is an underlying motivation in much of adolescent peer interaction. It should not be ignored, but information about sex should not be titillating. Too often children want to experience what is talked about.

Application

All children over the age of 12. A modified programme should be used for children under 12 where:

1.   insufficient age-appropriate information exists and/or
2.   sexually related problems are presented.

Measures

1. Positive self-statements.
2. Positive peer (both sexes) interaction.
3. Amount of inappropriate sexual 'acting out'.

Procedure

This technique is done on either a one-to-one basis, or in small groups conducive to easy communication and discussion. Preferably the parents should be present for all sessions.

1. Obtain a baseline estimate of the child's present information and attitude towards sex.

2. Explain why, what and how to the parents. Obtain their consent and note it on file.

3. Give the child and his parents an opportunity to sit in on your discussion with a child who is able to talk fairly freely about sex.

4. Begin with a general discussion of boy–girl relations, feelings and conflicts.

5. Outline age-appropriate basics of human anatomy and physiology; male and female. Emphasise the effect of hormones in producing strong feelings and drives.

6. Discuss the basics of courting, matching, mating and the ingredients of a good-enduring relationship.

7. Discuss the importance of child care and the need for commitment. Give the child a fertilised egg to mother for two days.

8. Give a brief outline of contraception methods. Give them honest answers to questions about abortion, including the hazards and complications. Emphasising the seriousness of the issue.

9. Discuss self-image in terms of patients' own sexuality. Assertiveness Training to be able to maintain decisions in the face of peer pressure should be given. Show how to use distraction with other activities when under pressure to perform sexually.

10. Teach parents how to answer questions comfortably. Emphasise the importance of their demonstrating how men and women should interact.

11. On follow-up, make notes of the child's sexual talk or behaviour. Don't hesitate to bring up the subject again.

Untoward Effects

Too detailed information to a child who is not ready for it can cause shock or disgust. A child might interpret information as a licence to be promiscuous or want to experience what he has heard about.

Charting Requirements

Document any films or books used. Any concerns and the answers given are to be charted.

Shaping (S) — 'Shaping up'
Technique — Second Level

Rationale

Children will repeat behaviours that are reinforced. Often these behaviours are maladaptive because parents attend to behaviours that they cannot ignore. They inadvertently pay attention to the behaviours that irritate them most. Attention is one of the most powerful reinforcers because it has survival value.

In order that the child may learn a new behaviour by shaping, you must first break each new behaviour to be learned into small steps. Through successive approximation, each step is reinforced. Begin with those behaviours that the child already possesses that most clearly resemble the final desired behaviour. Once the step is learned, the reinforcement is terminated so the child will explore and eventually discover the next behaviour. Cueing is used to help a child see the next step.

Application

Shaping is used with almost every kind of problem, at any age and with any condition. Retarded children, very young children, enuretics, encopretics, stutterers, anorexics, compulsive eaters, autistic children, phobic children can all benefit.

Measures

Graph each 'target response', the number of times reinforced, and when there was a change in reinforcement.

Procedure

1. Obtain a baseline both at home and for two days on the ward.

2. After the family and the treatment team have agreed on the goals, give the child and his parents a careful explanation of the procedure.

3. Demonstrate how adaptive and maladaptive behaviour is reinforced whenever adults pay attention.

4. Clearly label and identify each step of the new behaviour.

5. Work out what are good reinforcers. Try to use natural reinforcers (hug, praise) rather than tokens, stars, etc.

6. Reinforce each step until it occurs frequently.

7. Gradually diminish the reinforcement and watch carefully for the behaviour that is slightly more similar to the goal. Use cueing sparingly.

8. Repeat this procedure until the 'target response' is achieved and

is occurring frequently.

9. Put the child on a variable ratio reinforcement schedule.

10. Teach the parent how to become the reinforcing agent. It sets a positive framework for learning other skills and allows an easy transition from non-social to social reinforcements.

11. Teach the parents the technique you have been using. Make sure they are doing it smoothly before the child leaves hospital.

12. On follow-up, make sure the parents are forging ahead.

Untoward Effects

Shaping requires great patience. If that patience is not demonstrated, it could increase the child's tension, decrease his spontaneity and inhibit exploration.

Charting Requirements

Chart the 'target response'. Chart each step that makes up the 'target response'. Chart reinforcement used. Graph as in measures. Chart any unusual response from the child. Chart teaching given to the parent and what the parent has been able to demonstrate to you that he can perform.

Sphincter Control (SC) — 'I can hang on or let go when I want to' Technique — Second Level

Rationale

Some children during their natural drive for autonomy encounter parents who demand sphincter control in the way and at the time they prescribe. If the child doesn't comply, he may be punished and so becomes fixated by a conflict. By interfering with the child's drive for autonomy, parents may produce considerable aggression in the child, a fear of his own impulses, and a demand for unnecessary control in other areas of his life.

The child should be helped to gain self-control and autonomy. To do this, the child needs a better understanding of the dynamics involved. The underlying aggression should be diverted away from the problem area by training in assertion.

Application

Enuresis, encopresis, constipation, stuttering, etc.

Measures

1. The interval between involuntary releases.
2. The amount of urine voided or size of stool.
3. The amount of conflict surrounding the drive for autonomy.

Procedure

1. Obtaining a Baseline. Discuss the problem with the child and demonstrate an easy control, e.g. 'Now I'm going to the bathroom because I feel I should.'
2. Explore the child's anger, previous coercion, and his reaction to it.
3. Help the child first express anger in a non-verbal way, e.g. mud-throwing or mess therapy.
4. The child's anger should be directed to a verbal expression of anger as in Feelings Rehearsal or Assertiveness Training.
5. The child should be told that we want him to gain self-control by listening to his body and making up his own mind when he needs to go. If the child is old enough, get him to count his impulses to void.

Enuresis.

1. The staff should teach start-and-stop exercises with the explanation, 'they make you shut off muscles more strongly'. During micturition, get your patient to show you how often he can stop then start again.
2. Bladder stretching should begin by reassuring the child that his bladder will not burst. Encourage the child to drink large volumes of water. Measure his output and reinforce him for larger amounts of urine or for longer intervals between urinating. Make sure he is not diluting his sample.
3. Reinforce enuretic children for dry nights or for longer periods of dry sleep with a happy face or token.
4. If you can detect when he usually wets, get him up just before that time.
5. A wet alarm can help teach a child to wake up when he needs to go.
6. Give him the responsibility of changing his wet bed and rinsing out wet sheets.

Encopresis.

1. Give encopretic children considerable reassurance about not falling into the toilet.
2. Read to or otherwise entertain children while they sit first with

the lid down then with it up.

3. Sit encopretics on the toilet after meals when the gastro-colic reflex is more likely to function.

4. Reinforce any production in the toilet but don't show any negative effect if he does nothing. Remind him it's entirely his business.

5. If there is soiling, give the child an opportunity to change himself and wash out his own underwear. If there is underwear-hiding, don't give additional clean clothes.

Sphincter Control should be part of an encopretic child programme (refer to Chapter 5).

Untoward Effects

If staff efforts are coercive, there will be increased anxiety and confusion and the encopresis or enuresis might worsen.

Charting Requirements

Chart measures and a flow chart for bladder stretching and reinforcements.

Therapeutic Wrestling (TW) — 'Grunt and groan'
Technique — Second Level

Rationale

When children are overwhelmed by a violent, uncontrolled, aggressive adult, particularly a parent or caretaker, it produces an 'aggressive imprint'. The child is immobilised by anxiety, confusion and despair. He cannot run, he cannot fight back and he cannot object. From that time, children tend to re-enact the trauma by fighting with siblings and provoking other adults. They are trying to understand the rage that keeps boiling up inside them.

Therapeutic Wrestling is designed to:

(1) Allow free expression of feeling during an aggressive interplay, and to work through that initial trauma.
(2) Reassure children that adults can control their aggression.
(3) Give children the feeling of both victory and defeat, so that they will be less afraid of their impulses.
(4) Help children express their feelings about both of these.
(5) Help children learn to limit their own aggressiveness.

Application

Battered and criticised children, obsessive-compulsive and angry children, fearful, weak children may benefit. Don't use TW in situations of sexual abuse or incipient homosexuality.

Measures

Record the number of times therapeutic wrestling is done, the duration, and how much fear, eager or passivity is expressed by the child during TW.

Procedure

1. Baseline: Observe your patient fighting with other children and how he/she reacts to an angry adult.
2. Explain: 'We are going to learn how to get angry properly.' Reassure parents about injury.
3. Demonstrate to parents and child with another child.
4. Start with arm wrestling, Indian wrestling, then try pushing over on a mat, pillow fights or boppers, holding down (staff not astride the child), holding down and twisting a limb to create some discomfort.
5. Model and encourage much grunting. Increasingly loud, ambiguous expletives should be used, progressing to clear words, then shouting.
6. Encourage the child to use more controlled force. Match his effort. When he gets into it, he should both threaten and counter-threaten with 'I am not afraid' or other 'I am . . .' assertive statements.
7. There must be an equal number of wins and losses. The child must not be overwhelmed.
8. After the wrestling, spend time talking about how it felt. Model some emotional experiences, e.g. 'Wow it sure feels good to win', or 'I was afraid you were going to tear my arm off.'
9. Help your patient remember the times when he was attacked or beaten. Ask him about fantasies about getting even, etc.
10. On successive occasions, as the emotional tension subsides, make the wrestling more of an athletic competition.
11. Get the non-aggressive parent to wrestle with the child until both are comfortable.
12. Very gradually, start short sessions of wrestling between your patient and the aggressive or abusing parent. Make sure both are able to maintain control.
13. Provide plenty of opportunity for the child to express his rage and fear to an abusing parent.

14. Work towards some non-aggressive, competitive activity between child and aggressive parent.

15. On follow-up, stage a few competitions to ensure child and parent are still controlling their aggression.

Untoward Effects

If child or adult loses control the whole process becomes more complicated.

Charting Requirements

Note the child's reaction with each type of wrestling.

Time-out (TO) – 'Doing time'
Technique – Second Level

Rationale

Many people inadvertently reinforce a child's maladaptive behaviour (IRMB). They attend to the very behaviour that irritates them most. They inadvertently reinforce disobedience by patiently asking a child to do something 'for the ninth time'. Thus, the child's most irritating behaviour increases, making parents increasingly irritable and alienated from their child.

Not only do adults inadvertently reinforce maladaptive behaviour, but children reciprocally condition their parents (RCPB). They do so by reinforcing their parents with quietness or compliance for attending to their maladaptive behaviour, e.g. the child may comply with his mother's repeated requests and thereby reinforce the mother's nagging behaviour.

Both the child's and parent's mutually conditioned maladaptive behaviours are reinforced on a variable ratio reinforcement schedule. This ensures the more irritating behaviours are the most thoroughly fixed and difficult to change.

Time-out allows extinction to occur by withdrawing any kind of social reinforcement that may be maintaining a behaviour. During extinction the behaviour will get worse before it gets better. The amount it gets worse will depend upon the amount of time it has been conditioned and the previous reinforcement ratio. To ensure no one inadvertently reinforces a behaviour with attention, a barrier between the child and any social contact is required. This could involve a parent putting himself in time-out.

Time-out has some adaptive qualities:

(a) Time-out provides security, allowing a child to explode with pent-up aggression and not hurt himself.

(b) Time-out provides isolation which lessens the probability of aggression being initiated by other patients. It prevents the contagion of aggression.

(c) Time-out allows time for both parent and child to reflect on what happened, restructure their defences and come up with other ways of interacting.

Application

Time-out can be used for almost any maladaptive behaviour, but usually for aggressive and destructive behaviour. Do not use it for claustrophobic children. The amount of time-out depends on age: two minutes for children up to six years, plus thirty seconds of quietness if the child is still carrying on; five minutes for children beyond six years, plus one minute of quietness before they are allowed out.

Measures

Measure the number of time-outs and the total duration in time-out. Report the child's behaviour before, during and after the time-out.

Procedure

1. Give the child a detailed explanation of the time-out procedure and the rules for which time-out will be used. Demonstrate time-out by putting yourselves in time-out and ranting and raving about injustice a little. Get a child to demonstrate self-imposed time-out.

2. Preferably, ask the child if he will go into time-out on his own. If not, lead him gently. If that does not work, he should be marched in with a staff member holding stiffly onto his arm on either side. This technique prevents the child from both hitting and kicking as he must walk to maintain his balance.

3. You can place a ball, chalk or cardboard box in with the child to provide him a medium to express any aggression.

4. When any infraction justifying time-out occurs, don't hesitate or explain, usher the child straight into time-out.

5. Let the child see you set the timer. He should be able to see a clock so he can keep track of the passage of time.

6. When the child has done his time, explain why he went in and ask him about his feelings in time-out.

7. Make it quite clear to the child that the relationship between you and him is still OK.

8. Staff may accompany the child into time-out for special purposes, e.g. a fearful child.

9. Teach the child how to give himself time-out. Reinforce justified self-imposed time-out with shorter periods inside. This can be started by giving the child a cue, e.g. 'OK you know what happens when you do that.'

10. Show the child an accumulative record of his time-out each week.

11. Teach parents how to use time-out. If no room is available, they can place the child outside. Emphasise the fact that frequent, short time-outs are better than long ones, and that parents should keep their cool.

12. Check the parents' time-out record when you go for follow-up visits.

Untoward Effects

It is possible to increase claustrophobia and/or anger. Too frequent time-out can cause a child to feel he cannot win or as though he's in an invisible prison.

Charting Requirements

Note measures and emotional responses. Note the number of time-outs for the unit as a whole. The ward time-out rate is an indication of how tense the unit is becoming. The time-out cubicle should be almost indestructible, lined with plywood, vented with a strong grate, and not be so large that the child could hurt himself by throwing himself about or so small he can't move around. It should have a plexiglass window through which the child can see a clock or timer. To avoid the possibility of forgetting the child in time-out, there must be a warning light which is switched on by staff whenever anyone is in time-out.

Aversive Conditioning (AC)
Technique – Third Level

Rationale

This is used to extinguish repetitive, persistent, maladaptive behaviour that interferes with the child's life. The derision and teasing that the child receives is usually more aversive than the aversive stimuli received in treatment. Children readily accept well-controlled aversive therapy to become free from embarrassing habits.

Application

Tics, smoking, fetishes, glue sniffing, Tourette's Syndrome, thumb sucking, hair pulling, nail biting, pica, bed wetting, atavisms.

Measures

Note the response rate prior to treatment, once a week during treatment and at follow-up. Use subjective measures of how the child is feeling about himselt at every session.

Procedures

1. Obtain a baseline of at least two days under difficult conditions.
2. Give a detailed explanation to the parents and the child and obtain specific consent.
3. Deal with all the child's fears.
4. Obtain a special informed consent from parents and child.
5. Use yourself as a subject to show how the intensity of the aversive stimulus can be varied.
6. First apply the stimulus that is most effective, least painful, most natural, most immediate and most easily applied on a continuous basis, i.e. every time the response occurs. If the treatment involves an electric stimulus, the procedure should be carried out for about half-an-hour two or three times a day until the habit is extinguished.
7. Once the response rate has lessened, a variable ratio schedule should be instituted.

Many aversive stimuli can be used: loud sounds, shouts, an elastic band, mild electric stimuli. The Farrell Company make an electric stimulus device which can be remotely triggered.

Untoward Effects

This procedure may interfere with a psychotherapeutic relationship. Generally another staff member should do aversive conditioning. If other underlying problems are not dealt with, the child may substitute another symptom.

Although aversive therapy is seldom necessary, staff have great difficulty bringing themselves to hurt children in any way. It is important to obtain good counselling and careful supervision in which your ambivalence and conflict can be discussed.

Charting Requirements

Informed consent signed by parents should be in the file. Objective measures graphed and subjective measures charted in the 24-Hour Progress Note. Also chart any signs of untoward reactions.

Biofeedback Training (BT) — 'Bells and buzzers' Technique — Third Level

Rationale

Overt behaviours are affected by their consequences. This applies to relatively covert physiological responses as well. Feedback or knowledge of results about one's internal state is sufficiently reinforcing to many people to enable them to modify their bodily states with practice. The body seeks homeostasis to conserve energy. Unfortunately, many people have been taught to ignore their own inner feedback. A display of physiological fluctuations helps to reinstate self-awareness. Children are very curious about their inner functions and want to learn greater self-control.

Applications

Children with anxiety, psychosomatic complaints, impulsivity and some epilepsy may benefit from biofeedback.

Measures

Measures of physiological responses (EEG, EMG, electrodermal activity, skin temperature, etc.) are provided by the apparatus itself. In addition, it is helpful to monitor behavioural and emotional correlates of bodily states, e.g. anxiety, tension, fatigue, headaches.

Procedures

Staff members must be checked out on the equipment by the Biofeedback Committee. Written consent of the child's parent or guardian is also required. Explain and demonstrate the procedure to parents and the child. Biofeedback usage requires staff training beyond the scope of this manual. Basically, though, the principles involved are:

1. Discrimination of physiological states, e.g. tension versus relaxation.

2. Shaping, e.g. progressively recalibrating the equipment so as to change the operational definition of, say, relaxation.

3. Fading out the apparatus.

4. Learning to observe and respond to natural internal messages.

Untoward Effects

There is difficulty in maintaining treatment gains in real-life stress situations without the apparatus. Children become too self-conscious.

Charting Requirements

Measures only necessary.

Brief Insight-oriented Psychotherapy (BIP) – 'Why I worry' Technique – Third Level

Rationale

Although insight may not cure a problem, everyone can benefit from knowing about themselves. Insight may occur only after behaviour changes; even then it is beneficial. In talking to children, point out that they can benefit from understanding their own life-history. They can learn from their past just like the world can learn from its history. Insight will give them the ability to discern their attitudes and responses in a given situation, making it possible to redirect their behaviour. In knowing about themselves they can anticipate and avoid future problems.

Insight provides a greater freedom of action. Insight increases responsibility. People who know about themselves can be held more responsible for their own actions. Insight is a way of overcoming hang-ups. It helps children find ways around the obstructions that interfere with their development.

Insight can free emotional energies. It provides children with an opportunity better to utilise their mental processes for more constructive activities. When there is less energy involved in futile conflict-solving mediation, children are more vigorous and better balanced. If there is a traumatic event in their lives they can better sustain the disequilibrium and adjust to major life changes.

Measures

Make a verbatim recording of the beginning and ending sentences of a session. Note your intuitions and statements. The therapist should record the child's effect, the setting and any transference or counter-transference. Record your observations and hypothesis. Note the child's response to empathy and insight.

Procedures

Psychotherapy with children is one of the most difficult techniques. It takes years of experience and supervision to acquire competence but these are some of the basic components:

1. Explain to the child in words he will understand, e.g. 'I want you to understand yourself better so that you can drive your machine more safely.' Awareness of the mental mechanisms gives him a better control over his own life. Running his own life more efficiently prevents people from wanting to take charge of him.

2. Any topic is self-revealing. Children cannot lie, whatever they say is typical of themselves and can be used in psychotherapy. Children are more relaxed about talking if they are doing something with their hands. How they play is often very revealing of how they think. Avoid crashing the problem. Give the child plenty of opportunity to discover for himself. Interpretations should be infrequent and well timed.

3. Concentrate on areas which are effect-laden or often repeated.

4. Avoid asking questions. Rather, use your intuition to guide you into areas that are more fruitful. Observe, hypothesise and test with tentative interpretations.

5. Watch for displacement but use your own emotions to help you understand what emotion the child is experiencing.

6. Work at defence mechanisms but don't destroy them.

7. Empathetic statements help clarify and encourage a patient by letting him know you understand.

8. Interpret resistance and transference when it becomes a resistance. Interpretation should include comment on the impulse, the anxiety and the defence in the context of the genetic, economic and transference components in a therapeutic relationship.

Untoward Effects

Anxiety may increase during psychotherapy. Defences which are determined too rapidly occasionally precipitate a psychosis or the emergence of new symptoms.

Charting Requirements

Measures to be recorded on the 24-Hour Progress Note.

Giving Medication (GM) – 'Yech!'
Technique – Third Level

Rationale

1. Medication can decrease the presence of impulses.
2. Medication can lessen the consequent conflicts that anxieties create.

3. Medication can diminish the psychic pain so that a child can exercise his mind, engage in psychotherapy and continue to function in school. It is like giving an analgesic so that someone can exercise a sore leg.
4. Medication can alienate the depressing effect which inhibits mental energies.
5. Methylphenidate can decrease distractability and impulsiveness of some hyperactive children.
6. Antidepressants can help establish a more hopeful outlook on life.

Application

1. Psychologically and physically traumatised battered children.
2. Psychotic or borderline children whose incipient psychotic break may be detected because of their excessive dreaming.
3. Depressed children.
4. Hyperactive children.
5. Obsessional, phobic and other very anxious children.

Measures

The child's baseline responses can be used to determine the rate and extent of change. Measures of sadness, hyperactivity or time-lag in response can be used. Physiological measures, blood pressure, pulse, etc., psychological measures of performance on tests and subjective measures, e.g. dreams, should be recorded.

Procedures

The following order could be used:
e.g. Methylphenidate	e.g. Antidepressants
Week 1 — Baseline	One week — Baseline
Week 2 — Medication	Two weeks — Medication
Week 3 — Baseline	One week — Baseline
Week 4 — Medication	One week — Medication

Two days' baseline. Three days' medication if effective.
1. Baseline measures.
2. Give a careful explanation, e.g. 'This is to help you control yourself', 'We are not trying to take over your responsibilities', 'If you don't like it after trying it, we will talk about stopping'.
3. Demonstration: Another child who has had medication can be asked to testify to its beneficial effect. If the child is very suspicious, the staff might bite off a bit of the pill or take some of the elixir themselves.

4. Explore all the child's and the parents' anxieties about taking medication. The pill and the effects of the pill have many meanings. The meanings of the pill arise from the parents' and the child's previous experience with medication and doctors. The energising or quietening effects may not always be felt to be beneficial.

5. After the medication has been started, the staff must take time to explore the effects, e.g. 'How does it feel?'

6. Check with the attending physician who will advise regarding the possible side-effects.

Untoward Effects

There are side-effects that can be very frightening to children. They worry about losing control and may even use the medication to explain why they are increasingly aggressive. The loss of drive might be felt as a passivity tantamount to feminisation in adolescent boys.

Charting Requirements

Follow hospital policies regarding the charting of each medication, its results and any untoward effects.

Grief Facilitation (GF) — 'I guess she's really gone'
Technique — Third Level

Rationale

People have difficulty engaging in a new relationship until they have said goodbye to some old ones. The grieving tends to be put off or prolonged by many unconscious mechanisms which interfere with the normal processs. Ambivalence in the relationship with some desire to terminate the relationship, or wish that the person die or move away, increases the difficulty. It is much harder to grieve for the person who dies after a prolonged illness. It is harder for children who are trying to protect others from the expression of their feelings. Society and parents may discourage children from grieving, sometimes because it makes the adult sad to see the child mourn or because it makes them feel guilty.

Children who have experienced losses early in life may need to grieve three or four times as they mature. Each experience helps them gain a better understanding of the significance of their losses. Unresolved grief may result in an overt or masked depression.

Grief facilitation is an attempt to help the child and/or parent go through the process of grieving by helping them identify their feelings and conflicts.

Application

Children who have unresolved losses of significant people, places, pets or parts of a body can be helped. Parents who have lost a child in fact or in fantasy, e.g. a handicapped or retarded child, should be helped to mourn.

Measures

Subjective
(1) The ability to talk about the loss with appropriate effect.
(2) The ability to make new attachments.

Objective
The increase in the number of smiles, self-care and hopeful statements.

Procedure

1. Make baseline observations in the natural environment of home or school before admission.
2. Give a careful explanation of the whole process with words and concepts appropriate in the child's level of development, e.g. 'I would like to help you say goodbye to . . .' Comment on the inevitability of grief, the ambivalent feelings of sadness and anger, the natural progression of events and advantages of a new attachment.
3. A child or adult who has gone through the whole process may be able to describe what it was like.
4. Help the child understand by giving a case illustration or story. Recount:
    (a) The events surrounding the loss.
    (b) The events in detail.
    (c) The events in eliciting feelings that others had about the situation.
    (d) The events with the patient's own feelings, especially those of ambivalence.
5. Help the child to describe both good and bad features of the lost person or place. 'If they were alive or here now, what would you tell them? What would they say?'
6. Visit the grave, place flowers on the grave, throw dirt on it. Write a letter saying goodbye. Rehearse saying goodbye with all its nuances.

If parents are living but the child is not living with them, arrange a visit so that both can say goodbye. Meet with the child and the parent to ensure no double messages are given.
7. Talk about the future and people who might replace the lost

person. Say hello to the new parent, child or place by getting to know them, thinking about them in detail. Deal with the desires for reunion.

Untoward Effects

Grieving releases the pressure of feelings but if the whole problem is not dealt with the feelings will build up again. It will then be more difficult to resolve the next time.

Charting Requirements

Chart subjective and objective measures. Narrative charting on 24-Hour Progress Note, stating the stages dealt with and the child's reaction to them is necessary.

Hypnotic Therapy (HT)
Technique — Third Level

Rationale

Hypnosis is more frequently used as an aid to treatment rather than treatment itself. It can overcome ambivalence and provide motivation. With children it can be effectively used to clear up questions in an otherwise faulty history.

There are ambivalent feelings in almost everyone about everything. This means that although most people want to control themselves they also have a tendency to regress and allow somebody to take control. Thus, it is possible to hypnotise everyone to some extent. Though people are hypnotised to the extent that they co-operate, it is possible to obtain co-operation in almost everyone with subtle suggestions.

Story-telling is a kind of hypnosis. With a setting described in compelling detail and a spell-binding plot, very few people cannot pay attention. In a similar manner, the hypnotist with a good descriptive vocabulary and an understanding of his patient, can gain the patient's interest. The quality of the hypnotist's voice, his own apparent relaxation and his convincing manner, all help to relax the patient and encourage him to co-operate.

Like other relaxation techniques, good feeling arises from two sources:

(1) During the time the patient is hypnotised, the focus of his attention is outside of himself. Physiological studies have demonstrated that when we think with concentration about something or somebody other than ourself, our blood pressure is lowered,

our muscle tension decreases. When our mind is fixed upon ourself, it is not long before it is in conflict, debating pros and cons
of various decisions.

(2) Everybody wishes to have control of their own mind. With hypnosis, it is putting the control of your own mind in the hands of
somebody you trust. The good therapist, however, convinces his
patient that he is really doing it himself.

There are many common features to all relaxation techniques:

1. Follow the Leader: 'I will show you how to get it' For group
survival there is a tendency on the part of everyone to allow someone
to direct their lives. Hopefully the leader will bring them to a desired
goal which they could not obtain on their own. This tendency implies
that people have already had good experience in being led. Others who
have no experience in being led are more suggestible. Those who have
had bad experiences are usually more resistant.

2. Homeostasis: 'Let me help you with that load' Any technique or
any person that helps prevent fatigue is appreciated. Everyone would
like to be able to do the required work with less effort. A convincing
offer of help and support is almost always accepted.

3. Biorhythms: 'Follow the beat and take it easy' The body seeks to
relax in order to conserve energy. The monotony of the intoning voice,
if well fitted to an individual's biorhythm, tends to reinforce that
rhythm. Without increasing attention to that rhythm, a good hypnotist
can pace his statements to the patient's slower breathing, heart beat,
etc.

4. Immobility: 'Stay still and you will be all right' All species tend to
remain immobile when under overwhelming attack. In the young this
serves to help them remain unseen. It also helps diminish the attacker's
aggression and makes the victim look appealing.

5. Regression: 'It's okay now, I will look after you' In all people
there is a tendency to return to infancy when care is provided with very
little appeal or effect.

6. Focusing Attention: 'It's very important to watch this carefully'
When the body is scanning the environment or concentrating on a
problem, most physiological processes will revert to more relaxed
states, e.g. blood pressure is lowered. It is part of the organism's need to
solve puzzles.

7. Problem-solving: 'Let me figure this conflict out for you' All
humans are problem-solving in order to become more efficient. Offers

of help to solve problems are almost always accepted.

Hypnosis emphasises relaxation, reassurance, abreaction, suggestion, concentration and an ability to remember.

Application

Hypnosis is useful for traumatised children and those with psychosomatic disorders, obesity, habit disorders.

Measures

You can use the Stanford Scale for Depth of Hypnosis. Before and after behaviour, subjective responses and the frequency of target behaviours should be measured.

Procedure

1. Baseline: Before beginning and over two days, measure target behaviour and the ability of the child to relax.

2. Explanation: It is important to deal with common fears associated with hypnosis, i.e. the loss of control, the possibility of doing something foolish under hypnosis, the fact that it might not work, the fear of post-hypnotic suggestion, a concern about being assaulted under hypnosis. The patient must be reassured that the hypnotist cannot hypnotise him against his will or persuade him to do something stupid against his better judgement.

3. Demonstration: Use a willing child who is a relatively good hypnotic subject or another staff member.

4. Relaxation: Teach the patient to inhibit anxiety through the reciprocally inhibiting stimulus of relaxation. Teach him to breath deeply, tense his muscles and then concentrate on the feeling of relaxation as he allows the tension to diminish. Help the child to master simple techniques of relaxing himself.

5. Induction: Use the arm falling, fixation or rhythm contradiction techniques to help the child become slightly hypnotised. Then describe with his concurrence a very relaxing scene. This may be on a beach, in a mountain meadow, or curled up on a leather chair in front of a crackling fire while the wind blows the rain against the window, while one is reading an intriguing story and Mozart is playing in the background. (The child should be asked on a previous occasion what he finds one of the most relaxing situations.) All directions must be given in a positive statement.

6. Memory Illumination: As a patient is more deeply hypnotised he can be asked to remember some event in some particular time in his

life. With a pre-arranged signal he is awakened and asked to recall the event.

7. Suggestion. Use a trigger stimulus in the environment that will help the child perform the kind of behaviour that he had found difficult to manage in the past. During this time, the therapist uses the patient's chosen scene and develops one of his own he feels the patient would enjoy. He may describe a scene concentrating on specific elements that hold people's attention such as changing colours, twinkling lights, spiral staircases, etc. It is important to take into consideration the patient's preference of posture and what phenomena they would like to experience. Most hypnotic suggestions have to do with helping patients overcome ambivalence. One should suggest that the patient will not remember elements of the session. Suggest a trigger stimulus that will enable him to become more rapidly hypnotised in the next session. The therapist should not openly concern himself with how deeply the patient is hypnotised.

8. Awaken. Make sure the child is fully alert before he leaves you. Bring the patient back to a completely awakened state with the assurance he can stay relaxed as long as he wishes.

Untoward Effects

In many children there is a post-hypnotic daze and passivity. To overcome this a fellow staff member should engage the child in arousing kinds of play activity. In some children there is an exaggerated beneficial response which belies a more long-term effect.

Charting Requirements

Narrative documentation in the 24-Hour Progress Note and further reading.

Name Change (NC) — 'I would like to be called'
Technique — Third Level

Rationale

Everyone identifies with his own name. Unfortunately, many children have bad associations with the name they have been given. This may occur if they are given an awkward name which is easy to ridicule. Sometimes their name has a bad association with an unpopular uncle, etc. Sometimes the name is very confusing because it is similar to that of a sibling. Sometimes a child would rather be spoken of as a more adult person. Frequently, children's names are changed when they become part of a new family, i.e. with a stepfather. The name change may be the first name, the surname or both names.

Name changes may accompany and reinforce the change in a child's identity and personality which results from treatment. The wish to get rid of a name may indicate the child's desire to end a bad relationship or association.

The process of changing a name is similar to the process of changing an identity — it requires saying goodbye to old associations and old attachments before new ones can form. The child, in selecting a name, usually has a new identity in mind. This should be explored.

Application

Fearful, anxious children who are often teased about awkward names, children adopted by a stepfather, children who need to accept the non-legal use of the mother's new husband's name and children with a big shift in their identity should be given the opportunity to change their name.

Measures

1. Obtain before and after treatment anxiety levels which arise when the child is called or teased by his old and new names.
2. Note the frequency with which the child uses his new name for himself.

Procedure

1. There should be extensive discussion with the child and the child's family about the need to have a new name. The child should be given the opportunity to select a new first name, but it should first be checked out with the parents. They have their own good and bad associations to certain names.
2. Baseline: Measure the child's reaction to the use of his old and new names. The child should be asked to report all his associations to both names, e.g. 'What does Smith make you think of?'
3. Explanation: The child needs to be told what is involved in letting go and accepting a partially new identity. He should be reassured that this is not his whole identity but only a piece of his identity that will change.
4. Demonstration: The staff can be used as a model with the child's therapist asking, 'What was your name and what is it now?'
5. Description: Give the child every opportunity to describe his identity. Help him become aware that his personhood is distinct

from his name, but his name is part of his identity.

6. Tell the child, 'If you are not "Johnnie Smith" anymore, I guess it's goodbye to your old name.'

7. The child should practise saying, 'I am not Johnnie Smith anymore, goodbye Johnnie Smith.'

8. A ritual goodbye: the child should be encouraged to write down on paper his old name and then bury or burn it. This should be made an important occasion with witnesses present.

9. Ask the child, 'Who are you?' Then encourage the child to use his new name and to write a description of himself on paper.

10. Formal introduction: Once a child has practised using his new name and feels comfortable with it, he should be formally introduced to his family, a group of peers and the staff, e.g. 'Ladies and Gentlemen, I would like to introduce Johnnie James.' There should be a party to celebrate the occasion.

11. Ask the family to have any legal documents recording the changes ready for the child to read and, if possible, sign. Make sure the school is informed. The whole class should be drilled on the use of the child's new name.

12. The group should respond to the occasion by asking him what his new name is. Once he has become adept at responding comfortably, they should shout, 'What is your name?' He should reply with a shout, 'My name is Johnnie James.'

13. The staff should say, 'Your name is Johnnie James. I want you to write your name on paper.'

14. Everyday use: If, in the course of everyday communication, you make a mistake and call the child by his wrong name, you should wait for the child to correct you. If he does not, you should state, 'I'm sorry. That's not your name is it? Tell me what it is.'

15. Check on follow-up to see how much and how comfortably everyone is using the new name.

Untoward Effects

Children with poor identities can be confused with a new name. The process must be gradual, and the staff must make sure that the child wants and accepts his new appellation.

Charting Requirements

Record the name and personality changes. Note any untoward reactions.

Parent–Child Contract (PCC) – 'It's a deal'
Technique – Third Level

Rationale

When a child's parenting has been inconsistent or interrupted because of divorce, finances, illness, or any other reason, the child becomes fearful of attaching himself to any adult who parents him. Step-parents tend to be viewed as bad (the wicked stepmother of fairy tales), because it seems they have driven away the parent to whom the child was at least partially attached and to whom they struggle to stay loyal.

This fear can demonstrate itself in many ways, some of which may look as if the child is rejecting the parent. The child indeed feels that no one loves him enough to care for him or to be with him all the time. Once the child knows the parent will love him, care for him and provide a home for him, regardless of his behaviour, then the child can relax and let the relationship happen.

Parents who state or imply that their care of the child depends upon the child's good behaviour may only see the worst side of their child. The child in his anxiety may try so hard he always makes mistakes. He may be so angry at the threat of losing his support, he may unconsciously wreck his best attempts at being good. A contract signed in the presence of the child is a visible demonstration of the parents' determination to care, even if they aren't always pleased with their child.

Application

Children who benefit are those whose parenting has been interrupted, especially children of divorced parents who have to spend time living with both parents.

Measures

Note changes in the child's relationships, spontaneity and body tension. Objective measurements of these to be determined for each individual child.

Procedure

1. Obtain a baseline and give a careful explanation and demonstration to the parents and child.

2. Help the parents gain a full understanding of their ambivalence to the child and its effect on him.

3. A firm decision as to permanent placement of the child must be

made prior to this technique.

4. Recount the child's past experiences of parenting and help him deal with feelings from it.

5. Parents should role-play the commitment with staff prior to making a contract with the child. If they can't make a duration of the child's life contract, negotiate for as long a period as they can sincerely give.

6. The child should have an opportunity to say goodbye to other parents he might have had.

7. Parents should commit themselves to care for the child in the presence of staff. All members of the family should be present. A contract should be signed and sealed with an embrace.

8. A new parent could also give the child some symbol belonging to the family, e.g. family crest, photo album, ring, cross or family name.

9. The child should now understand he has a right to be in that family. His presence and care does not depend upon his being wanted. Help him practise defending that right.

10. On follow-up, check to make sure no one is breaking the contract.

Untoward Effects

A contract broken by insincere or irresponsible parents may destroy the child's already shaky trust of adults.

Charting Requirements

Detailed narrative charting of each session to be recorded in the 24-Hour Progress Note.

Play Therapy — Interpretative (PTI) — 'How and why'
Technique — Third Level

Rationale

Like adults, children internalise unresolved interpersonal conflicts. As a result, they engage in maladaptive behaviour which gets them into more trouble. By repetition–compulsion or the re-enactment of old conflicts, children attempt better to understand themselves. Internalised conflicts drain a child of energy so that he is unable to concentrate on the task at hand. Because he is functioning less effectively, he gets into further trouble even when he tries to please.

Children have a limited verbal facility and are unable to express many feelings, memories and perceptions with words. Instead of free association, children are encouraged to play freely with a wide variety of media. In their play they portray the components of internalised conflicts that they cannot otherwise express. This gives the therapist opportunity to understand and interact with the child.

Application

Every conflicted child, except those who cannot tolerate lack of structure, can benefit from insight gained in play therapy.

Measures

1. Make descriptions of the child's play, indicating the kinds of emotions involved and areas of major preoccupation.

2. Note the duration of play on a particular theme and the child's attempt to involve the therapist.

Procedure

1. Obtain a baseline of play activity without interpretations being given.

2. Explain to the child and his parents the purpose of psychotherapy and briefly outline the process. Show him the toys and indicate both the guidelines and limitations. These are:
   (a) A time limit of 45 minutes. It may be more depending on the child.
   (b) He cannot destroy toys or attack the therapist.
   (c) He cannot take the toys with him.
   (d) What he talks about is confidential unless it is very important for the parents to know, e.g. the child is suicidal. Encourage the child to tell his parents. If not, tell the child what you are going to report to the parents and if possible, speak to them in front of the child.

3. Demonstrate using another child or possibly an adult.

4. Provide bendable human figures, toy animals, furniture, a limited number of mechanical toys and sand or water. Introduce the materials by pushing them about in the sand yourself and then sit back and allow the child to play as freely as he wishes.

5. Observe for themes or conflicts that are repeated, that have strong emotion, that are obviously conflicted and those that the child is trying to avoid disclosing.

6. Make empathetic statements, e.g. 'I see you are very worried about your father leaving home.'

7. Interpret resistances first. This allows the child to overcome the inhibitions to expressing himself. Interpret major conflicts by pointing out the underlying impulse, the consequent anxiety and the favoured defence. When these are sufficiently engaged, suggest alternative behaviours. Interpret the transference when it becomes a resistance.

8. Timing is very important. Interpretations made too quickly increase resistance.

9. Observe, hypothesise and test once again.

Untoward Effects

Interpretations made too early or too frequently confuse the child. The child can develop a transference neurosis which, if not resolved, leaves him in a worse state. Therapists may find themselves involved in a destructive counter-transference. For this reason, they must have a supervisor.

Charting Requirements

Measures only are charted.

Psychological Testing Interpretation (PTI) – 'Puzzles and problems' Technique – Third Level

Rationale

Behaviour is the outcome of an interaction between the child's enduring traits, acute states and the social environment (other people). Hence, an assessment of traits and states may be useful.

Ideally, a psychological assessment ought to be both prescriptive of treatment and predictive of outcome. Repeated measures on parallel forms have more predictive power than single tests.

Testing

A comprehensive IQ test battery (for example, WISCR, WPPSI, Stanford-Binet) represents the state of the art of psychological assessment. Under the right conditions, IQ tests are the most reliable, valid and useful tests available. The IQ can be a handy measure of developmental level, scholastic aptitude (as distinct from achievement), ego strength, right versus left hemisphere function, capacity for insight, ability to process auditory versus visual information, test anxiety, self-esteem, etc.

IQ	Classification	Percentile	Per cent of children
130 plus	very superior	98–100	2
120–129	superior	91–97	7
110–119	high average	76–90	16
90–109	average	26–75	50
80–89	low average	10–25	16
70–79	borderline	3–9	7
69 minus	retarded	0–2	2

Interpretation of subtest scores is tricky because each subject measures diverse abilities. Diagnoses are made on the basis of the configuration (profile) of subtest scores.

Personality Testing. Children vary in their temperamental make-up along such dimensions as labile, stable, intro/extroverted, antisocial/tenderminded, etc. Questionnaires are available which purport to measure these dimensions. In practice, however, there is probably no substitute for the observations by the child's nursing staff.

Vocational Testing. Adolescents may be assessed to determine their vocational interests and aptitudes. Obviously these tests become less valid with younger children, but they may be useful in steering a child towards a long-range life goal. Vocational tests are computer scored and thus, feedback of results takes a few weeks.

Neuropsychological Testing. Children with soft neurological signs or a history of brain injury may benefit from special-purpose testing by the neurophysiometrician. Consult the psychologist about a referral.

Application

We believe that though test results have limited validity and may be open to misuse, parents need the information better to determine how to nurture and guide their children.

Feedback

Parents and children can use information about their abilities and aptitudes. Realistic assessments can be the basis for realistic expectations.

Procedure

1. Obtain previous test results and how the family have used any information they have obtained of these results.

2. Explain how the tests are administered, what they mean and their limitations.

3. Show a video tape of previous testing and giving feedback.

4. Bring the child together with his parents for a feedback session.

5. Watch the non-verbal interaction even as the psychologist gives the feedback. Be an ego auxiliary to whoever needs it.

Untoward Effects

Psychological test scores may have limited validity because of the child's depression, psychosis, malingering, distractibility, etc., or because of limitations inherent in the tests themselves. Some scores, such as a low IQ, may be potentially depressing or stigmatising. For this reason, test results may not be disclosed without the consent of the psychologist.

Charting Requirements

Results of the tests must be filed in the child's chart. Feedback given to parents and child is charted in the 24-Hour Progress Note.

Rage Restraining (RR) – 'Lion taming'
Technique – Third Level

Rationale

Under certain conditions it is necessary to remove a child against his will. Whenever someone's actions frustrate, hurt or anger a child, you should be prepared for a free flow of aggression and hostility. Staff should not wait until the child is out of control to remove him, but do it as a preventive step. The staff must know ways that they can control the child and remove him without risk to themselves or the child. Staff should not respond to anger, but learn to approach such a situation with a non-threatening, non-punitive, non-judgemental attitude. Helping a child control himself while maintaining an open, caring attitude will set the climate for the future therapeutic staff–patient relationship.

Application

1. When normal perceptions of danger limits are lost, an enraged child presents a physical danger to himself, other children or staff.

2. When the group tension between a child and the rest of the group is becoming so threatening that it might lead either to withdrawal or loss of control.

3. When it is necessary to 'guarantee behavioural stoppage' of a child

in order either to maintain the therapeutic milieu or to meet the clinical objectives for the child.

Measures

Staff should analyse the situation in retrospect, including antecedents and milieu, in order to increase insight and knowledge and to prevent a recurrence.

Procedure

1. When observing a situation in which a child needs to be removed, the staff should ask themselves:
   (a) Can I do it safely?
   (b) What should happen to the rest of the group?
   (c) What happens to the child after removal?
   (d) Do I need assistance?

Once these questions have been answered, staff should approach the child in an understanding manner so that the rest of the 'lifespaces' is filled with acceptance. The child should be able to control and release immediate frustration.

2. Staff breathing should be controlled. Inhale deeply as you begin the approach and exhale sharply as you begin a critical action.

3. Move as you speak to the child. Moving and walking as you talk makes it difficult for the child to anticipate your actions.

4. Make sure that you are strongly balanced from side to side so you can resist a push. Feet are shoulder width apart, the forward foot points in front of you, the rear foot is approximately at a 90° angle to the forward foot.

5. Eye contact is extremely important in anticipating the action of the child. The child will shift his eye to the area he intends to attack you.

6. Restrain the patient with another staff member and move to the designated area (side-room or time-out room). Use the straight arm lever restraint or underarm restraint. Once the child has been removed, give the child time to regain control. It is the staff's clinical judgement to determine if each individual child can be alone.

7. If staff decide to stay with the child, it should be that staff member that has the best relationship with the child and who, at that time, is in control of his own anxiety and anger.

8. Staff then can choose suitable activity and/or dialogue to help the child gain insight into their encounter. Explain:
   (i) The reason for the removal or stopping behaviour that he could

not stop, to help him avoid worse trouble.

(ii) The precipitating factors in the provoking situation. Listen to the child's interpretation first, then slowly explain your interpretation of the situation. Ask the child how he can avoid this provoking situation the next time. Have suggestions for him.

(iii) It is important that this discussion be entirely free of anger so it cannot be confused with punishment, revenge or rejection.

(iv) Interpret this situation in the light of difficulties that the child experiences in peer or family relationships.

9. Explain how you will deal with a similar situation in the future. The child should rejoin the group as soon as he and his staff feel he can handle the situation.

10. Teach the parents to use the technique with which they are most comfortable.

Untoward Effects

These include injury to staff or child or destroying a therapeutic relationship. The rest of the children may identify with the removed child. They may misinterpret staff actions as aggression or punishment. They may make a 'hero' of the child and split the therapeutic milieu into a 'we' and 'they' situation.

Charting Requirements

Narrative documentation of measures, untoward effects and recommendations for the future.

Rebonding for Battered Children (RBC)
Technique – Third Level

Rationale

Some battered children have never had a proper bond established with either mother or father. Bonding makes a child an extension of a parent. It tends to inhibit the expression of those occasional rages or tendencies to neglect that all parents have. Children that are not bonded are seen as distant, sometimes foreign bodies that are much easier to hurt. In some children a tenuous bond has been broken by separation. In other children an episode of trauma, especially being beaten, breaks a bond which results in a vicious cycle of abusing.

Being beaten produces a situation of aversive conditioning whereby anything from the parents is seen as painful. This increases the child's resistance to the parent's direction, which increases the parent's annoyance towards the child and results in more battering and pain. Eventually, both the child and the parent become aversively conditioned to each other. The fear they feel in each other's presence results in more of the irritating behaviour that stimulates rage or neglect.

Application

Battered, assaulted and deprived children.

Measures

Heart rate, pupil size and emotional reaction as a function of distance between parent and child. Record the parent's statements while responding to the child, especially when holding him.

Procedure

1. Baseline: Physiological and emotional responses at different distances, parent from child.

2. Explanation: The child should be helped to understand about his fear of the parent. The parent needs the process of bonding and aversive conditioning explained, ending with 'We don't want you to be afraid of each other'.

3. Demonstrate with other children and parents who have graduated from the programme.

4. Parent and child should be taught relaxation.

5. A two-way mirror with parent and child either side of each other with one staff member with each. Good and bad points should be pointed out and discussed.

6. Parent and child should be on opposite sides of the room and gradually brought together. The staff may model giving and receiving verbal and physical strokes.

7. Holding hands.

8. Cuddling and rocking with spontaneous positive statements reinforced by staff.

9. Parent hugging and taking the whole weight of the child.

Untoward Effects

If it is done too quickly and clumsily, the sensitivity of child to parent will increase.

Charting Requirements

Measures plus document when light and sound are introduced. Chart summary of each session in the 24-Hour Progress Notes.

Secret Disclosure (SD) — 'Who knows what I know?'
Technique — Third Level

Rationale

There are few secrets in a family. Most that are thought to be secrets are at least known about, sometimes unconsciously. Adults should keep some things from children, particularly those things that would make them worry and about which they can do nothing.

Legitimate secrets are those such as finances, parents' sexual life, previous affairs, possible moves, worries about the world situation, etc. To know about these tends to make children feel tense. They may desperately want to do something but they are so small and the problem so big they feel helpless. By trying to keep a secret, children become tense, worried about an uncertain future and alienated from peers or siblings. Sometimes secrets are gradually disclosed but the piecemeal disclosure makes the child even more uncertain and sometimes more curious.

When secrets are disclosed there is often a much better relationship, more communication and a decrease in activity. Secrets regarding death, adoption, parenting, divorce, treatment, IQ test results and moves when they are about to occur, should probably be disclosed. Secrets that tend to make people want to give up should not be disclosed unless there is something else to hope for.

Application

Families where there is child abuse, alcohol and drug abuse, epilepsy, retardation, learning disability, criminals, adopted children, fostered children, children with mixed racial origin or hereditary disorders, can benefit.

Measures

Measure the child's level of tension. Note the nature of the relationship between the child and those significant others that he has or has not shared the secret with.

Procedure

1. It is important carefully to determine the advantages and disadvantages prior to embarking on this technique.
2. Obtain a baseline, recording the level of tension.
3. Discuss with the parents what you intend to do. Obtain their informed consent.

4. Role-play how the child may react once he is told.

5. Hint at the subject to see if the child can fill in the pieces once he has been reassured that it is all right to do so. If he does not respond, the child should be told of the secret by the parents, plainly and frankly.

6. Then give him lots of opportunity to react. Often there is a period of disbelief, then a feeling of shame, or guilt, leading to anger and sometimes fear towards the parent.

7. Encourage the parents to explain why there has been a secret for so long.

8. At the end of this, the parents should be encouraged to put their arms around the child and reassure him that the relationship is still there.

9. During follow-up, hint at the former secret and see if the family can still talk about it openly.

Untoward Effects

It might harm or disrupt a relationship. The child might become increasingly anxious or demand more knowledge than the parent is prepared to provide.

Charting Requirements

Chart the level of tension in the child. Once the secret has been told, write down exactly what the child was told, how it was described, his reaction to it and questions he had about it.

Systematic Desensitisation (SD) — 'I'm not afraid'
Technique — Third Level

Rationale

A phobia is inadvertently reinforced by parents and other people who are significant to the child, whenever they give attention to a child while he is avoiding the anxiety-producing situation. Children also reinforce themselves with the relaxation that occurs as they walk away from the phobic situation. This can happen either in action or in fantasy.

The phobia may begin with a sudden fright or be learned by modelling a parent. It may be a fear of a real threat or symbolise an anxiety created by a conflict. In treatment, one must deal with the three components: the feared object, the reinforcers and the underlying conflict.

The fear is usually more extensive and intensive than it first appears.

The child may seem calm and symptom-free until near the phobic situation, then may panic. In other children, the phobia may interfere with many aspects of their lives.

Application

Almost all phobias, e.g. school, confined spaces, open spaces, elevators, insects, snakes, criticism, can be treated. More symbolic fears of people and the child's own impulses can also be treated.

Measures

Take physiological measures of anxiety: respiratory rate, heart rate and pupil dilation. Measure the proximity of the anxiety-producing stimulus and the amount of anxiety as a ratio, e.g. heart rate/distance. Make subjective measures of the child's expressions.

Procedures

1. Make baseline measures before hospitalisation.
2. Explain carefully to parents and child the whole procedure.
3. Demonstrate the technique using another child.
4. Obtain a hierarchy of fears. List and rank order the anxiety-producing stimuli, such as elevator, fire, noise, etc. Then list and rank order under each object which situation is most frightening, e.g. old elevators, new elevators, elevators with no one in them, elevators with just one person inside, etc.
5. Try to find the fear beyond the fear: 'So if that happens, then what?' If an old elevator with no one in it was the greatest fear, what does the child think would happen if he got in it?; then what and then what . . . ?
6. From the list, determine what is the most probable symbolic component.
7. Teach a relaxation technique that can be easily self-initiated and which quickly produces self-control.
8. Determine if, by imagining the situation, the child exhibits anxiety. If not, try and reconstruct the anxiety-producing situation and keep it handy.
9. Arrange a subtle signal that the patient will use to indicate when his anxiety level gets too high.
10. Induce relaxation then get the child to imagine the anxiety-producing stimulus in its mildest form.
11. Maintain relaxation through the successive approximations to more intensely anxious situations. If at any point they signal that they

are too anxious, turn off the imagination and concentrate on relaxation.

12. Practical Restraining: Use the same technique that was used in step 11 but this time, do it in an *in vivo* situation. Accompany the child, moving slowly into closer approximation of the anxiety-producing stimulus while remaining relaxed.

13. The end result should be to have the child in the most intensely anxious situation and be completely relaxed or at least, in control. Once the programme has been engaged in, it must continue in a predetermined progression of events. Backing away or stalling will increase the patient's anxiety. The therapist's self-assurance will enhance the child's progress.

14. Make sure the child can handle all his phobias before discharge but make a careful check on follow-up.

Untoward Effects

Sometimes the child will appear to be progressing well and then may panic. It is important to continue even at this point of panic or you will reinforce the phobia.

Charting Requirements

Chart measures and the hierarchy of fear. Each list and its extension is to be charted in the 24-Hour Progress Notes.

Chart which relaxation technique is used and what level of control the child has on this technique. Also chart what 'signal' the child is to use when his anxiety level gets too high.

4 GROUP TECHNIQUES

Assignment of Levels

Group Techniques — First Level (Low Risk)

Messy Play
Strength Bombardment

Group Techniques — Second Level (Moderate Risk)

Anatomy and Physiology Training	Role-playing
Home Maintenance Skills	Sensitivity Exercises
Kangaroo Kort	Social Skills Training
Limit Challenge	Teaching Parents Skills
Negotiating Guidelines and	Tradition Engendering
Consequences	Ward Control
Recreation Introduction	

Group Techniques — Third Level (High Risk)

Family Counselling

Messy Play (MP) — 'Messy stuff'
Technique — First Level

Rationale

Some children have been taught to avoid playing with dirty things, partly for hygiene reasons but also because some parents believe if the child's interest in mud is not curbed he will never want to be clean. Although there is an ancient and useful fear of anything that might be contaminated with faeces, many children's obsessive fear of dirt is quite unnecessary and may be very inhibiting. Without permission or opportunity to explore with messy things, areas of the child's developing intelligence are inhibited. Because many emotions are tied to what one does with dirty things, not being able to mess about will inhibit the expression of some emotions.

The objects of messy play are:

(1) To introduce messy situations as enjoyable and acceptable but with limits, guidelines and appropriate clean-up.

178

(2) To desensitise those children with strong aversions to messy or dirty situations and to disinhibit unnecessary repression of emotion.

(3) To help a child sublimate his interest in messiness and demonstrate how creative he can be with it.

(4) To show parents and siblings that their fear of dirt is unfounded, that the patient can benefit from enjoying his messy play and his expressions of messy feelings.

Application

Those children who are encopretic, phobic to 'dirt', anorexic, depressed, autistic, obsessive–compulsive and passive–aggressive can benefit.

Measures

1. With encopretic children record the number of soiling incidents.

2. With compulsive children record the number of impulsive or spontaneous activities.

3. Note the child's level of anxiety while he is getting messy and also the parent's reaction.

Procedure

1. Obtain a baseline by giving the child access to messy media and standing back to watch what he does with it.

2. Explain to parents and child the benefits and procedure.

3. Demonstrate how enjoyable it can be to play with messy stuff and how important it is to express many feelings. Don't get too carried away. Make sure you show how easy it is to get cleaned up again.

4. Introduce messy media in a positive, matter-of-fact manner. You can use papier mâché, glueing, baking, gardening, finger paints, clay, soap, slime or mud.

5. The therapist should model appropriate behaviour and expressions of feeling for the patient. In the case of a non-verbal or very behaviour-inappropriate child, use verbal mediation.

6. Do some mud slinging with children who have repressed anger. It sometimes helps to draw a picture of the person they would like to get at and allow them to throw handfuls of mud at the picture while using appropriately angry expletives, e.g. 'Take that!'

7. Once the child is thoroughly enjoying the messy play, encourage him to do something constructive with it.

8. End the session with a good and satisfying clean-up. Don't do too

much of it yourself.

   9. Show the parents the child both enjoying the mess and cleaning up on his own.

  10. Encourage parents to join in.

  11. Check on follow-up to ensure parents haven't become inhibiting again.

Untoward Effects

   1. Pushing a 'fragile' emotional child might lead to excessive anxiety and/or increased repression.

   2. Poor choice of messy activity could increase phobic reactions rather than result in desensitisation.

   3. Therapists should be aware of small cuts or scratches on hands of patient; inadequate washing might lead to minor infections.

Charting Requirements

Record the child's communications and feelings.

Strength Bombardment (SB) – 'Stop it. I like it'
Technique – First Level

Rationale

The frequent onslaught of criticism that disturbed children often receive increases their poor self-esteem. Their unhappiness interferes with the motivation and energy the child needs in order to adapt and learn. When children perform less well at school they are more likely to be criticised.

When things go wrong in a family, children tend to blame themselves. For this reason they are more likely to expect criticism than praise. They tend to amplify the negative things that are said about them, and less frequently notice the good comments. Even in the best of households the criticism usually exceeds the praise.

Parents tend to believe that a child should know he is appreciated without having to be told: 'After all we look after him all the time.' Adults too often think children should not have to be praised when they are obedient, just criticised when they are failing and punished if they are disobedient. When children are too frequently criticised they give up trying to please, but they still need attention. They then go about getting this attention with negative behaviour.

Strength bombardment is an opportunity for the child to hear from friends, foes, family and staff the good things they detect in him.

Hearing of his strengths from people important to him produces, at least, a momentary improvement in self-concept which can reverse a cycle of negative self-image-provoking criticism. When the child feels better about himself, he will use more appropriate ways of trying to please those who are important to him.

Strength bombardment can teach children both to hear and accept compliments. Over a period of time the good things they feel about themselves become more firmly established. 'My nurse keeps saying I'm pretty smart and I trust her. Maybe I'm not so dumb after all.' With an improved self-image, children are able to reject criticism that is not in keeping with the good things they know about themselves.

Application

There are very few children who cannot benefit, but depressed, negative and apathetic children need it most.

Measures

1. Count experiences of self-worth, before and after strength bombardment.
2. Record the child's ability to accept and give appropriate praise.

Procedure

1. Baseline: Obtain measures on the child prior to and just after hospitalisation.
2. Explanation: Let the child know that you do not intend to make him conceited. Convince him that the comments are genuine. Explain to the group who are providing strength bombardment that the comments must be based on fact. They should emphasise personal qualities, rather than appearance. There should be no overriding qualifiers.
3. Demonstration: The child should have an opportunity to be part of a group which gives a bombardment prior to being on the receiving end.
4. Round 1: With a few staff the child is given some comments on his good qualities. The emphasis should be to teach him how to accept compliments, e.g. 'Thank you I appreciate having you say that.' He should be taught how to use appropriate modifiers, e.g. 'That's true but I also lose my temper too often.' Give the child an opportunity to summarise at the end — 'I have learned these are my good qualities, but I can't agree with you when you say this and this.'
5. Round 2: This should be done by a group of ward peers and some staff.

6. Round 3: A group of family and a few staff give the child strength bombardment.

7. Round 4: Ward peers and staff should feed back both strengths and a few weaknesses.

8. Round 5: Family and a few staff will comment on both strengths and weaknesses. The child should be enabled to accept and reject appropriately those characteristics that he can and cannot accept.

9. Teach the family how to do it for every member.

10. On follow-up, check to see the family is sticking with it and not using strength bombardment in a manipulative way.

Untoward Effects

It is possible that the child will become conceited. It is more likely he will reject what is said about him.

Charting Requirements

Measures only.

Anatomy and Physiology Teaching (APT) − 'How my body works' Technique − Second Level

Rationale

Many children are unaware of how their bodies function. Pain may mean damage is occurring to their body. Uncontrolled reactions are frightening to children. Children who have an awareness of how their individual body works are in a better position to regulate their functions and to monitor their own emotional changes. When they understand that pain is sometimes the result of tension arising from conflicts, they can better deal with the source of the problem.

Knowledge of how their bodies function can reassure anxious children. Children with psychosomatic and tension states can better understand the effects of tension. Children are who engaged in sex education can greatly benefit from understanding their physiology and anatomy. Children struggling to attain an autonomous control of appetites and sphincters need the information.

Application

1. Psychosomatic problems: The emphasis should be on physiology, and the effects of anxiety and conflict which result from ambivalence and unexpressed feelings.

2. Enuresis, encopresis, articulation difficulties.

3. Anorexia, obesity.
4. Autistic and psychotic children.
5. Children with habit spasms, tics and trichotillomania.

Measures

Give a brief 'before and after' A & P quiz. After instructions, ask the child if he is satisfied with what he has learned. Make a statement regarding some of the child's own emotional reactions.

Procedure

Obtain a baseline from the A & P quiz. Ask the child to do a careful drawing of his body. Give a brief explanation of the teaching that is involved and a demonstration in which another child or staff is given some of the same teaching.

Introduce the subject by asking 'Have you ever wondered about your body and how it works?' Use your own enthusiasm and wonderment, for example, 'Boy, when I found out . . .'

Focus on the area of greatest concern only after other areas of physiology have been talked about. Answer as many questions as the child asks. Do not titillate a curiosity that is not there. Eventually the child should be asked to do his own drawing of the area discussed and to describe how it works.

In teaching anatomy and physiology, make liberal use of colour prints, slides or movies. Sometimes a visit to the hospital autopsy lab. is indicated.

Untoward Effects

By teaching the child more than he is prepared to learn, the child may be overwhelmed or become bored. In the area of sex, the child's latent curiosity and desire for stimulation may be unnecessarily titillated so that he desires to experiment without having an understanding of the implications.

Charting Requirements

Only measures are necessary unless the child has been given literature to read, then the title of the literature is to be documented in the 24-Hour Progress Note.

Home Maintenance Skills (HMS) — 'Chores'
Technique — Second Level

Rationale

Parents appreciate children who help with the chores, duties and responsibilities around the house. All parents want their children to help willingly with home maintenance but some have no idea how to teach the necessary skills, how to encourage getting started and how to reinforce the ongoing appropriate behaviour. Many parents have difficulty with their child's negative attitude towards the task. They feel that since they work hard for the child's benefit, it is only fair that the child should help around the house without having to be continually reminded to do so. The co-operative carrying-out of functions that make it easier for everyone to live in the house is one of the most joyous aspects of family life. Unfortunately, many people have been conditioned to think of this as 'chores'. There must be an 'attitude' change and a 'behavioural' change.

Application

This technique is very useful for children who come from chaotic homes or homes with one or more obsessively tidy parents. Children whose parents continually complain about their lack of co-operation around the house can benefit. It is very useful for children of a single parent whose time is already spread very thinly and for children in homes below the poverty line.

Measures

Measures on number of activities, number of compliances and agreeable attitude in doing home maintenance should be made at home prior to treatment.

Procedure

1. Obtain a baseline.
2. Explain the objects and procedure to the child and parent.
3. Ask another family to describe it works with them.
4. Obtain from the parents a list of:
(a) Self-care behaviours.
(b) Home maintenance activities done by the child for the benefit of the whole family.
(c) Home maintenance activities to be done with one or more members of the family.

5. Start with the self-care skills. Do not choose more than three.

6. Model tasks for the child, do them with him, or be with him when he does them.

7. Reinforce each step (depending on assessment of his developmental level in each skill). For example, most children need help in organising and sorting out their clothes and the appropriate drawers for them. After they have done this with an adult who explains what she is doing and why, they may be better able to repeat the function. A younger child can manage to keep his drawers clean and organised for some time after this demonstration but will need help again when reorganisation and sorting are necessary.

8. Praise the child for each new skill. Younger children can be started on a 'star' or 'happy face' chart.

9. Next work on the functions that a child is to do for the benefit of other members of the family. Some of these may need to be taught. For example, setting the table, preparing vegetables, unpacking the groceries, baking, operating the vacuum cleaner and the lawnmower, or chopping wood. The staff should perform this task on the unit as similarly as possible to the way it will be done at home. If this is not possible, the staff and the child should go home to carry out the task. It is most important that the staff visibly enjoy doing home maintenance. They should be singing, humming or communicating their enjoyment in non-verbal ways.

10. Use verbal statements about how happy it will make the other members of the family. Reinforce each step of the learning process. More importantly, admire and praise the completion of the task.

11. Use modelling and mediational modifications to obtain a smooth level of home maintenance.

12. Move to the one or two home care functions selected for the child to be done with one or more members of the family. This is to be one the parents or a sibling will readily do jointly with the child. The function chosen should be one that the parent usually enjoys doing, e.g. gardening, repair work, painting, baking, sewing, mending, preserving.

13. Review parental expectations of the child's performance. If necessary, alter them to an appropriate level for the child's development.

14. The main purpose is to teach the child to enjoy working with someone for the benefit of the family, not to get a perfectly iced cake or perfectly symmetrical hedge. This concept is especially difficult for the compulsively tidy parents. Within the home the primary care

worker needs to provide directions and feedback, using role-reversal and reinforcement in order to establish co-operation.

15. Negotiate guidelines and consequences for all the home maintenance activities the child can perform. Make sure these are written and signed prior to discharge, with copies to all concerned.

Untoward Effects

Frustrations increase when expectations are too high. Parents may feel the effort to get things going is so much greater than doing it themselves that they give up and then blame the staff for spoiling the child.

Charting Requirements

State the functions and the level to be achieved. Note any resistance or problems encountered.

Kangaroo Kort (KK)
Technique – Second Level

Rationale

Children are very adaptive. Even the most seriously disturbed can take advantage of a new environment to suppress old conflicts. When emotionally ill children are hospitalised, they often adapt so well that there is little evidence of the severe symptoms they exhibited at home. If you try to talk about their conflicts, they resist. They would much prefer to forget about their troubles.

Kangaroo Kort is a kind of psychodrama for children. It is intended to reawaken common, familiar family conflicts and provide a forum in which the child can gain insight and new coping skills. Kangaroo Kort precipitates an encounter with the emotions of familiar conflicts so that the child may find new ways of coping. We present a variety of conflicts in which we assume the child has probably been involved. We re-enact these conflicts in such a way that the child is drawn into re-experiencing them, and then we use his stirred up emotions to get him thinking and working at a solution. It is called a 'kort' because we encourage the child to make a decision about who is right or wrong. In order to make a judgement it is necessary for him to consider both sides of the conflict.

This technique can be used in conjunction with social skills training.

1. To Heighten Awareness. The entire series of Kangaroo Kort illustrations should encompass most of the children's common conflicts.

Seeing them demonstrated heightens the children's awareness and allows them to verbalise their feelings.

2. To Express Awakened Feelings. When feelings are heightened, it is easier to express them. The staff model the expression of feelings so that the children become more adept at finding the right words for their feelings.

3. Identify Ambivalence. Conflicted children need to become aware that they have mixed feelings about their life experiences. They should be helped to identify the elements of their conflicts — the pros and cons, the hates and loves that they feel towards their parents.

4. To Observe Interaction. In Kangaroo Kort the staff have an opportunity to observe the interactions and emotional responses that they wouldn't otherwise know about unless they were in the child's home during a major family conflict.

5. To Model Adaptive Responses. In Kangaroo Kort the staff have an opportunity to show that there are specific ways of handling emotions even though children cannot do much to resolve the conflict themselves. Each session should have some time devoted to the staff giving specific suggestions and modelling skills in conflict resolution.

Application

All children except those with poor impulse control or fragile egos.

Measures

Objective — estimate the amount of an individual child's participation.
Subjective — record the child's emotional reactions.

Observations

The staff must be careful to observe the child's reactions to the simulated conflict. While one staff member is watching the child who is speaking, other members must be careful to observe the other children in the group. The primary therapist should take the opportunity of helping the children to verbalise their conflicts. The auxiliary therapist should continue to keep the level of conflict relatively high by holding opposing positions regarding elements of the conflict.

Procedure

If possible each child should first observe one to three sessions through a one-way mirror. Obtain measures during the child's first session as a baseline. Carefully explain the procedure and goals to the child and parents.

Staging.
  1. Psychodrama presentation by the staff.
  2. Examples of previous patients (well camouflaged to ensure confidentiality).
  3. Personal examples described by a child.
  4. Films of common family conflicts.

Surprise is an important element in selecting which method to use. Mix the methods. Selection of the topics can be rotated. Once emotions are stressed, continue unless a child's reaction is uncontrolled. If it is, he should observe the session from the other side of the one-way screen. Then pose the question of who is right and who is wrong. Gradually shift the discussion from impersonal to personal, e.g. 'What's it like in your house?'

Phases.
  1. Embroiled. During the first phase, the children are embroiled vicariously in the conflict which is acted out by the staff. The auxiliary staff should attempt to sit behind the children.
  2. Feelings Expression. During this time, each child is given an opportunity to express his/her feelings. Differences of opinion are pointed out. Children are helped to put their feelings into words and speak them with the intensity that they feel.
  3. Decision-making. The children are given plenty of time to make up their minds about who is right. Then the decision is put to a vote.
  4. Staff Skills Required — ability to:
  (a) Empathise with children's feelings.
  (b) Model ways of handling conflicted feelings.
  (c) Dramatise conflict situations.
  (d) Observe interaction and coping mechanisms.
  (e) Interpret the basis of conflict.
  5. Resolution. During this time, staff members should bring forward a variety of suggestions for handling the conflicts in which the children are passively involved. The child is encouraged to choose what he sees as the suggestion appropriate to his situation and then to practise this resolution.

Identify the effective component of the conflicts in the children themselves. Having identified them, allow plenty of time for abreaction. Then make tentative group interpretations. Identify the usual conflicts, impulses, anxieties and defences.

Week 1	1. Teasing
	2. Authority
	3. Adoption or separated parent
	4. Marital conflict
	5. Leaving hospital
Week 2	6. Affection
	7. Feeling lonely
	8. Theft
	9. Anger
	10. Suspicion
Week 3	11. Being humiliated
	12. School, homework
	13. Beatings
	14. Drunken father
	15. Death
Week 4	16. Sibling rivalry
	17. Praise
	18. Unjustly accused
	19. Moves
	20. Scapegoating
Week 5	21. Danger — thrill vs fear
	22. Food — deprivation, control
	23. Growing up
	24. Busy parents — no time with children
	25. Sick parents

Untoward Effects

Increased anxiety and increased conflict could get out of hand.

Charting Requirements

Measures only.

Limit Challenge (LC) — 'Trying my best'
Technique — Second Level

Rationale

Many children don't know themselves. They are unaware of or mis-represent their strengths and weaknesses. They may live in a protected and protecting environment because their parents consider them weak and vulnerable. Some parents cannot acknowledge the child's strength because that implies the child is becoming independent more quickly than the parent may appreciate. Other parents cannot recognise the child's weaknesses because that has the connotation of dependence or that there has been a lack of parental training.

Many children identify with television and comic superheroes. They half-believe that, just like their hero, they can do anything if given the opportunity. They are glad that the occasion to test this illusion never really does arise. The other half of them knows full well that they are weak and vulnerable. They are afraid to examine that weakness in case they become more afraid of their vulnerability.

Some children are afraid of the natural environment. Modern stories tend to depict a child, together with his friendly robot, pitted against the vagaries of natural elements and forces. Forces of wind and temperature appear to be enemies which they hope to overcome rather than to understand and use.

Children need an opportunity to test themselves and to evaluate their capabilities in an environment of supportive permissiveness. Much of this is best done in the wilderness. Given an opportunity to challenge their limits, they can change their self-concepts and their peer relations.

Children are tested against their own assessment, not in comparison with other children or with standards set by adults. It must be done safely. In the process, the child should have the opportunity to learn to endure discomfort and to overcome his unrealistic fears. The emphasis is on courage, stamina and perseverance rather than on skill. These characteristics should help him deal with the discouragements of a conflicted family life.

Application

This technique is most useful for those children who are over- or under-confident, e.g. bullies and wimps. It is useful for all children who have grown up in a restricted environment.

Measures

1. Record the child's assessment of his ability before and after the test.

2. Note this behaviour before and after each challenge.

Procedure

1. Baseline: Obtain measures without the child observing.
2. Explanation: Provide the child with a clear idea of what is involved.

Reassure the parents with respect to safety. Help them deal with their own inability realistically to assess their child.

3. Demonstration: The adult may demonstrate the test involved, but he must go only part way. This is to avoid the tendency of the child to make unfavourable comparisons.

4. Make the challenge clearly: one of the child pitting himself against his estimate of his abilities. List all the possibilities he is interested in. 'How fast could you run around that track?', 'How much do you think you can lift?', 'Can you climb that mountain?', 'How far can you swim under water?'

5. Obtain a carefully described estimate from the child of how long it would take him or how far he might be able to go. Record this and ask him to sign it.

6. Trial: Give the child a good opportunity to show his best. Give plenty of encouragement. Stay with him, just behind not assisting.

7. Re-estimation: Each child should give another estimate after the trial. If it is markedly different from the first one, show him the difference. Ask him how well his parents could do at the same activity.

8. Re-trial: This time with no encouragement.

9. Feedback: 'Well, I guess that's the best you can do. It's not as good as you thought, but you really tried. At least you know you won't fall apart if the going gets rough.'

If the child can accept his limits, then respond with, 'Shall we try something else?' If the child cannot accept, respond with, 'So you still don't believe it? Maybe we should talk about it.' Spend some time analysing the child's expectations of himself and where these come from.

10. Re-trial: Try once again under conditions set by the child. Persist until the child is able to acknowledge both his strengths and weaknesses.

11. If he is within reach of a reasonable goal, encourage him to train and keep trying.

12. Do this in the presence of parents.

13. Show them how best to encourage or reassure their children.

Untoward Effects

There are real dangers about which the parents must know and the staff be able to deal with. If the child fails too miserably he may not want to try again.

Charting Requirements

Measures, tests and results.

Negotiating Guidelines and Consequences (NGC) — 'Rules and rewards' Technique — Second Level

Rationale

Children need guidance and the security of consistent guidelines and consequences. Parents who demand control are often fearful of their own poorly controlled impulses or conflicts. Parents who can use more democratically determined control usually have more adaptable and innovative children. Children who have some say in the rules that govern their lives are more inclined to abide by those rules. Children who learn from the consequences of their decisions tend to be more responsible for themselves.

Parents may interfere with the natural consequences which would govern the child's behaviour. They may inadvertently reinforce the child's non-compliance by repeated admonitions. Reciprocally, they may be reinforced for nagging by the child's eventual compliance. Continual pressure by the parents often produces a counter force, the resistance of which is expressed in anger, delayed compliance and disinterest in the activity.

Enormous amounts of energy may be consumed in running a household when there are hassles about routine tasks. This usually means parents have less time to play and communicate with their children. Having controls always imposed on him the child has less self-control and is less sure of his decisions and impulses when he grows up. When parents have an easy control, the children look upon them more benignly, try harder to please them, are more likely to interject a good 'object' and more inclined to imitate good parenting behaviour.

The process of negotiating is time well spent. It encourages communication, teaches democracy and helps children learn to express their point of view clearly. Any habitual area of conflict is an appropriate area to negotiate. It is wise to start with small problems with few emotional conflicts, so that the family learns the process and gains confidence.

Potential Parent Worries About This Technique.

1. Parents may fear allowing their child too much freedom which they might use destructively.

2. They may fear losing respect in their child's eyes.

3. Negotiation may also be seen as a compromise and, therefore, as 'being weak' or backing down on principles.

4. Negotiation may also be seen as taking too much time.

5. Some parents believe they are always wiser than their children and therefore should make all decisions.

6. Parents may feel that their child is too young to understand the process of negotiating.

Responses to the Above Problems.

1. Loss of Control: This approach helps the child gradually to assume greater responsibility for his own behaviour, an attribute which every adult needs.

2. Loss of Respect: One cannot demand respect. This technique allows the parent the opportunity to 'earn' the respect of his child.

3. Weakness or 'Giving In': No one is giving in. The guideline doesn't need to be less than you want. Negotiating is reaching a mutually agreeable solution.

4. Too Much Time: It does take time but once the solution is reached, the problem is solved for a long time.

5. Wiser: The parent is wiser in many areas but not in all areas concerning their child. A child may have a lot of insight into his own problems. He should contribute to the solution.

6. Too Young: Even young children realise the benefits of consistent, reasonable guidelines in their world. To stop the constant nagging or punishments, children will happily work on the solutions.

Application

Any area of child or family behaviour which is continuing to create unnecessary friction with no movement towards a solution.

Measures

Record the time spent in negotiating. Record results of negotiations in two columns — tentative and final guidelines and consequences. Note the percentage compliance on each, both in hospital and at home.

Procedure

During weeks one and two, discuss with the family the problems they are having at home and what they see as viable alternatives. Provide realistic parental feedback to their ideas and suggest the idea of negotiation.

Once you are familiar with the child's viewpoint, begin the first pre-negotiation session with the parents, representing the child's point of view.

Having accomplished your goals in the pre-negotiation session with parent and child tackle the negotiation session with the family. By conducting negotiations during week three you can enable the family to have some guidelines in effect for the first and second weekend pass. This will be helpful to establish a definite pattern with the child and siblings prior to discharge. It provides two weeks to work out any unforeseen problem areas.

For the negotiating sessions, include the whole family, i.e. everybody in the household. Begin with the easiest, least important problems first, and work your way up to the most difficult ones. Set a specific time period for which these guidelines and consequences will be in effect, i.e. for 3, 6, 9, 12 months, at which time they will be open for re-negotiation. This date for re-negotiation offers the child an element of hope that things will change. It also offers the parent a chance to update the guidelines so that they better fit the increasing maturity of the family. Choose a comfortable place and convenient time for negotiation.

1. Obtain a baseline estimate of compliance in problem areas.

2. Parents and children should be asked to list all areas of persistent friction.

3. Each person must rank order in importance these problems.

4. Explain and model the negotiation procedure. Explain why parents will not lose control or respect. Point out advantages, e.g. the children learn more self-control, they learn the exercise of democracy, etc.

5. Begin negotiating with the least important behaviour. Staff should act as mediator whenever parents and children get stuck on a particular behaviour.

6. Encourage children to state their own arguments as clearly and as eloquently as possible. Encourage parents to listen and counter quietly, praising the children for any good arguments they make.

7. In the first negotiating sessions, settle on two behaviours; one the parents want to see more of, and one they want to see less of.

8. Try out each guideline and consequence on the ward. If they work, encourage their use at home during the weekends. Guidelines and consequences need to be clearly written and signed by both parties.

9. Obtain a record of the trial use of the guidelines and consequences.

10. Work towards more difficult behaviours.

11. Gradually hand over the mediating to the head of the house.

12. Remember this document should be POSITIVE. At least half the consequences should be rewarding. Wherever possible use natural consequences.

13. Check during follow-up to see if parents are being consistent.

Specimen of Guidelines and Consequences

Guideline	Consequence
1. In bed 8.30 p.m. weekdays, face washed, teeth brushed, PJs on, lying down, light may be on	If on time three of five nights, may stay up until 10.00 p.m. on Friday and Saturday evenings. If late, get up ½ hour earlier
2. Set table every evening by 6.00 p.m.	Receive 10¢ of earned allowance if on time
3. Take laundry to laundry room by 9.00 a.m. on Saturday	Mom will wash laundry. She will not wash anything that arrives after 9.00 a.m. on Saturday
4. No temper outbursts longer than 60 seconds	A star on a chart for each ½ day and each evening there are no tantrums. With six stars, say, father will take child fishing. If outbursts longer than 60 seconds, must go to room for 15 minutes
5. On time for meals	Get the full meal. If late, get cold food, no dessert

Untoward Effects

Parents may give up in disgust when they find they can't be consistent or the child's behaviour doesn't change fast enough. There is a possibility that no consequence in the parents' repertoire or within their financial means will have any effect.

If negotiating is handled improperly, future discussions between parent and children become more difficult. It is important that all agree and are able to carry through their part of the agreement.

Charting Requirements

Measures plus a final copy of the guidelines and consequences should be placed in the child's chart for reference during follow-up care.

Recreation Introduction (RI) – 'I never knew it was so interesting'
Technique – Second Level

Rationale

Children with limited experience in life have limited expectations, delayed development and fewer social skills. Limited experience limits intelligence and learning skills. Without a few bright experiences in their lives, frustrated children tend to give up hope easily. With reduced hope, there is reduced biological drive to survive. With limited experiences of life, children are afraid to engage the real world. They are more likely to participate passively in other people's experience, especially television.

Recreation introduction is designed to:

1. Increase the child's awarenes of what is available to him and his family.

2. Decrease the fear of unknown places and unfamiliar activities.

3. Increase the child's desire to try new adventures, look for new things to do and explore the world.

4. Increase the child's reliance on adults who can teach him new skills or assist him when he becomes anxious in new situations.

5. Increase the child's resistance to advertising and high-cost fun promulgated by the media and, thereby, decrease the child's demand that his parents provide passive fun, e.g. movies, hockey games, etc.

6. Teach parents how to introduce and encourage a child in a new activity.

7. Show parents how to play with their children and at the same time be teaching them life skills.

8. Help children explore the full range of their emotions and capabilities.

Application

For all children, especially those children with limited experience, fears and deprived backgrounds.

Measures

List the child's interests, experiences and skills in recreational settings. Compare the child's new and old interests on follow-up.

Procedure

1. Record as baseline all the activities the child and his family

presently engage in and enjoy.

2. Explanation, e.g. 'We want you to have fun and to learn at the same time', 'These are some things you might get your mother or father interested in . . .' Staff should reassure parents about their own anxieties regarding costs, time and acccidents. Tell parents that this is healthy for them as well as their children.

3. Take your patient's family along on some outing with another family that already enjoys exploring together.

4. Describe new situations and activities beforehand. Once they are there, describe the environment, e.g. 'Did you see?', 'Let's stop and investigate'.

5. In making a decision on what to do, encourage a child to voice his fears. The staff can model the mental process in making those decisions, the fears and hopes of the outcome. Discuss a child's previous failed attempts.

6. Encourage them to persist when they are finding it's not fun. To begin with, get them to measure their own physiological reactions so that they feel inclined to push the limit and not fear they will collapse.

7. Show children and families how to observe. Show them how to listen, look, feel, etc. and to check out simple hypotheses by simple experiences, e.g. 'that if we did this . . . then we would probably find that . . .'

8. Following a vigorous activity, encourage them to sit back and enjoy the view while observing their own feelings of relaxation.

Try this sequence:

   (i) 'This is what we are going to do and this is how we are going to go about it.'

  (ii) 'Hey, let's find something to do.'

 (iii) 'What do you suggest we do?'

 (iv) 'Why don't you phone your folks and see if they would like to go with you?'

  (v) 'Let's see if the family can plan the next outing.'

9. It is important that the parents be involved in recreational activity. Explore with the parents their reticence and disappointments with unenthusiastic children.

10. On follow-up, check to see how many new activities your patient's family has tried, who initiated it, and what was enjoyed most.

Untoward Effects

Increasing fears of how to ask parents could occur.

Charting Requirements

Measures only necessary.

Role-playing (RP) – 'Acting'
Technique – Second Level

Rationale

Role-playing can be an extension of play, or an extension of real life. It provides a laboratory for the child and the therapists to experiment, observe, react, analyse and learn. Role-playing, particularly when roles are reversed, is an effective tool in developing a sense of empathy in children. Stage props, costumes and make-up help children get into the act.

Application

All children can benefit, especially those needing to make profound transactional behavioural changes.

Measures

Note change in level of anxiety (pulse, pupil dilation) during conflictual transactions and changes in key behaviours.

Procedure

1. Obtain a baseline while observing the child in his home or at school.

2. Explain to the child and parents how people learn about themselves by stepping out of character.

3. It helps the child to give it a try, by watching how it happens with some other child.

4. Start role-playing the least conflicted situation then work gradually towards areas of intense emotion or conflict.

5. After selecting the scenario, let the child pick out clothes, props or make-up, that will help him get into the role.

6. Observe and assess the child's feelings, fears and behavioural reactions during the conflicted transaction with you. Repeat it at least once more, giving added weight to the feelings discussed.

7. Discuss with the child these feelings, fears and behavioural reactions.

8. Re-enact (with child's knowledge) the conflicted transaction but with reversed roles.

9. Discuss feeling, fears and behaviours after role reversal.

10. With each transaction provide the child with alternative transactional patterns.

11. Role-play selected alternatives under increasingly provocative and anxiety-producing situations.

12. Teach the parents when and how to role-play.

13. On follow-up try one transaction to see if they can still do it.

Untoward Effects

There may be some decrease in spontaneity of relationship but this is usually only temporary.

Charting Requirements

Chart measures plus narrative on each session.

Sensitivity Exercises — 'Getting to know you' Technique — Second Level

Rationale

The following exercises are designed to meet the need of developing awareness of self and beyond, among children on the Child and Family Unit. The format for the exercises is based on the regular five-week admission and the broad goals associated with each successive week. Because admissions and discharges occur each week and only two children out of ten are at the same point in the progression at any one time, each week contains the exercises covering an entire five-week period. For example, every Monday's exercises concentrate on 'establishing rapport', while each Tuesday 'communication' is emphasised. Each successive Monday, for a five-week period, the 'establishing rapport' exercises will vary and similarly for the other four days of the week.

The exercises contained here have been tested and tried by the hospital staff under a variety of conditions and combinations of diagnoses, age and sex categories and have proved relatively successful, despite the handicaps such variety produced.

The emphasised value of these exercises is the improvement in the child or parent's awareness of his own feelings, the world around him and how he responds to each of these. Each week of his admission the child is encouraged to focus on a different aspect of his world. There is considerable overlap among these aspects and the exercises are formulated to account for this fact.

During the first week of admission the patient is required to interact with six to nine new children as well as a greater number of adults. These interactions will likely be a new experience for most children due to the therapeutic nature of the environment. He must learn to trust the people with whom he will be spending much time. This involves letting go of old defences and taking risks. This trusting process also involves sharing his ideas and feelings, and listening to and observing others around him. The theme of the first week is therefore 'establishing rapport'.

By the second week the patient has already begun to talk about himself and his concerns. During this week he will be encouraged to become increasingly aware of his feelings and how they are expressed. Emphasis here is on listening, understanding and sharing thoughts and feelings. 'Communication' is emphasised this week.

'Solving problems' is the primary concern of week three. The patient is encouraged not only to look at himself closely but also to strive to change those areas that are a hindrance to successful functioning. He will be looking closely at what kind of person he is; how he interacts with others; and how he handles frustration. He will be encouraged to become aware of others' points of view and how to deal with these. He will become aware of his need to seek and accept assistance from those around him.

'Being a success' for most of these children is a new experience. During the fourth week they will be encouraged to see their strengths as well as limitations. Differences between people will be seen as valuable. Feeling good about themselves is an important goal at this time.

The last week of admission involves 'saying goodbye' to the new friends they made and looking ahead to being back in the 'real' world. The young patient must grapple with strong emotions of anger, sadness and fear associated with saying goodbye. He must look back at what has happened recently and look forward to what he might expect to happen.

Parents should move along the same progression with their children. Some exercises have been suggested to help them become aware of themselves and their world.

We found that the children respond best when there is a certain amount of playfulness and fun involved. Games work very well. We also found that discussion following an exercise was not necessary for the point to be understood by the children. You should be able to capitalise on spontaneous expressions by the children during the exercises. Often the most helpful thing the leader can do is simply introduce the point of the exercise before or during the period and allow the children to absorb the lessons from there on. Guidelines as to purposes for each exercise should be briefly stated prior to each exercise. Leave a short time following each exercise for discussion by staff, regarding the variations and modifications possible for each exercise.

Application

All children on the unit unless they are too ill to endure the trauma of the interactions.

Measures

Make before, during and after observations on the number and quality of child–child and child–staff communications.

Procedure

Week One.
1. Monday

Purpose: to clarify perceptions of people. Provide one sheet of drawing paper and one felt pen for each person in the group. Have each person write his or her name on the paper and place it where others can draw on it. Each person then moves from one sheet to another and quickly sketches some aspect of the person whose name appears at the top of the page. It is important that this exercise be done fairly quickly so that drawing itself does not become the important issue.

A variation of the above exercise involves each member drawing himself as his favourite animal. Other members then try to guess who each drawing represents since no one has put his name on his drawing.

2. Tuesday

Purpose: to give and receive messages. Have the group divide themselves into teams or simply proceed with individual volunteers. The volunteer is given or chooses a popular TV programme or movie or even other people in the group. The rest of the group try to determine who it is by interpreting the volunteer's body movements. As a contest, one team gives a member of the opposing team a title, that he must get his team to produce. It is also possible for a volunteer or group of volunteers to act out some recent incident on the ward and have the rest of the group guess the nature of the incident.

3. Wednesday

Purpose: to understand non-verbal communication. 'No Spicka da

Language': The group is divided into two teams. A delegate from each team comes to the worker who gives an order to be bought in a foreign store. Items may be a pound of coffee, two cows, four yards of lace, a used camel, etc. The delegate goes back to his group and pantomimes the order until someone guesses what he wants. No talking or forming of letters is allowed. The first group to guess gets one point.

4. Thursday
Purpose: accepting praise and strengths with Strength Bombardment. The group is asked to sit in a circle. One member is chosen or volunteers and each member in turn states one thing he likes or thinks is a strength of that person. This procedure continues around the group until everyone has had a turn. Encourage members to look at the person about whom they are speaking. Focus on children about to be discharged.

5. Friday
Purpose: sensory awareness. Before the exercise commences collect at least four small and common articles. Place each object in a separate cloth bag and pass them around to each group member. The members attempt to identify the objects by using all their senses except sight. Try doing it in semi-dark and have the children whisper in staff's ear what they have.

Week Two.
1. Monday
Purpose: letting go and being together. 'Electricity': ask group to sit in a circle on the floor. They should all join hands and close their eyes. The leader should then start a current going by gently squeezing the hand of the person on his right. This person passes the current on to the next person and so on around the entire group. The procedure can be varied by increasing the speed of the current or trying to change the direction of the current. As a game have one person leave the circle and when he returns shortly he must try and guess the exact location of the current.

2. Tuesday
Purpose: communication and role-playing. Play charades or get the group to form themselves into a standing circle and members join hands. Members are then instructed to walk into the centre of the circle and try and get as close to it as possible. Do this part as quietly as

possible. This is done several times to get the group used to the process. When the group seems ready have each person yell his loudest yell. Do this several times.

3. Wednesday
Purpose: co-operation and observation. A large number of different objects are placed for one minute in the centre of the group. After a minute remove all the objects. The group should attempt to write down all the objects they can remember. If this becomes too easy have them recall the characteristics of each object.

The exercise can be varied by placing a dozen or so objects in the circle and then asking one member to leave the area while one object is removed from the circle. When the member returns he must try to recall the missing object.

4. Thursday
Purpose: gaining positive feedback. Ask each group member in succession to describe another group member in positive terms only, without mentioning his or her name. The rest of the group tries to guess whom he is talking about. A variation to this exercise involves the member describing another in terms of skills, likes, dislikes, personality, and the group guesses who it is.

5. Friday
Purpose: recall past events and friendships. Provide the group with construction paper, newspapers and magazines. Ask the group to construct a collage or goodbye card that contains references to the things the group has done together and reminders of themselves for the member who is leaving.

Week Three.
1. Monday
Purpose: to let go and observe. The group is asked to form a group machine. One person begins by making repetitious movements with his hands and accompanying this with some suitable sound. The rest of the group attaches themselves by doing their own movements and sounds. Decide on what kind of machine first.

2. Tuesday
Purpose: to understand how communication becomes distorted. The leader asks for three volunteers. Two of these people are sent out of the

room while the third stays. The leader then pantomimes a situation such as changing a baby; building an igloo; washing an elephant; or some such elaborate story. The first volunteer has watched the whole thing and must now repeat the performance for the benefit of the second person who is called in from outside. This person in turn repeats it for the third person.

The group sits in a circle and the leader begins some message by whispering it in the ear of the person sitting to his right. This person then whispers it to the person on his right and so on to the end of the circle. The message is then revealed by the last person and changes noted.

3. Wednesday

Purpose: identifying feelings. Collect a series of pictures depicting a variety of feelings and emotions. Show each individual picture to the group and have the group members identify the feeling portrayed and construct a story that might fit the picture shown. You can use 'feeling and emotion' pictures.

4. Thursday

Purpose: more careful observation. The leader should select some common article before the session begins. This object is then passed around the group and each one makes some observation about the article that no one has made before. Encourage the use of all five senses. A variation involves passing the object again but this time the person is to imagine he is the object and to state, 'The worst thing that could happen to me is . . .', or 'The best thing that could happen to me is . . .'

5. Friday

Purpose: to remember and note changes. Ask each member of the group to tell the rest what his best experience was while on the ward. The worst thing that happened could also be included.

Have each person recall his first impression of the person sitting to his right. Then have him state how this impression has changed since they first met. The exercise might be introduced by using a large interesting picture and have the children give an immediate impression of the picture.

Week Four.

1. Monday
Purpose: getting better acquainted. Ask one member of the group to volunteer to be the 'celebrity'. The group could imagine themselves on some kind of talk show. The group then asks the 'celebrity' questions about what kind of person he is. Another way of doing this is to have one person act as a 'reporter' with a tape recorder and he interviews the rest of the group who are all now 'celebrities'.

2. Tuesday
Purpose: awareness of body-language. 'Mirroring': ask the group to find a partner. Ask member A to mirror all the movements made by his partner B. The movements will be quick at first but with time and encouragement they will slow down and it will be hard to tell who is leading. The next step is to ask A to mirror everything that B says and how he says it.

3. Wednesday
Purpose: co-operation. 'Who am I?': slips of paper with very familiar names of nursery rhyme characters or members of familiar TV characters or animals are pinned on the back of each person. Each person must find out who he is by asking questions of the others. The questions can only have 'yes' or 'no' answers.

4. Thursday
Purpose: to learn to take a risk and that risking involves trusting. Arrange the group in a circle, and ask for a volunteer who feels he can trust you. Ask the volunteer to walk across the circle to you. He takes your place; you take his. 'Was that hard to do?' Ask him if he is willing to try something harder. If 'no', accept that, enlist a new volunteer and start again. If 'yes', ask him to close his eyes, walk across the circle to you; assure him you won't let him bump into anyone. As he walks, give verbal reassurance, and reach out when near to make physical contact. Do this with one or two others. Have the group consider the degree of risk involved now. When ready, invite group members, one at a time, to choose anyone in the circle whom they can trust in doing a blind walk. When appropriate, discuss experiences and feelings.

5. Friday
Purpose: identifying feelings. A deck of cards is compiled with the name of different emotions such as anger, sadness, loneliness, etc.

written on them. There will be several cards with the same emotion on them. The cards are then dealt to all the group members. The person on the right of the dealer then picks a card from his hand and expresses the emotion shown through pantomime. The rest of the group looks through their own hand to find the matching emotion card. All cards are then placed face down on the table until all have decided. The cards are then matched with the actor's. Those whose cards match are permitted to place them in the centre of the table; those who fail to match their cards must pick up another from the pile in the middle. The winner is the person who gets rid of all his cards first.

Week Five.
1. Monday
Purpose: to experience trust. 'Swizzle stick': the group members form a tight circle around a volunteer. Ask the volunteer to close his eyes as you gently twirl him around. Suggest he allows himself to fall forwards or backwards keeping his knees straight. The group then catches and passes him around.

'Hammock': as each volunteer finishes the above exercise have the group join together in supporting the person into a horizontal position and lifting him to waist height and gently rocking him back and forth for several moments. Gently lower to the floor.

'I'll catch you': ask the group to pair off or into groups of three. One member then allows himself to fall into the arms of his partner(s). The distance to fall can be gradually increased as trust between members increases.

2. Tuesday
Purpose: better communication. The group is asked to move freely about the room. As they do this call out different characters and ask each one to pretend he is that person. Characters such as: a sad old man; a worried mother; an excited teenager; a shy child; an angry father; a school principal; or their best friend, are good examples. Suggest that there is no talking while this is going on.

3. Wednesday
Purpose: seeing others' point of view. Provide the group with an interesting and familiar situation such as family suppertime with one child who won't eat his potatoes and another who is being messy. Have some members of the group volunteer to role-play the characters and then, following the first attempt, have the roles switched.

4. Thursday

Purpose: co-operation. One person is chosen to be IT and leaves the room. The rest of the group then decides on some simple task they will get IT to perform (e.g. write on the blackboard or untie John's shoelace). When IT returns he walks around and the group claps quietly when he is far away from the correct task and louder as he approaches the task required. Humming, chanting 'hot', 'cold', 'warm' can be substituted for clapping.

5. Friday

Purpose: anticipation and recall. The group sits in a circle. The first person begins by saying, 'When I leave here I hope . . .' and finishes with some short statement that is appropriate. The next person repeats the phrase and the person's statement and then adds his own statement and so on around the circle. The player who forgets must move to the end of the line.

For Parents

Week One.

Ask each parent to construct a list of his expectations of himself, of his partner, of his child, and of the staff. They can then decide if these expectations are realistic or not.

Week Two.

Have both parents and the child sit five or six feet apart and work at developing an argument. Allow them to generate some 'heat' then stop them. Move them closer together and ask them to continue the argument but under these conditions; they must maintain eye contact and each person must paraphrase the other's statement to the latter's satisfaction. Statements should be kept short.

Week Three.

Have each partner take the usual role of the other or the child. Choose a situation that is fresh in everyone's memory and have the persons rehearse the scene again.

Week Four.

Ask both parents to compile a list of at least ten strengths they and their partner have. This can be complemented with a similar list of five weaknesses.

Week Five.

Get the parents to dream up an ideal two weeks holiday for themselves. Then ask them to work on one holiday for both of them which is a compromise. This will provide plenty of opportunities to talk about how they deal with disappointments.

Untoward Effects

If not carefully conducted with enthusiasm, children become bored and won't want to attend.

Charting Requirements

Chart measures each day.

Social Skills Training (SST)
Technique — Second Level

Rationale

Children don't always learn social skills without help. They may lack basic interpersonal skills sometimes because of deprivation or lack of good models. Sometimes children have little opportunity to engage in social skills activity because they are so preoccupied with just surviving. Some children are too sensitive and take almost any response from their peers as negative. Some have bad social experiences because of the poor neighbourhood they grew up in. Some never get the chance to establish some social skills because they are moving so frequently. They eventually become afraid to relate to people.

Since all children need social skills they try to engage in social activities appropriate to their level of development. Without skill they may be so socially clumsy, they are ignored, teased or ostracised. Their resulting anger or withdrawal increases social deprivation which heightens the need for social interaction. So they try again; usually with no more success than the first time. If they are anxious they engage in silly attention-obtaining behaviour. If they are angry they get into fights.

Children with poor social skills eventually give up or develop ties where they are accepted. Occasionally this is with delinquent sub-groups.

The object of this technique is to teach children when and how to interact. The child must be able to empathise with the feelings and reactions of others. To focus on the experience of other children helps them become less preoccupied with themselves. This technique requires setting up probable interpersonal situations, role-playing and re-enacting conflicts which reactivate the child's emotions, then practising new skills.

Application

All children who are awkward in groups, especially anorexics, compulsives, depressives, delinquents and psychotic children, will benefit.

Measures

Make before, during and after measures on:
  (i) Positive and negative peer relations.
  (ii) The level of anxiety while interacting.
  (iii) Verbatim statements of the child's experience.

Procedure

A. Components
  (a) sociodramatic – 'Wow, she sounds just like my old lady'
  (b) feeling release – 'It feels good to let it out'
  (c) insight: individual – 'Now I know why I keep going it'; group – 'They sure can make it hard for me'
  (d) imitation, modelling – 'It works for him so I'll try it'
  (e) mediational – 'I tell myself to keep cool'
  (f) practice: conditioned inhibition – 'It's boring'; successive approximation – 'I'm getting it'
  (g) crisis repeat – 'OK, now I know what to do, I don't need to be so scared'

B. Model.
1. crisis → 2. feelings expression → 3. feelings rehearsal

8. practice   4. individual and group analysis

7. mediational ← 6. practice ← 5. modelling staff then child

1. Obtain two days of baseline measures on the child under the usual ward conditions.

2. Provide the child and the parents with a full explanation emphasing the parents' later role.

3. The child and parents should stand behind the one-way mirror and watch the other children and the staff training children.

4. To arouse the child's feelings and precipitate participation and evoke feelings, traumatic situations can be role-played by the staff.

5. Use your experience with other children to tell a fictitious case history or dramatise a story, e.g. 'I once knew a boy who . . .'

6. Each crisis situation should present a conflicting situation fairly typical of the child's own experience. Possible scenarios are:

(a) accusations – 'You did it, didn't you?'

(b) loss – 'I am sorry but I have to go away and won't see you again'

(c) teasing – 'You are mental, stupid, retarded, etc.'

(d) criticism – 'Why are you so dumb all the time?'

(e) new friend – 'Hi! What's your name?'

(f) punishment – 'OK, you're gonna get it'

(g) embarrassment – 'Hey! Your fly's open'

(h) parents fighting – 'Shut up you stupid bastard!'

7. Feelings Release: At the end of the role-play or story of a crisis situation, give all the children an opportunity to discharge a portion of their emotional tension. Help them talk about their feelings with whatever language they wish. Model some of the feelings release statements a child can use appropriately. Encourage those non-verbal expressions which would naturally accompany the feelings expressed, e.g. 'It makes me so mad I could scream' (jump up), 'I can't face it' (bury face in hands), 'Shut up, shut up, please shut up' (hands over ears), 'Please don't go away Daddy' (reaching out to grasp).

Feelings release will discharge a portion of the tension thereby gaining a relative state of well-being and gratitude. At the end of this phase the child should be able to comment on the difference in tension states so the child will be motivated to find a skill to bring it about himself. Use some feeling rehearsal to make sure feelings are expressed, 'OK, let's all say it together – please leave me alone.'

8. Analysis: Give the child an opportunity to explore and express his ambivalence about the situation. He is bound to feel two ways, at least, about each situation, e.g. 'Please don't go', 'I hope you get run over when you do'; 'Shut up', 'But don't ignore me'.

Explain some of the effects of the conflict, e.g. 'When you are mad at your Mum you feel like hitting her but she is a lot bigger and she might hurt you, so you run away.' During the analysis of the conflict the child should be given an opportunity to comment on how the group affects his behaviour, e.g. 'When Johnny got mad the rest of you started picking on me.'

9. Modelling: Make is easy for the child to identify with you by

telling him something about your own experience, e.g. 'When I was a kid I had big, fat freckles and the kids all called me "Blotchy".' Begin by expressing the dilemma that is engendered by the conflict 'I didn't know if I should hit him or hide.'

10. Provide the child some of the fruitless advice that they probably get, e.g. 'My mother said I should ignore him but I couldn't help hearing what he said and it hurt.' Mediate the solution, 'So I said to myself — why not say something back, I might get a black eye, but that's not so bad as the shame and humiliation.'

11. Set up a practice situation with two staff members, one as the provocateur and the other as the respondent. Model the above with increasing emphasis on the final stated solution, e.g. 'You are blotchy yourself.' After modelling a few variations ask the star pupil in the group to model the response. Commend him well for his efforts — 'Say, that's really great' — 'Try it again, only look him right in the eyes this time.'

12. Practise the Solution: Each child should practise final statements. Give them quiet direction, cues and reinforcements for success with approximations to the model's behaviour, e.g. 'Try not to look away.' 'That's much better.' Use videotape so a child may watch himself and comment on his performance. Videotaping or filming can also be used to reward children who really try, e.g. 'You are a lot better now. We will make you the TV cameraman.'

13. Practise Mediation: Model the thought processes behind the final response, e.g. 'When he does that I feel like running away but that's no good', 'I figure if I just stand there and say something back he will probably go away', 'I don't want to look scared and so I'll say the same thing back to him', 'I must remember not to look scared', 'Here goes . . . "Get lost kid" . . . Say that wasn't bad', '. . . I really did OK, good for me'.

14. The use of praise builds the child's confidence but it can't be phoney. You don't fool kids.

15. Final Practice: Give each child an opportunity to practise a series of statements gradually saying them more quietly but no less emphatically to himself. Finally do a slowed then more rapid practice of both mediation and expressive comments to a final social situation, e.g. 'OK, when I run into this situation the first thing I should remember is, don't over-react', 'He isn't as tough as he sounds', 'You are blotchy too', 'This is stupid, why don't we become friends?'

16. Crisis Re-enactment: Provide a brief re-enactment of the original crisis during which one therapist expresses his/her reaction, mediates

aloud, and models the appropriate final response. Coach the children in their reaction, e.g. 'I am getting really mad but I am thinking to myself I can handle this', 'So I say to myself, OK buddy, let's try this', 'You're blotchy!'

17. The trainee should be encouraged to respond and the staff reinforce him with 'You are thinking that way too, aren't you?', 'OK let's hear what you would like to say', 'That's really good'.

18. Reassure all of the children regardless of how well they did. Advise them not to try it at home before they have really got it down to a fine art.

19. Homework: Ask the child to:
(a) Count the critical social situations that occur each day.
(b) Make a special effort at a quarter of them, gradually increasing the percentage.
(c) Report their successes to the group.
(d) Pick a partner to rehearse both mediation and final statements with.

Test him a few times to see how he responds to staff, other patients, siblings and parents.

20. Make sure you demonstrate to other family members what your patient can do now. If any other family members have a similar problem, offer to teach them also.

21. Check the child's social skills during follow-up by watching him in the school playground during breaks.

Untoward Effects

Before a new social skill is well practised, children may get themselves into more difficulties. Suggest they wait until they have been given a stamp of approval by the staff.

Charting Requirements

Briefly describe the scenario used, your patient's more intense responses and his emotional state at the end of the session.

Teaching Parents Skills (TPS) — 'School for parents'
Technique — Second Level

Rationale

Every parent hopes that they will provide their children with a better childhood than they had. Most of the parents of child psychiatric patients feel extraordinarily guilty about the harm they have done to their children. They yearn for ways of doing things differently and undoing any harm they may have done. They have usually found the advice they were given by relatives and friends didn't work, or was impossible to carry out. They understand that the reason for their difficulties is their own personality. After repeated frustrations they give up. It may be hard to rekindle their hope and give it another try. Yet most parents learn to change a little and even a little change can go a long way.

It is our hope that every parent can become sufficiently good at parenting that they will enjoy it. For if they enjoy being a parent, then children will enjoy being children.

Unfortunately, many parents have forgotten what it was like to be a child. Though there is part of them that is still child-like, they have generally lost a child's point of view and are ignorant of child development. Without insight and an understanding of parent skills, parents tend to treat their children as they were treated. By repetition–compulsion, they tend to transact with children to recreate unsolved problems out of their own childhood. The child may represent a figure from their past with whom they try to work out a problem. Unfortunately, in doing this, they project onto the child characteristics which are not true of them.

Parents sometimes do not want to make an extra effort. They feel that they are already drained of all the energy they have, by repeated attempts to manage their children. It is hard to persuade them that the expenditure of a little extra effort now will have large dividends in their child's future. Yet if the staff can help change the parents' skills, the child will change and this will make being with him more enjoyable for the parent. The added enjoyment and success will stimulate them to put out more effort. If nothing else, the next generation will benefit.

Application

Since every parent hopes to be a better parent than their parents were, every parent can benefit from learning better parenting skills.

Measures

1. The amount of time parents spend with their children and a verbatim report of feelings.

2. Parents' report of the perception of the child — are they more objective?

3. Measures of behaviour — parents of each other, e.g. the frequency

of praise or criticism directed at children.
  4. Rates of target child behaviour.

Procedure

  1. Baseline: Make measures of the family at home prior to admission.
  2. Explanation: Emphasise that the responsibility remains with the parent.
  3. Demonstration: Parents should join ward skill training groups prior to their child's admission. They should watch staff work with another family on at least one occasion.
  4. Awareness: Parents need to be objective observers of their own children. Using a one-way mirror or video, parents should watch their own children interacting with other children. Give them specific guidelines on what things to look for.
  5. Once they have been able to comment generally, teach them to make behavioural counts. If the observations are done with two parents on two children of separate families, get them to compare notes. They may find they tend to view the other parent's child more objectively.
  6. Evening parent training seminars in objective observation and seminars in seeing the world from the child's point of view, emphasise the importance of seeing children objectively.
  7. Give special demonstrations which provide parents with an opportunity to watch the staff observing children. Staff and parents can compare notes.
  8. Continuously model objective observations, comment on the child's behaviour in the context of everyday routines sufficiently loudly so that the parent standing nearby can hear.
  9. Using seminars, special demonstrations and continuous modelling teach parents how to:
  (a) Listen to their children.
  (b) Give 'I' messages.
  (c) Avoid projection.
  (d) Work co-operatively on problems.
  (e) Respond with empathetic statements.
  (f) Provide an optimum learning environment.
  Spend time helping parents negotiate guidelines and consequences with their children. Teach parents how to reinforce adaptive and ignore maladaptive behaviour.
  10. Teach parents the necessary elements of the other techniques staff have found useful.

11. During follow-up ensure parents aren't forgetting what they have learned.

Untoward Effects

If parents have not been given sufficient understanding or practice, they will fail and tend to give up. Parents who have had some training tend to be much more difficult to train than those who have had none.

Charting Requirements

Chart measures, plus brief explanation of teaching given.

Tradition Engendering (TE)
Technique — Second Level

Rationale

Family traditions serve many purposes. Unfortunately, they tend to be discarded in favour of a family's greater flexibility and mobility. Flexibility may provide more immediate pleasure but it creates an expectation of the continuing pleasures which ultimately results in disappointment. More important, gratification can produce increasingly demanding children.

Traditions are useful because:

(i) They help families deal with major life transitions, e.g. death, moves, graduating, retiring. 'In our family the first thing we do when we move is . . .'

(ii) They are direct pointers. They indicate what behaviours are expected at certain ages or how to react in difficult circumstances. 'Once you get to 16 in our family you can . . .'

(iii) They provide anticipatory pleasure which helps children endure boredom or anxiety. 'One of the best things about Christmas is when we all sit around and play . . .'

(iv) They are stabilising. They produce a predictability to future events that diminish uncertainty and anxiety. 'The world may fall apart but I can count on my family always . . .'

(v) They engender family togetherness and promote extended families even if for brief periods. 'Grandpa and Grandma always visit at Easter.'

(vi) They foster communication between siblings, and peers, e.g. 'What are you doing at Christmas?' 'I remember when . . .'

(vii) They provide an added value to the older generation. Old people are revered because they hold the traditions and can explain the origins. 'Granny can tell such great tales of the horse and buggy days.'

Traditions can be restricting. For that reason each generation should be free occasionally to modify traditions or add to them. This technique is designed to provide a family with an opportunity to consciously examine their traditions, pick out the desired components of their regular life-style, enshrine them to a certain extent and develop new ones. A tradition is defined as a special event which has a predictably unique routine for that family. There is usually an expectation that everyone will be there and participate even if it is inconvenient.

Application

All families who have had frequent moves or have few ties with the community or have had little continuity.

Measures

1. The number of verbal exchanges divided by the number of people in the family during a randomly selected, 15-minute period of family togetherness.

2. The number of times the family refers to a past or future get-together.

3. A description of present family traditions.

4. The degree of agreement between family members when they describe what usually happens.

Procedure

1. Baseline: Take the measures on two occasions in both the home and the clinical setting.

2. Explanation: Give a full explanation to the whole family of why traditions are important. Remember to deal with the disappointments surrounding previous traditions.

3. Demonstrate: Ask another family how they went about gathering traditions.

4. Enumerate celebrations the family has or would like to observe:

   (a) Religious holidays and services.

   (b) Life events — birthdays, homecomings, past occasions.

   (c) Major transitions, e.g., passing school.

5. Assign roles to each family member, e.g. at Christmas Dad always hands out the presents.

6. Ritualise unique routines, e.g. how the family typically hangs up a child's toothbrush or where they usually go to celebrate, following a review of a child's recently obtained report card.

7. Give the family an opportunity to describe how they would like to deal with major transitions, moves etc., e.g. 'Let's pretend we're in Ottawa and it's 50° below.'

8. Role-play with staff and the family both the old and new traditions.

9. Rehearse some of these when you visit the family during follow-up.

Untoward Effects

You might pick something alien to that particular family's culture.

Charting Requirements

Measures and family interactions should be recorded.

Ward Control
Technique — Second Level

Rationale

It is very important that the ward milieu be maintained as optimally therapeutic with the minimum amount of staff effort. Too frequently staff have been so occupied in maintaining control over the children's behaviour there is insufficient time to get on with individual treatment. This results in frustrated staff and frustrated patients. If control becomes the major preoccupation, the ward is no longer therapeutic but custodial.

To avoid custodial care:

1. The ward must be sufficiently well staffed that there is the maximum amount of individual or group treatment leaving little opportunity for problems of behaviour.

2. Staff must concentrate on individual or group treatment. If there are problems of control, those problems should be left to the staff who are involved with those particular children only.

3. Staff must work on continual refinement and elaboration of treatment techniques and milieu programmes that provide for smooth ward control without much staff involvement.

4. Ward philosophy emphasises that within certain limits the child is allowed a choice of activities. This emphasises the need for each

individual to become responsible for himself in a world that provides constraints and limited alternatives.

5. Staff must make attendance at school or treatment sessions as attractive as possible. They are encouraged to play non-distracting games, e.g. draughts, during individual sessions and to end group sessions with a hand out of fruit, etc. Sweets or nuts may be available in the office for children to obtain on a non-contingent basis.

The ward has compulsory activities:

1. Attending school.
2. Most individual and group treatments. Exceptions are provided at the discretion of the therapist.
3. Group recreational activities. The optional activities are certain recreations and free time activities.

Application

All patients and siblings.

Measures

It is important to measure the child's total time in time-out and the amount of work he is accomplishing. It is mandatory to measure and graph the total time-out used on the ward each day. The graph provides very rapid feedback on ward tension and staff morale.

Procedure

Although it is hoped the children will gradually gain greater control over their own lives, many children will become anxious with greater responsibility and others will almost automatically rebel against environmental restraints. When the child does not choose to comply with the request of staff or the programmed activity, they are given a series of alternatives. These become increasingly less enjoyable to the child. At each step a choice is provided and time to choose.

1. If the child does not automatically comply with the programmed activity, request that he does so. If he does not, repeat the request once only and remind him of the alternatives and consequences.

2. Give the child two minutes to choose. Back away and give him space in which to decide on the alternatives without making the decision a power struggle.

3. If the child does not choose, spend five minutes with him discussing the conflicts and repeat the request. Give him two minutes to

choose. If he still does not choose, or if he declines in the first instance, face him with the first consequence.

4. The first consequence is that the child is force-marched to treatment (not school). If it is possible, carry out the treatment, such as psychotherapy, wherever the child is, so that he will gradually become aware of the fact that the confidential nature of the things discussed, are more appropriately dealt with in the seclusion of the therapist's office.

5. Once the child is located where the treatment is taking place, back away and give him five minutes to involve himself without being under pressure.

6. If the child does not involve himself, request that he does so, outline the alternatives and consequences and give him two minutes to choose. If he fails to choose, spend five minutes talking over his difficulty in making the choices and the conflicts surrounding those. If he still does not choose or if he declines, face him with the second consequence.

7. The second consequence is to provide him alternative work. This is preferably X number of squares of rug hooking which would, according to his age and ability, involve him for approximately 20 minutes. Point out to him that the rug once hooked, will be sold and the proceeds go towards ward outings. If he prefers rug hooking to therapy sessions or school, allow him to continue until he is thoroughly bored and tired.

8. After completing X number of squares of rug hooking (no reminders to continue working), request the child returns to school or treatment and give him two minutes to choose. If he does not choose after this, he is force-marched to the treatment situation. If he chooses not to be involved in school work or treatment, or if he declines to do the required amount of work, face him with the third consequence.

9. The third consequence is cleaning, sweeping, washing walls or windows, of the required amount that would occupy him for approximately 20 minutes. Once this is completed, request that he returns to school or treatment and if he does not, after two minutes, during which he is allowed time to choose, he is force-marched back to treatment and the above procedure repeated.

10. After 10 minutes of non-involvement at school or treatment, face him with the fourth consequence which is five minutes in the large time-out. Provide him with a cardboard carton on which to scribble or which he may tear apart in frustration and anger.

11. The above procedure is repeated each time, lengthening the

Standard Nursing Care Plan for Runaways for Child and Family Unit

Depressed or psychotic children who may be at risk to themselves or others will have a special regime.
Children who run away from the Child and Family Unit require a different treatment approach than prescribed for adult patients.
Frequently the 'running away' behaviour is what the community has asked us to deal with and formulate a treatment plan for them.

Usual Patient Problem	Expected Outcome	Chart	Nursing Action
1. HABIT — Some children have habitually run when under stress. They don't understand other options	The child will identify stressors and use alternate ways of coping	PRN	Follow-through nurse: Relief staff: For All Problems: Explain to the child the consequences of running away but no specific containment procedures are employed to prevent the runaway behaviour as this would be antithetical to treatment Implement Feelings Rehearsal Techniques Observe and record antecedent behaviour to running away Help child identify what occurs prior to their run and what his feelings were at the time, so he can learn why he runs Help him develop realistic alternatives to running away Once the child demonstrates an understanding of why he runs away and the alternative choices he has, set up a routine of consequences for the community to follow whenever this behaviour occurs When an elopement has occurred the nurse will: 1) Notify the building charge nurse and 2) Notify the physician and obtain consent for a police search
2. FEELINGS OF OVERWHELMING FEAR AND/OR ANGER — Impulsive reaction	The child will identify a variety of feelings, use a wide variety of expression for these feelings and know how to appeal for help		
3. PROVOCATION — An angry statement by the children made against the unit and for their family	The child will recognise his anger and needs and verbalise these to the adults caring for him. The adults will recognise the child's needs and and provide him with an opportunity to demonstrate positive behaviour		
4. ATTENTION-SEEKING			

Problem	Goal	PRN
5. PEER INFLUENCE — Some children who will not run alone, but will run with someone else. Other children inspire group action in order to avoid individual responsibility	The child will take responsibility for his own actions. He will evaluate the suggestions of others before he runs away. He will be less dependent on peer approval	(Sometimes the physician may give the child discretionary time to return on his own.) Most children are given half an hour to return. Small, suicidal, delirious or psychotic children are sought for immediately 3) Notify the parents and obtain a witnessed consent. Parents usually agree to an additional half hour before contacting the police 4) Assist primary care workers in giving complete description of patient to police 5) Complete an Unusual Occurrence Report 6) Document on chart details of behaviour prior to elopement
6. CONFUSION — Seriously ill or handicapped children may not understand what they are doing or what are the usual guidelines and consequences	The child may require frequent careful instructions. He may respond to lines on the floor which he is not supposed to cross	
7. FEELINGS OF LOW SELF-ESTEEM — 'I'm bad' — and feelings of fear of abandonment	The child will develop increased self-esteem and an increased sense of security in the home and on the unit	7) Document all contacts or communications made or received re. runaway Hospital and nursing administration are to be informed of all contacts and information regarding the runaway and his whereabouts On return to the unit after runaway, inform the child all unit privileges are lost for 24 hours and clothe in hospital pyjamas
8. SUICIDE — A few children are depressed or desperate enough to want to kill or harm themselves	Children this depressed require special nurturing until they have regained trust in the unit and hope in the future	

If running away becomes a continuous problem with a child, he must then earn his clothes back on a trust basis, one article at a time. The last article to be earned back are the shoes.
The decision to earn back clothes is to be a team decision involving both the primary worker and the physician.

period of time-out by five minutes.

12. The small time-out is to be used for aggressive or destructive behaviour.

13. Inter-muscular chlorpromazine is only to be used for uncontrollable rage or anxiety. It is not used to control behaviour. It is used to treat acute psychiatric turmoil.

14. There are special procedures for children who run away (see Standard Nursing Care Plan for Runaways).

Untoward Effects

Rebellious and obstreperous children will often choose to work through their major conflict with authority in the area of compliance, treatment and school. If this occurs, it may take two to three weeks before the child learns that he is making choices and that the only person he is really hurting is himself. If, however, staff become too authoritarian and do not allow the child the opportunity to choose, rebellious behaviour and non-compliance may continue. It is vitally important to know whether the child has claustrophobia, in which case, he should be isolated in his bedroom rather than the time-out room.

Charting Requirements

Each time-out must be charted, together with the reason it was used and the child's response during time-out and immediately after.

Family Counselling
Technique — Third Level

Rationale

The problem child is almost never the only problem in a family; the difficulties he experiences are both cause and effect. As stated in the second law of thermodynamics, the behaviour of one particle depends upon the behaviour of all the other particles in the same system. The child, being part of a family system, behaves in a way that is dependent upon and contributes to the behaviour of all his family members.

By seeing the family together, it is possible to obtain a more complete and objective view of family interrelationships, individual psychopathology, modes of communication, typical transactions, areas of major anxieties, family and individual strengths and behavioural contingencies. Not only is seeing the family together a benefit to more correct understanding of the child but insight is gained much more rapidly.

Interpretations may be individual, insight-oriented, group dynamic, transactional or behavioural. The therapist may quickly become a component of the dominant dynamic and be drawn into its neurosis. Family interpretative psychotherapy is more efficient. In the family context it is much easier to point out when miscommunications occur.

In family counselling, it is important to include all those within a household, including grandparents, live-in babysitter and any infants.

Application

Family counselling is applicable in almost every family. It is less useful where it might disrupt tenuous relationships or overwhelm a borderline psychotic child with anxiety or create such stress as to precipitate a psychosomatic disorder.

Measures

Write a brief description of the family history and present dynamics, transactions and behavioural contingencies. Note changes in interaction patterns and communication. Record the explanation or interpretations you give to the family.

Procedure

1. Baseline: The family should be seen in the context of their own home. If that is not possible, they should be given a particular task or game to play such as 'Aggravation' which will stimulate their usual interaction.

2. Explanation: This should include the process and the rules governing the session. The family should commit themselves to a series of interviews of a certain length. The rules include:

   (a) It is better to talk out the problem than to act it out.
   (b) Do not make any major decisions during family counselling.
   (c) Secrets between family members, apart from the parents' personal, sexual or financial concerns, are discouraged.
   (d) There must be no retaliation. The parents cannot express their anger towards a child for what he might expose within the counselling session.
   (e) Confidentiality: What is talked about in the session should not be talked about outside the session without all the others' permission.

3. Demonstration: Reassure the family while showing a videotape or a role-play of the family counselling interviews.

4. Therapists should remember that:

   (a) People cannot not communicate.

(b) Every subject is useful material.

(c) The family should express freely whatever is on their mind.

(d) The therapist should concentrate on whatever is repetitious and whatever communication provokes a high level of effect.

5. The procedure is to observe, hypothesise, clarify the hypothesis and make an interpretation. The therapist should use his/her own feelings as an indication of the emotions being dealt with, but he/she must be aware of counter-transference.

6. Do not repeatedly ask questions but rather request information, e.g. 'Tell me more about your grandfather.'

7. Discourage discounting of feelings or discrediting of observations.

8. Defend those children that are the underdogs and explain what you are doing.

9. Voice your observations, especially those that are empathetic. This helps the family feel that they are being understood.

10. When your hypothesis has been repeatedly confirmed, make an interpretation of the impulse, anxiety and defences in the genetic, economic and transference areas. In pointing out games, indicate when parent, adult or child is engaged, what are the pay-offs, and what are alternative ploys. Interpret behavioural settings and discriminative, reinforcing and punishing stimuli.

11. When interviewing, keep a rough measure of the number of times you:

(a) question;

(b) empathise;

(c) request;

(d) use an interpretative probe.

Too many questions in proportion to the others means the interview is not going well.

Untoward Effects

Strained relationships may be further strained and marriages can break up. The family may be made defensive and less inclined to communicate. Anxiety can overwhelm fragile egos.

Charting Requirements

Measures, hypothesis, interpretations given and how received.

5 SPECIFIC PROGRAMMES

Programmes

Abuse Programme
Anorexia Programme
Autism Programme
Conversion Reaction Programme
Depressed Programme

Encopretic Programme
Fire Lighters Programme
Incest Treatment Programme
School Phobia Programme
Weight Control Programme

Introduction

Having assessed the child prior to admission and having determined which of our staff or community workers, with what skills, are available, we work with the parents to construct a programme. We usually manage to enumerate the problems, identify key conflicts and decide on what techniques will be used by which staff, for how long, all at the admission conference. The following are some of the programmes we have developed. They are intended to be used as guidelines around which you will construct your own programmes with a different combination of techniques depending on the individual children and their families.

The suggested amounts of time and the staff members will vary with who is available. We have been well blessed with staff having numerous skills. In our unit everyone works hard and the workload is evenly spread. If it appears from our suggestions that one professional group is more skilled or works harder than the others, please be assured that it is not the case. They have different professional and individual skills and tend to specialise, but no skill is valued less.

Abuse Programme

Children are abused, molested and neglected for a wide variety of reasons, but there are enough common elements to the problem to enable us to design a programme. This programme outline will provide some guidance but the combination you use will depend upon the type

225

of abuse and the family constellation. The most important components of this programme are:

(1) Individuation and rebonding to ensure the parent is appropriately attached to the child as he is and not just as the parent perceives him to be.

(2) Nurturing the parents in order to give them rest and reassurance and to put them in touch once again with their own more child-like needs for care and comfort.

(3) Teaching child handling and communication skills so the parents don't feel trapped into violent or demeaning attempts at management.

(4) Helping the children work through a previous trauma so they are able to stop provoking parents into a repetition of tragedy.

It is necessary for the parents to abreact any trauma from their own childhood. A large number of abusive parents were abused themselves as children and until such time as their pain and suffering about this can be felt and heard, they cannot be free to feel and hear their child's distress. Once parents have abreacted their own childhood and the lack of nurturing given them as children, they can see what would have been 'good care' for them when they were children. This work with parents could start prior to admission of the child.

It is difficult for parents who have not been nurtured as children freely to give to or easily withhold from their own children. Neglected children who become parents tend to vacillate between being strict and punitive and being overprotective or permissive. This confuses children who are not sure how to ask or when.

A number of abusive parents rely on their children to satisfy many of their needs and to boost their self-esteem. Assist the parents in having their needs met through other avenues such as study, hobby, career or adult relationships. Some parents have not become adult and cannot respond to their children's needs because they are locked into child-like dependencies with their parents. Help them to evaluate these relationships, improve them or terminate them if necessary.

Classes in parenting techniques are given to provide understanding of child development, observation skills, communication abilities and child management techniques. These growing skills are practised on the ward. Once the parents can feel more confident about their ability to parent, they are encouraged to participate in the management and treatment of the child on the unit.

Frequently, parents' expectations are above their child's capabilities. The parents, who are soon disappointed, express their frustration in rage or criticism. Having clear, easily attained expectations makes life smooth for both parents and child. It is important for the parents to know what 'irritants' in their children's behaviour evoke unwanted, uncontrollable impulses in them. Once these 'irritants' are identified, the parents can learn adaptive ways to control their reactions.

During nurturing the parents, you should get a full and complete story of how and when the parents have mistreated their children. 'I can understand how irritating Johnny can be and I can see why you can lose your cool. Please tell me about all the things you have done which have hurt him.' Once all the details have been disclosed, the parent has nothing to hide and is much more open to insight-oriented therapy. We have found that parents are much more likely to give a complete story at the beginning of treatment, especially during nurturing when they feel rested and supported.

It is important to have the child abreact the trauma of his abuse or neglect. During the child's nurturing, you should review the abusive incidents and help the child express all the mixed feelings of fear, anger and hate. The child then must mourn the loss of the idealised parent. 'OK, Mummy shouldn't have done that, I guess she isn't the best Mum you could have. She is trying to change.' Even young children have an awareness of what they need and how they should be treated. They tend to expect their parents to be all things, to have total patience and tolerance and meet all their needs. It is important that these children hear such statements as, 'Sometimes after work Daddies are really tired and grumpy. That's when you've got to be careful not to bug him.'

Most abused children have developed conflicts which they may unconsciously attempt to solve by provoking a re-enactment of the abuse. Individual psychotherapy and Therapeutic Wrestling are necessary to free them of a compulsive repetition of the conflict.

Teach the child to identify his parents' 'red' and 'green' buttons. The 'red' buttons are behaviours such as, whining and swearing, that make parents angry and begin to lose control. The 'green' buttons are behaviours like 'please', 'thank you', picking up clothes, that make parents feel happy, warm and loving. In this manner the child learns that he has contributed to the relationship and can make things go better.

Put the child on a delayed gratification and a compliance programme in order to teach him how to wait to have his needs met and also to do what is requested of him. These two skills greatly improve the parent/

child relationship. By making the child easier to handle, his parents are more likely to want to spend time with him.

Frequently the abused child behaves in an inappropriate manner in a variety of social situations. Accordingly, give him Social Skills Training and Sensitivity Training. Once a child begins to understand his feelings and needs, give him Assertiveness Training. He needs to know how to express his anger about frustrated needs in a way people are best able to hear him.

Systematic desensitisation of child to parent, and parent to child, should occupy the main focus. This is achieved by the rebonding technique which makes extensive use of the one-way viewing mirror. Begin with individuation, so that parent and child have a clear, reasonably objective perception of each other. Once the desensitisation has been accomplished, work with the parent and child together on mutual needs identification and clarification, mutual nurturing, constructive feedback, and negotiating guidelines and consequences.

Likely Problems

 1. Difficulties with the control of emotions, child's and parent's.
 2. Child's high level of anxiety and consequently impaired learning and development.
 3. Poor self-esteem, parent's and child's.
 4. Child's oppositional, irritating behaviour.
 5. Impaired relationships, child–parent and parent–friends.
 6. Child put down by siblings and peers.
 7. Child's poor academic and social skills.
 8. Intergenerational dependencies.
 9. Family's social isolation and disadvantage.
10. Frequent shifts and changes.

Goals

1. Help parents develop greater skill in their use of discipline.
2. Assist in appropriate expression of feelings.
3. Assist with more effective relationships.
4. Help obtain satisfaction from co-operative efforts.

Key Conflicts

1. Parents' immaturity from their own deprivation and abuse.
2. Poor parent–parent and parent–child rebonding because of unresolved losses.

3. Child's propensity to provoke a re-enactment of previous trauma in an effort to solve major conflicts.

Nurturing of Child

1. Three days of rest in bed.
2. Child not included in the regular unit routines.
3. One-to-one staffing.
4. Lots of tender loving care.
5. Review his history (excellent if photo album and baby book available).
6. Build relationship between staff and child.

Individuation and Rebonding Timetable

Day 1–4	Period of separation of parent and child (length of time varies with age of child).
Day 1–3	Nurturing of child.
Day 5–7	Nuturing parent.
Day 7–8	Teach relaxation exercises to parents.
Day 9	Have the parent first describe self then the child by use of a personality rating scale. Start one-way viewing of child with the parents without sound. Allow negative verbalisation. When parents start to make some positive remarks, begin to model positive statements.
Day 10	Have the child first describe the parent and then self, using the same personality rating scale.
Day 11	Using the personality scale, staff describe their view of the parent and the child, first to the child alone, then with the parent. Introduce sound. Reinforce all positive moves and statements. Ignore negative comments.
Day 14	Introduce two-way viewing.
Day 16	Introduce two-way sound.
Day 17	Introduce supervised short visits. Keep up positive statements. Model physical affection. Assist both parent and child to show physical expressions of affection. During the time parent and child are together, help them describe first their common then different characteristics to each other.
Day 18	Short unsupervised visit and three-hour pass out together.
Day 19	Weekend pass.
Day 21	Teach assertive response to each to use when the other is

Table 5.1: Abuse Programme — Suggested Techniques

Techniques	Time	Goal	Suggested Staff
1. Abreaction	2 hr/day 1st 5 days	No difficulty remembering traumas and attached emotions less intense	Primary worker
2. Amorphous Blob	2 hr/wk	Ego identification	Primary worker
3. Assertiveness Training	2 hr/wk last 2 wks	Can deal appropriately with put-downs	Primary worker
4. Brief Insight-oriented Psychotherapy	3 hr/wk	Some insight into major conflicts	Psychiatrist
5. Compliance Training	wks 2-4	85 per cent on request	All staff
6. Delayed Gratification	3 hr/day	Time depending on age, approx. 1 min/6 min	Primary worker
7. Ego Auxiliary	Daily wks 2, 3, 4	Able to deal with stress	Primary worker
8. Family Counselling	2 hr/wk	Able to identify conflicts and communicate feelings	Social worker or registrar
9. Individuation	2 hr/wk	An awareness of parent as separate and ability to identify self	Parent and primary worker
10. Kangaroo Kort	5 hr/wk	Able to identify personal and group ambivalence and conflict	All staff
11. Limit Challenge	3 hr/wk	Can push limits on realistic assessment	Primary worker
12. Negotiating Guidelines and Consequences	2 hr/wk last 3 wks	A complete working set before discharge	Primary worker
13. Nurturing, first child then parent	3 days	Identify needs and form close relationship	Primary worker or volunteer
14. Parent Training Sessions	2 hr/wk	Parents able to understand, communication with and gently, firmly guide their children	Psychiatrist/psychologist
15. Pushing Red and Green Buttons	2 hr/wk last 3 wks	Child's awareness of how he affects parent	Primary worker
16. Relaxation Techniques	3 hr/wk	Ability to relax when under stress	Primary worker
17. Secret Disclosure	2 hr/wk last 2 wks	No important secrets that are child's business	Registrar
18. Social Skills Training	Daily	Ability to make and break social relationships	Occupational therapist
19. Therapeutic Wrestling	2 hr/wk last 2 wks	Not afraid to win, lose or stress body	Primary worker
20. Time-out	Daily as required	Extinguish irritating behaviours	All staff
21. Tradition Engendering	2 hr/wk last 2 wks	Establish two happy family traditions	Social worker

	attempting to over-engage.
Day 23	Model disengagement.
Day 25	Disengage using art as a medium.
Day 28	Disengage usirg movement as a medium.
Day 30	Encourage separate interests and activities.

Negotiating Guidelines and Consequences with Older Children

1. Identify problem areas of home management with the children.
2. Identify privileges important to the children.
3. Identify problem areas of home duties and responsibilities with parent.
4. Explain and demonstrate the negotiation procedure to both.
5. Assist by mediating in negotiating, starting with the easiest point. Keep it positive.
6. Write down guidelines and consequences.
7. Have both parent and children sign written contract. It is preferred to have all family members involved in these negotiations.
8. Try them out on trial weekends to work out any irregularities.

With younger children one staff will represent the child to work out reasonable guidelines and consequences. Young children can benefit by watching the adults negotiate.

Anorexia Programme

Though the efficacy of varying anorexia treatment programmes are hotly debated, we believe ours has been sufficiently successful with young anorexics to warrant more general use. As with the other programmes in this book, it is based on the recognition of the many intense personal and interpersonal conflicts, distorted transactions, repetitious, maladaptive behaviours and biochemical abnormalities. The usual pathogenesis includes the following history.

The child is closely attached to her parents who provide her with a great deal of pleasure and approval. In order continually to please her parents as a young child, the patient suppresses her awareness of her changing body as she reaches puberty. Often the patient has been subtly seduced by the father who wants to maintain a relationship with his daughter as a little girl. There has been a minimum amount of physical punishment or pain. When the child reaches puberty and gains weight she becomes alarmed at the prospect of becoming mature and sexually appealing to her father. Because anorexics are sufficiently self-centred to believe that their parents want them in only one form, they try to remain child-like. On the other hand, part of them wants to grow up and become mature. They become involved in an intense struggle for control centred on eating.

Eating has been a preoccupation with parents of anorexics who have been on diets themselves. As their child loses weight the parents begin to realise their lovely child could die and they begin to panic. They push eating at any price. Their child picks up their anxiety and her anxiety increases her inability to detect her inner impulses or trust her desires to eat. The general practitioner soon becomes involved. He attempts to encourage the child or hospitalises her with the emphasis on making sure she eats. Later the family may be referred to a psychiatrist.

It is important when the psychiatrist becomes involved that responsibilities are clearly delineated and critical weight levels set. If the low critical level is reached the child is quickly hospitalised. Before that happens inpatient treatment may not be necessary, but a hospital programme can be more efficient.

Although most of the major conflicts with young anorexics can be dealt with there will still be a continuing struggle for self-control. As long as the patient does not go beyond the agreed limits, it is safe to let her continue to struggle and mature. In our experience there are few patients who have gone below or above the agreed limits, although they often approach them. In time these limits can be narrowed as a patient becomes less desperate in her struggle.

We have been impressed with the frequency of these key conflicts:

(1) The parents' inability to trust themselves with expressing feelings or following their impulses. As a result they continually correct their children. Eventually these children can no longer trust their own feelings of hunger and satiation. They try to regulate their body weight by counting calories and estimating fuel consumption from the amount of daily activity.

(2) The parents have been so indulging and kindly to the children that the children have become dependent upon an almost continuous stream of approval. This makes it difficult for them to voice their opinions, to assert themselves appropriately and to endure interpersonal conflicts. These children tend to remain self-centred people, who are afraid of discomfort that they do not impose upon themselves.

(3) The parent of the opposite sex has related to their pubertal

child with a large number of innuendos with sexual overtones which make the child very conscious of her sexual self. It is a type of psychological seduction or undressing which makes the child determined to maintain a privacy of her body and of her mind. The shyness about the body makes it difficult for them to look at themselves naked and their secretiveness inhibits them from disclosing their thinking.

(4) There are some iatrogenic components whereby physicians have inadvertently reinforced the maladaptive behaviour associated with withdrawing and not eating.

The anorexic wants self-control but is afraid of disapproval. By the time she becomes unwell, she is afraid to assume self-control because she knows that she cannot handle it very well. Parents panic when the anorexic becomes very thin and the doctor is frustrated. In this situation we have found it very important to assign two responsible people to manage the treatment: one, a physician, will take over responsibility of the patient's medical condition outside certain prescribed weight limits; he will maintain the patient's weight even if it requires hospitalisation and intravenous feeding. The other person is primarily responsible for psychological therapies and will deal with the parents' guilt, co-ordinate treatment programmes and do individual psychotherapy.

Critical Components of a Treatment Programme

1. Responsibility. The areas of the patient's responsibility, the physician's responsibility and the parents' responsibility must be clearly delineated. To release pressure and struggles for control, as treatment staff, you must take firm control of most of the disputed area, especially with the parents. You will find they initially resist your taking their responsibilities, then they relax and are glad to hand over.

2. Weight. The patient is told that she has full responsibility for her own weight within certain, agreed-upon parameters. If she goes below a certain critical weight, the physician will hospitalise or medicate her and attend to her nutrition requirements. If she goes above a certain critical weight, the physician will take charge and treat her. These upper and lower limits are set with sufficiently broad limits that the patient will in all probability stay within them. The lowest limit is set approximately a kilogram below the patient's present low weight, unless the patient is medically unwell. The upper limit is established as an area of obesity, where the patient appears not to be able to control her intake. In the middle of the graph, which the patient will keep, is the ideal weight, usually 90 per cent of the average body weight, or the weight at which menstruation starts regularly.

Teach the patient to weigh herself regularly and graph her weight clearly. Make spot checks for honesty.

Don't hassle your patient about how much, when or what to eat. Starving, gorging, vomiting, etc. are all ignored unless the patient's weight goes above or below the defined limits.

Join the patient at meals and talk quietly and pleasantly to her while she is eating. Do not talk about eating. If the eating stops look away. These mild reinforcements and punishments applied to eating behaviour can gradually make it easier for your patient.

3. Body Image. Ask your patients to describe themselves indicating their idealised image; body, mind and personality.

Lie them upon a piece of paper and outline their silhouette.

Get them to superimpose their ideal image over the silhouette.

Encourage them to stand almost naked in front of the mirror and examine themselves objectively, commenting on the significance of breasts and buttocks.

Aim psychotherapy at fears of being too attractive, or becoming pregnant.

4. Sexuality. Near the beginning of the programme teach your patient the rudiments of anatomy and physiology.

Then discuss sex education, emphasising the emotions.

Deal with fears regarding menstruation and pregnancy, emphasising fears of contamination, blood, dirt, etc.

Using insight therapy and systematic desensitisation, work on anxieties regarding post-pubertal sexual attachment to father or father figures.

Help father take the initiative in diminishing his attachment to his daughter. Encourage him to become increasingly critical and mildly teasing. Teach your patient how to assert herself and retaliate appropriately.

In Social Skills Training teach your patient about dating, responding to flirtation, etc.

Help her try more attractive dressing.

Encourage her to spend time alone with an attractive boy.

Independence

Early in the treatment programme the anorexic child is engaged in psychotherapy which focuses on fear of disapproval by parents, teachers and peers. The root of this is often a childhood filled with approval for compliance, good school marks, etc.

Start systematic desensitisation to parental and teacher criticism shortly after psychotherapy begins.

To test teacher and parental reaction to growing independence, the child is encouraged to skip school. Initially this is set up by arranging a treatment appointment at a time when the child should be in school. The teacher is set up to show disapproval which gradually diminishes as the child describes her predicament.

Encourage your anorexic patient to become increasingly involved in becoming independent of parents and not feel responsible for their happiness. Show the parents ways to find gratification or joy in activities independent of their anorexic child.

Explore the child's fear of loneliness. Let her spend reasonably long periods by herself. During follow-up encourage her to go on increasingly long trips by herself and eventually to summer camp. Teach the parents to endure the anxiety from wondering if their child will starve without them.

Obsessiveness

Early in the treatment programme involve the anorexic child in corrective play therapy emphasising the use of a variety of increasingly colourful or messy media.

Encourage your patient to dress in an increasingly sloppy fashion with considerable approval from members of the staff and disapproval from parents and teachers.

Involve your patient in body painting, initially just the fingers, and then increasingly larger areas of her body. Try getting her to throw moss at members of the staff, and then mud or sand throwing, or at drawings of those she dislikes.

Let her leave a mess behind and come back later to clean up.

Assertiveness

Early in the therapy give your anorexic patient increasing amounts of Strength Bombardment. Make sure it is true and accurate.

Teach her to respond with 'I'm OK' or 'I am' statements in response to criticism or derogatory remarks. Later, begin formal training in assertion aimed at authorities, parents and peers.

Use pillow fights, arm and Indian wrestling coupled with assertive statements or grunts to help your patient gain confidence in her body and its response to aggression.

Introduce limit challenge during the second week. Encourage them to push themselves in activities where they normally wouldn't find themselves and to be comfortable when they fail. Eventually your patients should have a very clear awareness of what they can and cannot do.

Self-control

Each anorexic child must learn to listen to her own inner impulses and not be afraid of responding to them. By the end of treatment your patient should be able to tell when she is hungry or full, tired or excited. In conjunction with A & P Training teach your patient using the Listen to your Body technique.

Take your patient to a lonely beach and encourage her to shout with anger, excitement, desperation or joy in order to test her ability to let her feelings out with gusto. Then into more public places like the town square and try the same.

Encourage your patient to over-sleep, over-weep or any other activities over which she is afraid of losing control.

Using role-play and free play acting gradually get your patient to express a wide variety of body movements and emotions. You will probably find that with make-up on she becomes much more expressive. With all these techniques, the object is to get your anorexic patient to hear her own body telling her what it needs instead of responding to her parents' conflicting messages or trying to decide what she needs by calculating energy consumption and intake. She must learn to assume confident control over her inner impulses and not be afraid of what might happen as her parents have inferred.

Conflict Displacement

It is very important to help the patient express major conflicts of independence, etc. in any other area but feeding. Choose some other function that a child normally assumes control of and create a conflict. This area should be safe but sufficiently irritating to the parents that they can get into expressing their displeasure without acting.

On our unit we use bedtime for conflict displacement. It isn't unusual for us to insist a 13-year-old be in bed at 7 p.m. In their usual compliant way anorexics usually comply, at least at first. After a while

Table 5.2: Anorexia Programme — Suggested Techniques

Techniques	Time	Goal	Suggested Staff
1. Amorphous Blob	1 hr/wk	Ego identification	Primary worker
2. Anatomy and Physiology Teaching	4 hrs 1st wk	Awareness of body and how it functions	Resident (registrar)
3. Assertiveness Training	3 hr/wk	Practical responses to put-downs	Primary worker
4. Biofeedback Training	2 hr/wk last 3 wks	Able to follow one's monitors	Occupational therapist
5. Brief Insight-oriented Psychotherapy	3 hr/wk	Some insight into major conflicts	Psychiatrist
6. Body Impulse Directing and Body Painting	2 hr/wk	Unafraid to view own body objectively	Primary worker
7. Conflict Displacement	7 hr/wk	Parents' ability to divert conflict away from critical areas	Primary worker
8. Family Counselling	2 hr/wk	Able to identify conflicts and communicate feelings	Social worker
9. Feelings Rehearsal	5 hr/wk	Able to identify and express feelings	Primary worker
10. Individuation	3 hr/wk	An awareness of parent as separate, and ability to identify self	Parent and primary worker
11. Kangaroo Kort	5 hr/wk	Able to identify personal and group ambivalence and conflict	Primary worker
12. Limit Challenge	3 hr/wk	Can push limits on realistic assessment	Primary worker
13. Listen to Your Body	Daily	To recognise and trust inner urges	Primary worker
14. Medicational Modification	4 hr/wk last 2 wks	Learn how to talk self out of temptation	Primary worker
15. Messy Play	4 hr/wk	Lose fear of primitive enjoyments	Occupational therapist
16. Negotiating Guidelines	3 hr/wk	A complete working set before discharge	Primary worker
17. Psychological Testing Interpretation	6 hr in 5 wks	Realistic expectations by patients	Psychologist
18. Self-control	3 hr/wk	Able to control impulses	Primary worker
19. Sensitivity Exercises	5 x ½ hr/wk	To perceive and exchange feelings	Primary worker
20. Sex Education	3 hr/wk	Understanding of basic physiology and emotions	Intern
21. Teaching Parents Skills	1½ hr/wk	Comfortable use of management skills with all the children in the family	All staff

she will begin to object. Then some of the staff will encourage your patient to protest and those representing the parents must keep up the pressure. The patient is encouraged to object when the staff demand that she goes to bed at unreasonable times until a full-scale conflict is created.

With insight-oriented psychotherapy the patient becomes increasingly aware of her conflicts over independence. As this displacement conflict begins to resolve you can gradually start role-plays depicting the central conflict over eating.

Instruction on mental mechanisms will help your patient become aware of why her conflicts have become expressed as anorexia.

Key Conflicts

1. Self-control. Difficulty perceiving inner physical monitors and the ability to trust a response to them because the parental and social controls dominate.

2. Sexuality. A fear of becoming sexually attractive because the sexual fantasies, evoked by subtle parental seduction, might become enacted.

3. Self-centredness. A pampered, greatly approved, successful child desperately tries both to maintain her image, and break free of the trap which limits her growth, but is afraid of anger or loneliness. She spends most of her waking day thinking about herself.

Common Problems

1. Fear of hurt and dirt.
2. Distorted body image.
3. Weight loss resulting in hormonal, electrolyte and homeostatic imbalances.
4. Demanding controlling behaviour with threats to use the weapon, 'I'll just starve myself to death.'
5. Sexual conflicts confused with other inner impulses.
6. Fearful and angry parents and professionals.
7. Fear of failure, disapproval and alienation.
8. Inability to assert herself appropriately.
9. A long history of inadvertently reinforcing maladaptive non-eating behaviour.

Autism Programme

Introduction

Childhood autism is one of the greatest enigmas known to psychiatry. Although an enormous amount of research has been done attempting to determine the cause or causes, we still know very little about why such beautifully formed, bright-eyed children never develop properly. Parents are caught up in debating with themselves, over and over again, whether these children are retarded, have language difficulties or just refuse to learn. Parents have good reason to suspect that they are intelligent. Autistic children have good memories. They appear to understand speech because when not watched too carefully, these children will whisper well-formed, clearly enunciated sentences. There is no apparent anatomical, genetic or neurochemical abnormality that would easily explain such huge behavioural and intellectual deficits in normal-looking children. Whatever the parents try seems to make things worse and eventually they tend to withdraw. As a result all the parents that I have encountered feel very guilty without real cause.

Autistic children appear to have biochemical abnormalities, possibly as a result of the high level of stress that they are experiencing every day of their lives. They have been found to have high levels of serotonin which, when reduced by fenfluramine, seems to enable them to become more relaxed and inquisitive about the environment. It is important that in giving the child medication, the proper procedure is adhered to. After twenty years of clinical work and research with autistic children I am still inclined to believe that there is very little neurophysically wrong with these children but that they have auditory hyper-acuity which makes them withdraw from the environment. Because they are so withdrawn, they eventually become linguistically and intellectually retarded.

The treatment programme outlined here is one that has slowly developed over a number of years. It attempts to deal with four critical difficulties found in autistic children:

(1) Lack of social interaction.
(2) Oppositional, non-compliant and non-imitative behaviour.
(3) Fear of the world resulting in so little exploring.
(4) Lack of directed, intentional communication.

Although parts of this programme will overlap, it should proceed in the following order.

Social Contact

As staff you should gradually bring the child out of his autism to the stage of intimacy, in which a very close bond is developed with one primary care staff member. The child and his primary therapist will then go through a stage of symbiosis towards individuation. Finally the child should develop an independent identity.

When approaching an autistic child do not look directly at him. Whenever talking with the child do so with complete language and speak softly. To begin contact you should sit beside the child, then after a period of time together, gradually place your arm around him. When the child is able to accept your encircling arm, gently squeeze him for short periods. If he appears to enjoy that, try tickling him. If the child appears to enjoy a gentle tickle, sit with the child rocking and crooning, sometimes singing. The child should then begin to allow you to feed and care for him without pushing you away. You can determine how intimate the relationship is becoming by watching how the child reacts when you approach him. They should glance towards you or possibly walk towards you when you enter the room. An indication of a more intimate relationship would be if the child walks towards you when you outstretch your arms or beckon him to come. Hopefully, by this time, the child will prefer you to anyone else.

In your conversations with other staff members or the parents try not to talk about the child as if he is not there. When you want him to understand what will happen to him next, carefully explain the programme in his presence to the parents. Don't hesitate to talk with the child but talk in such a way that you don't wait for a response. Show your appreciation quietly if he does speak.

As an intimate relationship develops you should begin to allow that relationship to become more symbiotic. Allow the child to do things for you. Indicate that you miss him when he is away or withdrawn. It may be possible to ask quietly whether he missed you.

After a period of symbiotic attachment, work towards individuation by engaging in many hellos and goodbyes. In order to help the child become more aware of himself get him looking at himself in the mirror. Describe the child to himself, noting the differences between you and him. About this time add anatomy and physiology teaching. Autistic children are very interested in what goes on inside them even if they don't clearly indicate it. Allow them to listen to their own heart and bowel sounds with a stethoscope. Draw a silhouette of the child on paper and then get him to help you colour it in.

As the child's individual identity becomes increasingly clear take photographs of the child and get him to pick himself out in a group. Allow the child to watch himself on a videotape. Label his clothes, toys, etc., and use his name as often as possible. Involve him in body painting and messy play. Ask him to point to various body parts as you name them. With the individuation form, help him describe himself in relation to some other child you are treating and his parents.

Compliance

Parents, teachers and therapists find it is very difficult to teach autistic children to comply and this has been corroborated in scientific experiments. Unless one obtains a reasonably high degree of compliance it is very difficult to teach the child anything. Part of the difficulty is finding a useful, easily available reinforcer. The best ones we have found are movement, spinning or rocking, music and some foods. Even if these are not reinforcing to the child, one can usually find a preferred behaviour, the access to which is reinforcing.

In obtaining a compliant behaviour, speak quietly and request once only. Wait for 15 seconds before showing a mild interest if the child is beginning to comply. On the completion of the compliance, give the reinforcement without too much enthusiasm. It appears that children have a great conflict in allowing themselves to comply. Somehow they don't like to be detected at it. Obtain an 80 per cent compliance rate before moving on to the next step. As the child becomes increasingly compliant he should be taught to imitate and then to model.

Use the compliant technique as described in this book. Make a hierarchy of one-step behaviours (those that require only one action) according to the probability of their being completed by the child. Beginning with the highest probability behaviour, state your request, wait 15 seconds and provide the reinforcement when the child complies.

When the child is able to do the least probable, one-step behaviours in your hierarchy, begin with behaviours that require two actions. When the child is able to comply at an 80 per cent level with the least probable two-step behaviours begin to teach him to imitate. When he becomes good at imitation he will gradually develop an ability to model your behaviour without direction. Begin the imitation training with a 'do this, do that' or a 'Simon Says' game, rewarding him for increasingly close approximations of your actions. Involving the other children you are treating, you can get your patient involved in 'follow the leader' games.

When an autistic child is dressed up, he becomes less conscious of himself and more free to become part of a group activity. Dressed as a clown, an autistic child becomes better able to imitate the activities of other children. When he is good at imitation involve him in the Child Free Play Acting technique.

When modelling has been well established encourage the child in imitating non-verbal and then verbal communication. If he becomes good at this you can teach him cognitive restructuring. These, however, are much more difficult tasks and should not be attempted until the other parts of the programme — exploring and directed communication — have also been well developed.

Directed Communication

Like everybody, an autistic child cannot not communicate. He actively distorts his communication as if he is afraid to be understood. It almost seems that he is afraid to elicit verbal interchange because vocal sounds have aversive qualities. Even though the autistic child communicates so infrequently, when he does he speaks very clearly, much to the amazement of therapists and parents alike. It seems as if once he decides to communicate he has no difficulty forming the words or structuring the language.

It is important to avoid speech therapy or procedures which attempt to teach speech by imitation. Assuming that there is no damage to the child's language centre or neurophysiological speech structures, the emphasis must be on encouraging the autistic child to feel free to communicate. The therapist should be as non-directive as possible. Your best chance of success with an autistic child is stubborn, patient persistence.

Teach communication by overcoming the child's resistance to use the communication he has. Begin with reinforcing eye contact for increasingly long periods of time, then reinforce eye contact which occurs with facial movement, especially those which are expressive of some mood or desire. Once eye contact with facial movement is well established reinforce eye contact which occurs with gestures, particularly when the child points to what he wishes to obtain. Once the child is pointing you can use that behaviour to establish other communication.

Now begin reinforcing vocalisations that occur with eye contact. Because autistic children will more readily learn speech which isn't meant to communicate, do not reinforce echolalic or parrot-like speech.

It is important to talk to him as if he understands at an age-appropriate level. Help him become increasingly aware of his conflict about communicating or not communicating. You can guess at his fears and if you guess correctly you will often find there is a sudden light of understanding in his expression.

You should now begin reinforcing any vocalisation which is an approximation of a word accompanying eye contact. You will find that sometimes if you are engaged in play that really absorbs the austistic child he will speak quite clearly, almost accidentally. Be prepared quietly and subtly to reinforce him at any time he communicates directly and purposefully. One should not engage in therapy for communication as a separate activity — it should go along with many others.

If the child is able to express himself clearly, encourage him to express himself with greater feeling and with greater volume. If possible the two of you should spend time on a beach or in a field shouting at each other, even if the words are relatively simple.

Now begin a question-and-answer dialogue reinforcing the child when he answers appropriately, especially if his response is more than an answer to the question. After a dialogue is well established, encourage the child to use personal pronouns.

Finally, encourage the autistic child to use expressions with descriptions and emotions, e.g. 'My goodness what a hot day. I am feeling pooped, how about you?' 'I'm very tired.'

Exploring

One of the main reasons that autistic children are so developmentally retarded is that they spend so little time developing their intelligence with exploratory, sensory and motor activity. It almost appears that autistic children are so afraid of the environment, they cannot follow their natural inclination to poke into things.

Once the child has a reasonable identity you should encourage him to explore. Support him with your presence but don't become too involved. Begin by hiding a favourite object or sweet so that he must turn things over or poke into things to discover it.

In a warm swimming pool or in a quiet environment engage in mutual exploring, as often as possible following his lead. As the autistic child becomes increasingly bold take him to a deserted beach and allow him to explore various kinds of tactile sensations. When he is familiar with a wide variety of surfaces encourage him to explore sights, shapes and weights. Finally, encourage the child to explore a variety of sounds.

Table 5.3: Autism Programme — Suggested Techniques

Techniques	Time	Goal	Suggested Staff
1. Anatomy and Physiology Teaching	2 hr/wk first 3 wks	Aware of body and its functions	Psychiatric resident (registrar)
2. Assertiveness Training	2 hr/wk last 2 wks	Can deal appropriately with put-downs	Primary worker
3. Biofeedback Training	2 hr/wk last 3 wks	Able to follow one's monitor	Occupational therapist
4. Body Impulse Directing and Body Painting	2 hr/wk	Unafraid to view own body objectively	Primary worker
5. Compliance Training	½ hr/wk	To overcome negativism	Primary worker
6. Family Counselling	2 hr/wk	Learning how to keep priorities straight	Social worker or psychiatrist
7. Feelings Rehearsal	5 hr/wk	Able to identify and express feelings	Primary worker
8. Giving Medication	1 hr/day	Accept with little protest	Nurse or primary worker
9. Individuation	2 hr/wk	An awareness of parent as separate and ability to identify self	Parent and primary worker
10. Limit Challenge	3 hr/wk	Can push limits on realistic assessment	Primary worker
11. Play Therapy — Corrective	3 hr/wk	Understand own ambivalence	Resident (registrar)
12. Recreation Introduction	last 3 wkends	Explore the environment	Secondary worker
13. Sensitivity Exercises	daily	To perceive and exchange feelings	Occupational therapist
14. Teaching Machine Instruction	daily	Enjoys operating	Teacher

Likely Problems

1. Parent-child conflicts over autonomous activity, eating, dressing, toileting, etc.
2. Lack of appropriate school facilities.
3. No peers to model or patient playmates to interact with.
4. A confusing array of would-be helpers who wish to rescue the autistic child.
5. Frustration over the child's determined non-compliance.
6. Atavistic, sometimes damaging, maladaptive behaviours, e.g. bashing his head.
7. The child's inability to show any appreciation for the efforts of the adults or therapists.
8. The child's very confusing communication with little or no show of inner feelings.

Conversion Reaction Programme

There is considerable debate regarding the causes and the treatment of conversion reaction or abnormal illness behaviour that manifests itself in immobility. It is apparent that once the symptom is established, there are powerful forces which reinforce the maladaptive behaviour. The underlying dynamics seem to indicate that the immobility is often an expression of conflict which cannot be expressed in any other way. The family and consequently the patient have difficulty in expressing their feelings directly. They are afraid to assert themselves or decline openly because they cannot upset the system. The family transacts to maintain the integration of the system, by having one individual who represents and expresses all the turmoil that cannot be expressed and conflicts that cannot be solved. The collective concern for the child's immobility usually represents many other issues which have not been voiced. There is often a powerful social component. Conversion reactions may represent fads in school or cultures and wax or wane in frequency depending on the peer pressures.

The treatment is difficult and requires considerable consistency and patience on the part of the staff. Medical staff have a strong urge to make the child move, lest the immobility result in permanent contractures or muscle wasting. In this way, staff may be drawn into perpetuating the very conflict or the abnormal illness behaviour they are trying to correct. It is understandable why the immobile child elicits sympathy — they are usually sad, helpless and readily appear as victims

Table 5.4: Conversion Reaction Programme — Suggested Techniques

Techniques	Time	Goal	Suggested Staff
1. Amorphous Blob	2 hr/wk	Ego identification	Primary worker
2. Anatomy and Physiology Teaching	4 hrs 1st/wk	Aware of body and how it functions	Registrar
3. Assertiveness Training	2 hr/wk last 2 wks	Can deal appropriately with put-downs	Primary worker
4. Brief Insight-oriented Psychotherapy	3 hr/wk	Some insight into major conflicts	Psychiatrist
5. Conflict Displacement	7 hr/wk	Parents' ability to divert conflict away from critical areas	Primary worker
6. Ego Auxiliary	daily wks 2, 3, 4	Able to deal with stress	Primary worker
7. Family Counselling	2 hr/wk	Able to identify conflicts and communicate feelings	Social worker or registrar
8. Feelings Rehearsal	5 hr/wk	Able to identify and express feelings	Primary worker
9. Individuation	2 hr/wk	An awareness of parent as separate and ability to identify self	Parent and primary worker
10. Kangaroo Kort	5 hr/wk	Able to identify personal and group ambivalence and conflict	All staff
11. Limit Challenge	3 hr/wk	Can push limits on realistic assessment	Primary worker
12. Mediational Modification	4 hr/wk last 2 wks	Learn how to talk self out of temptation	Primary worker
13. Messy Play	4 hr/wk	Lose fear of primitive enjoyments	OT staff
14. Negotiating Guidelines and Consequences	2 hr/wk last 3 wks	A complete working set before discharge	Primary worker
15. Secret Disclosure	2 hr/wk last 2 wks	No important secrets that are child's business	Registrar
16. Sex Education	3 hr/wk	Understanding of basic physiology and emotions	Intern
17. Social Skills Training	daily	Ability to make and break social relationships	Occupational therapist
18. Therapeutic Wrestling	2 hr/wk last 2 wks	Not afraid to win, lose or stress body	Primary worker

of mean parents.

Important components of this treatment programme include the technique of conflict displacement. The young patient is gradually encouraged to work out his difficulty in expressing feelings, asserting himself or declining openly in an area totally unrelated to his particular conversion symptom. We use a lot of pressure to try and make the child go to bed early and eventually they begin protesting. For the obsessively neat child we insist they produce an unreasonable number of finger paintings each day. To feel sufficiently well integrated to allow for some agitation within the system and to be able to reinforce mobility, the family must understand the extent and origin of their conflict. The child needs plenty of opportunity to learn how to make his own decisions and to become independent in his activity even though he may hurt himself or others. This usually means placing the immobile child in a situation where he must move himself a small distance or deal with a natural consequence, e.g. wheel himself to the toilet or table.

Key Conflicts

1. Fears of independence of action and thought.
2. Difficulty expressing feelings and opinions in an open manner.
3. Instability in the family situation.

Problem Behaviours

1. Unresolved, unspoken, marital conflict.
2. The child's high levels of anxiety associated with fears of upsetting the family.
3. The child's anxiety associated with being hurt or hurting.
4. Immobility in thought and action.
5. The child's difficulties in making decisions.
6. Poor peer relationships.
7. Low levels of energy, sometimes a major depressive episode.
8. The child's poor self-esteem.
9. The child's fears of disease or pain.
10. Very distorted ideas of the causes of illnesses.

Depressed Programme

Introduction

Although professionals have not been detecting many depressed children, there is reason to believe that the incidence of depression in children is similar to that of adults. Children are genetically the same as adults; they have similar biochemistry; they are as easily stressed by life events; they experience loss as frequently and are more affected by losing those they depend upon. It appears that 30 per cent to 45 per cent of the child who experience loss of a parent become clinically depressed. If up to 50 per cent of families are breaking up, the expected incidence of depression in children is 10–15 per cent. The reasons we have not recognised many depressed children may be:

(1) Their symptoms are somewhat different, they tend to be more active and aggressive.
(2) Depressed children don't often present as attempted suicides, more often as injuries as a result of a callous disregard for their own safety.
(3) Children mask their symptoms because they don't want to upset their families.
(4) Adults tend to overlook symptoms of depression because the child's sadness evokes a sadness in them that they may be trying to avoid.
(5) Adults may not want to recognise the depression because it reminds them of the guilt they feel having caused a family break-up or a move.
(6) Professionals tend to diagnose what they can best treat and that isn't usually depression; more often it is learning disability.
(7) We still have a cultural belief that children are sufficiently resilient that they should be able to endure losses.
(8) Adults believe that because they are little people it is only a small depression.
(9) A cultural belief that childhood is a happy time.

The components of a depressed child's treatment programme include dealing with his loss, sadness, debilitation and conflicts. Almost invariably loss evokes conflict and ambivalence in the child. The child needs to be helped to complete his mourning but wherever possible lost figures should be reinstated. Children tend to become depressed when their body malfunctions, so the children with intellectual disabilities, chronic pain or chronic illnesses need those aspects properly explained to them and treated. Children who have been deprived have a deeply rooted understanding that they have been cheated and because of this they have not grown into the type of child they have some impression they might have become. This sense of being cheated results in a

Table 5.5: Depressed Programme — Suggested Techniques

Techniques	Time	Goal	Suggested Staff
1. Abreaction	5 hr/day 1st 5 days	No difficulty remembering traumas and attached emotions	Primary worker
2. Amorphous Blob	1 hr/wk	Ego identification	Primary worker
3. Anatomy and Physiology Teaching	2 hr/wk	Aware of body and its functions	Resident (registrar)
4. Body Impulse Directing	2 hr/wk	Unafraid to view own body objectively	Primary worker
5. Brief Insight-oriented Psychotherapy	3 hr/wk	Some insight into major conflicts	Psychologist or psychiatrist
6. Corrective Feedback	Daily	Self-correcting	All staff
7. Ego Auxiliary	Daily wks 2, 3, 4	Able to deal with stress	Primary worker
8. Family Counselling	2 hr/wk	Able to identify conflicts and communicate feelings	Social worker or registrar
9. Giving Medication	1 hr/day	Accept with little protest	Nurse or primary worker
10. Grief Facilitation	3 hr/wk	Able to contemplate loss without fear and little sadness	Primary worker
11. Home Maintenance Skills	2 hr/wk last 2 wks	Sense of responsibility in the home	Primary worker
12. Kangaroo Kort	5 hr/wk	Able to identify personal and group ambivalence and conflict	Duty staff
13. Limit Challenge	3 hr/wk	Can push limits on realistic assessment	Primary worker
14. Mediational Modification	4 hr/wk last 2 wks	Learn how to talk self out of temptation	Psychologist or primary worker
15. Nurturing Child	first 3 days	A greater awareness of basic needs	Primary worker
16. Parent–Child Contract	3 hrs	Whatever parents can attain	Social worker
17. Play Therapy — Interpretative	3 hr/wk	Insight into major conflicts	Occupational therapist
18. Recreation Introduction	last 3 wkends	Explore at least three new free fun places	Secondary worker
19. Saying Goodbye	1 hr/wk	Ability to let go old relationships	Primary worker
20. Secret Disclosure	2 hr/wk last 2 wks	No important secrets that are child's business	Primary worker
21. Self-esteem	2 hr/wk	A feeling of I'm OK	Registrar
22. Sensitivity Exercises	Daily	To perceive and exchange feelings	Primary worker
23. Strength Bombardment	1 hr/wk	An awareness of strengths affirmed by peers	Occupational therapist
24. Teaching Machine Instruction	Daily	Enjoys operating	Staff and patients / Teacher
25. Therapeutic Wrestling	2 hr/wk last 2 wks	Not afraid to win, lose or stress body	Primary worker

deep-seated rage that they need to deal with. Children who have been abused may become depressed because they take the anger that was expressed to them and, multiplying it, express it against themselves. Children who have been severely criticised often have very damaged self-images. Depressed children usually have little energy for school work, sports or communication. Because they have failed in these areas they have little self-confidence. They need to learn how they can succeed and please people important to them. Parents may use a lot of corporal punishment on depressed children in an effort to make them more successful and less disagreeable. These children become increasingly aggressive. They need to learn how to control their rage, assert themselves properly and how to get the best out of their parents. Wherever the child has biophysiological changes as a result of his depression these need to be treated with the appropriate chemistry. A good anti-depressant can improve a depressed child's mood so he is more tractable and pleasant to have around. Because he gets more time with parents and more approval, his self-image improves.

Key Conflicts

1. Ambivalent feelings about losses, incomplete mourning, and a persistent hope of being reunited with the lost object.
2. A poor self-image as a result of scapegoating, excessive criticism or selfgoating.
3. A persisting family constellation which inhibits the expression of feeling and suppresses the appropriate expression of assertion.

Common Problems

1. Inability to deal with criticism and teasing.
2. Few friends and awkward social skills.
3. Poor self-image, ideas of hurting or killing himself.
4. Fears regarding the loss of present or future relationships.
5. Diminished psychic energy, seldom tries anything new.
6. Sad mood, irritable, isolated.
7. Inability to obtain affection with pleasing expressions.
8. Parents' inability to recognise sadness in child.
9. Parents' tendency to use excessive punishment or criticism.
10. Fewer social interests, declining group participation.
11. Poor school performance, difficulty in completing school work.
12. Psychological manifestations of disturbed neurohumoral rhythms; e.g. sleep loss, poor appetite, biochemical changes.

13. A depressing home environment.
14. Frightening dreams.

Treatment

Because we are so pragmatic, we use any technique in any combination (within the bounds of good ethics) that works best. Since the best evidence appears to indicate depression is on a continuum, we don't try very hard to separate out subtypes in order to decide which ones we treat with psychotherapy and which ones with antidepressants. We use biochemicals to help treat a child's depression when it appears from symptoms of biorhythms, or physiological change or from biochemical abnormalities, the depression has affected his body's ability to maintain its adaptive mechanisms. We have found tricyclics, tetracyclics and linoleic acid very useful.

The child's depression causes family turmoil but can itself be the result of family disturbances and often it is not possible to determine which came first. We have found it is important first to change the child's self-image and hopelessness. Once his mood improves the whole family tends to brighten up.

Encopretic Programme

Encopresis is the symptom of fecal soiling past the fourth birthday. It is defined as repeated, involuntary passage of stools into clothing or other inappropriate places without the presence of any organic causes to explain the symptom. All possible organic causes should be investigated prior to initiating this programme.

In encopresis the mother/child relationship is believed to be crucial. The mother is thought to be too coercive or permissive or both in her toilet training of the child. This may set up an ongoing struggle between mother and child as to when, where and if the child will comply, particularly by defecating the amount when and where the parent indicates. If there is a struggle for autonomy the child is left with a feeling of shame and doubt surrounding more issues than just the soiling. Parents become increasingly angry at the child's growing negativism. Some children with neuro-developmental problems and poor co-ordination are slow in developing bowel control which may initiate a grievance between the mother and child.

The child who fails to attain bowel control soon suffers hostile feelings from one or more family members. He may be ridiculed by peers and alienated from teachers. The child's awareness may become blunted to the effects of the symptom on others, but their negative attitude still affects his self-image. Many encopretic children seem to lack the sensory clues as to when they need to defecate. They have shut themselves off from natural feedback mechanisms, bodily and interpersonal, that would motivate and assist them in modifying their behaviour.

Soiling seems to be related to the child's inability to retain or let go of strong emotions that are bound with conflicts. Frequently this is anger. The encopretic child often does not understand his strong emotions and is fearful of his impulses. His passive compliance tends to make his parents believe that this child is wilfully disobedient.

Mothers of encopretic children are frequently depressed, and dissatisfied with their marriages and maternal roles. Her children find her emotionally remote. Fathers tend to be critical, emotionally distant, and absent physically or psychologically. There is some debate over whether these emotional responses in the parents are cause or effect.

Key Conflicts

1. Autonomy. 'May I and can I control myself?'

2. Hostility. 'I would like to shit on them (figuratively speaking), but they will get really mad.'

3. Parental Distrust. 'If I'm not careful with my feelings anything might happen. I must make sure Johnny learns to control himself.'

Likely Problems

1. Negativism: 'I won't and you can't make me.'
2. Hostility: usually expressed indirectly; swearing, breakages, writing on walls.
3. Non-compliance: usually less than the parents estimate.
4. Inability to express feelings.
5. Both child and parents' poor self-image.
6. Inability to deal with teasing, rejection.
7. Very little parental insight.
8. Frequent criticism, coercion or severe discipline by parents, or grandparents.
9. Parental conflict over discipline.
10. Parents' inability to enjoy playing with their children.
11. Little expression of warmth or approval in the family.

Table 5.6: Encopretic Programme — Suggested Techniques

Techniques	Time	Goal	Suggested Staff
1. Amorphous Blob	1 hr/wk	Ego identification	Primary worker
2. Anatomy and Physiology Teaching	4 hrs 1st/wk	Aware of body and its functions	Resident (registrar)
3. Assertiveness Training	2 hr/wk	Can deal appropriately with put-downs	Primary worker
4. Brief Insight-oriented Psychotherapy	3 hr/wk	Some insight into major conflicts	Psychiatrist
5. Compliance Training	5 hr/wk	85 per cent on request	All staff
6. Conflict Displacement	7 hr/wk	Parents' ability to divert conflict away from critical areas	Primary worker
7. Conjoint Marital Counselling	2 hr/wk	A working marital relationship	Psychologist
8. Family Counselling	2 hr/wk	Able to identify conflicts and communicate feelings	Social worker or registrar
9. Feelings Rehearsal	5 hr/wk	Able to identify and express feelings	Primary worker
10. Individuation	3 hr/wk	An awareness of parent as separate and ability to identify self	Parent and primary worker
11. Messy Play	4 hr/wk	Lose fear of primitive enjoyments	Occupational therapist
12. Negotiating Guidelines and Consequences	3 hr/wk	A complete working set before discharge	Primary worker
13. Nurturing (limited)	1st day	A greater awareness of needs	Primary staff
14. Relaxation Training	3 hr/wk	Ability to relax when under stress	Primary worker
15. Self-control	3 hr/wk	Able to control impulses	Primary worker
16. Self-esteem	2 hr/wk	A feeling of I'm OK	Primary worker
17. Social Skills Training	Daily	Ability to make and break social relationships	Occupational therapist
18. Strength Bombardment	1 hr/wk	An awareness of strengths affirmed by peers	Staff and patients
19. Teaching Parents Skills	1½ hr/wk	Comfortable use of management skills with all the children in the family	All staff

Treatment

Establish an environment where the child can be in touch with internal and external feedback in relation to his behaviour. This is accomplished by a selection of the techniques listed in Table 5.6 to meet his individual needs, in order to improve his self-image and learn self-control. The child is also put on an encopretic regime as follows:

1. Prepare a morning and bedtime hygiene schedule which includes five minutes of sitting on the toilet after breakfast and supper. This routine should be taped inside the closet door. While the child sits, entertain him with stories, jokes, etc., so his sphincter can relax and his bowels contract.

2. Encourage the child to show all bowel movements to staff. Staff should reinforce all bowel movements in the toilet (verbally, happy faces, token, milkshake made with fecal expanders, etc.). This reinforcement is noted on a chart.

3. Collect all underwear and do a pants count each shift. If the child soils, he is to clean himself up properly before he gets more clean underwear. No other negative consequence for soiling.

4. The child to have a bath every evening.

5. Child's diet should be high in roughage.

6. Chart antecedent events for all bowel movements (in toilet and elsewhere).

Individuation with one of the parents, marital therapy and communication enhancement are frequently necessary to provide a warmer family relationship. Teach parents each control and how to express their anger appropriately.

Assertiveness training and social skills development assist the child to repair his previous poor peer relationship.

Fire Lighters Programme

The symptom of fire setting is both dangerous and alarming to the community. It should be treated seriously whether the cause is lack of education, curiosity or individual psychopathology. Fire lighting may represent a form of hostility engendered by frustrations at home or school coupled with sexual arousal. It may become a habitual behaviour. It may be a form of excitement more or less sanctioned by the child's peers or subculture. This programme concentrates on conditioned inhibition but also uses dynamic interpretative and reinforcing techniques. Fire setting is often associated with enuresis in those children who are more interested in seeing the fire extinguished. Those children who are more interested in seeing the fire burn people are among the most aggressive and may also be cruel to animals. The child's hostility appears to come from three sources: frustration of desire for affection or approval; excessive or cruel punishment by parents; strong sexual urges stimulated by parents.

Fire setting in children is usually considered as: (1) an aggressive act aimed at some member of the family who refused to love them or was a rival to them; (2) normal fascination and investigation that is being ignored or inadequately handled by parents or caring adults; (3) early symptoms of pyromania. By far the majority of children that we see fall into the first two categories but since child psychiatry is a preventive field for adult psychiatry, we must review the symptoms of pyromania and as we see indications of them in our children, we build up their ego strengths in these areas.

Pyromania is a reoccurring failure to resist the impulse to set fires. There is an intense fascination with the setting of fires and seeing fires burn. There is sometimes a tremendous power associated with the extinguishing of fires. Prior to the setting of the fire there is a build-up of tension and once the fire is underway the individual experiences intense pleasure or release. Persons with pyromania frequently have histories of early rejection, severe deprivation, castration threats and accumulated rage over frustration caused by a sense of social, physical and sexual inferiority.

Society as a whole feels tremendous anger and fear over the death and destruction caused by fire. When children set fires they have these feelings projected towards them. This may cause a concerned or an overprotective response from parents which may at times be reinforcing to the behaviour and always helps reinforce a negative self-concept.

Key Conflicts

1. Fear of the expression of aggression.
2. Sexual identity and potency.
3. Need for warmth, attention and contact from parents and approval from peers.

Likely Problems

1. Parents critical and controlling.
2. Excessive discipline.

Table 5.7: Fire Lighters Programme – Suggested Techniques

Techniques	Time	Goal	Suggested Staff
1. Amorphous Blob	1 hr/wk	Ego identification	Primary worker
2. Assertiveness Training	3 hr/wk	Can deal appropriately with put-downs	Primary worker
3. Brief Insight-oriented Psychotherapy	3 hr/wk	Awareness of ambivalence and roots of conflicts	Registrar
4. Family Counselling	3 hr/wk	Communication skills and insight	Social worker
5. Feelings Rehearsal	2 hr/wk	Able to identify and express feelings	Primary worker
6. Kangaroo Kort	5 hr/wk	Able to identify personal and group ambivalence and conflict	All staff
7. Limit Challenge	½ hr/day	To know what is possible	Primary staff
8. Parent Counselling	2 hr/wk	Able to resolve conflict of control and aggression	Social worker
9. Self-control	2 hr/wk	Able to control impulses	Primary worker
10. Sensitivity Exercises	5 x ½ hr/wk	To perceive and exchange feelings	Occupational therapist
11. Sex Education	2 hr/wk	Understanding of basic physiology and emotions	Intern
12. Social Skills Training	Daily	Ability to make and break social relationships	Occupational therapist
13. Teaching Parents Skills	½ hr/day	Knowledge of child development	Consulting staff
14. Therapeutic Wrestling	1 hr/wk	Not afraid to win, lose or stress body	Primary worker

3. Parents' inability to express affection.
4. Child's poor self-image.
5. Child's inability to assert himself.
6. Child's lack of social skills.
7. Child's conflicts, own sexual identity and appropriate expressions of sexual interest.
8. Child's passive aggressive non-compliance.
9. Child's high level of preoccupation with inner conflicts and poor school performance.

Treatment

1. Start to explore with child any dreams or feelings about fire. Have him draw picture of fires and talk about dangers of fire. Discussion should include what gets burned, who gets burnt, anyone rescued and by whom. Ask which is more fun, to start fires or put them out.
2. Arrange a visit to the fire brigade and have a fireman talk to him in a very serious authoritative way about fires, the damage they do, that they make firemen angry, people get hurt, people die. Show him pictures of fires and the effects of fire. A staff member is to be with the child during this time but not to say anything until after presentation. The fireman should be very stern. (Until the fire brigade understands what you want in the presentation it is wise to meet with the fireman before the session to explain your needs.) Some pictures and films are too frightening. If the child is too sensitive or is having difficulty with reality testing, visit the fire chief before and select pictures to be shown and ask for a modified programme. If the fire chief demands a promise from the child not to set any fires or play with matches do not visit the fire station until the fire lighting sessions are completed. After the fire station visit there should be a debriefing process and talk about making a new start, forgiving and forgetting. The parents need to participate in a forgiving and forgetting session with staff prior to discharge. If the child has set damaging fires, work out a programme of restitution with the child, his parents and any victims.
3. After the visit to the fire station, spend time with the child drawing, painting and discussing fires.
4. Arrange a visit to a burnt-out home. Walk around the building. Talk about how it might have started and what and who might have been hurt or killed. Use support play to draw out more feelings and conflicts. Ask the child which is more fun, setting fires or putting them out and why.
5. To extinguish a habitual tendency to light fires requires great patience.

Buy with the child's own money, candles, matches and obtain a needle-less syringe.

(a) Light a candle and let the child put out the fire. Do this again, and again, until the child is totally wearied or bored with the process. Once or twice, you should let the match burn down and yell for the child to save you from burning your fingers (dramatise this part). Then get the child to put out the fire with water and syringe. Lead into a discussion about who gets hurt in fires (e.g. family, children, animals). Interpret conflicts and discuss controlling anger. This should be done for 2–3 sessions.

(b) Now get the child to light the candle after you strike the match for him. Let the child know what it is like to come close to burning himself and then you save him. Do not let the child strike the match when he is begging to. Wait until there are no more requests and then suggest it randomly. Use the opportunity to discuss the control of aggressive feelings. Make two sessions of this step. Have the child end-lessly light a match and candle. The staff will put it out by water and syringe. Immediately light again and again and again until the child is thoroughly tired of the process. (This takes at least half an hour or longer, with the child eventually begging to stop. This should be done for 3–4 sessions.)

6. Show a film of a forest fire to all the children on the unit. Discuss the effects on plants and animals in the environment.

Incest Treatment Programme

No one knows how common incest is but there is good evidence that as traditional family roles become confused, there is an increasing incidence of incest. Incest is more likely to take place between children and their step-parents, partly because the ancient taboo which restrains fathers and their children from having sexual relations does not seem to apply as strongly to step-parents. Although some professionals are calling for increasing vigilance and stiffer penalties, it appears that the victim–aggressor model does not adequately explain the complicated interrelationship. In fact, it is probably more accurate to think of a victim and a victim. This makes it difficult for the professional, who, on the one hand, has a strong desire to protect the child and even a strong sense of justice, but also has to deal with a need to understand the conflicts both in the child and in the adult. Invariably they end up with a feeling of compassion for both and become aware of the fact that it is unlikely one sex is more evil than the other. There is good evidence to suggest that the real tragedy lies in repetition–compulsion. Many incest victims tend to become involved in or repeatedly invite unpleasant sexual relationships. Children who have been involved in incest tend to become the parents of children who are involved in incest.

The trauma of incest creates a conflict because in nearly every instance the experience creates mixed emotions. Because of the intensity of the mixed emotions, the conflict is deeply fixed. Although a child experiences mostly fear, pain and disgust, there is some pleasure derived from the special treatment given. There are some moments of tenderness and affection that might not otherwise occur. The conflicts create questions that the child keeps asking her or himself:* 'Why, how, will it happen again, what's wrong with me, why did I let it happen and why didn't my mother protect me?' For those children who obtained more enjoyment an additional question is: 'Should I do it again?'

Children know basically what they need. That knowledge stems from an intuitive awareness of what they might become. The rage at being abused or deprived stems from an understanding that that abuse and deprivation will keep them from becoming what they may have become. Children are easily seduced because in looking for their basic needs, they must believe that the parent has their best interest at heart. They cannot believe the parents would take advantage of them. When the parent promises them something good they generally believe it, even if previous experience has taught them the parent will abuse them.

The conflicts use energy. The body, because it is a homeostatic organism designed to conserve energy, must resolve the conflicts. The conflicts may be resolved by private thought or by talking to someone. Unfortunately, the most commonly used method is to restage and replay the original conflict.

The real tragedy of incest is the propensity of a child to re-enact the problem in order to resolve the conflict. At first the child reluctantly becomes involved but may become increasingly co-operative or even seductive. It appears that once the child has been a victim it is easier to become a victim in the future. Thus the child may become an adult who is continually asking, 'Why does it keep happening to me?' If the history of the individual or of people, including nations, is to change,

---

* Incest victims can be either sex but since they are usually female, 'she' will be used to designate all children.

the victim and the aggressor must face each other. They need to change their transaction in such a way that neither will have to repeat the experience in order to learn from it.

The difficulties of incest victims in adult life are those in trusting, relating and sexual and marital conflict. Since incest tends to recur in families, many of the techniques used for the child can apply to the parents in treatment equally well. There are no shortcuts. The process is painful but must be completed if the individual is not to be hung up at a certain stage. If they become hung up, their behaviour becomes stereotyped and typical of that phase of the process. Parents and children need support as they are encouraged to go through each aspect of this progression.

These stages are not invariant. Sometimes people are in more than one phase at a time. However, it appears that the usual order flows from 1 to 6 below.

1. Recognise the Situation

(a) First encourage the patient to voice then answer these questions. If she hasn't already done so, she begins to see how she has been a victim and it raises more questions. 'What's been happening to me? Why does it keep happening? There's got to be a reason, it just isn't right.'

(b) It is important for the child and parent to recognise that they are a victim and that there is a continuity between the last incident and all those preceding it. It is important to get a complete history. 'I'm not surprised to find out it happened to me, my daughter and my mother.'

(c) The victim should be encouraged to express the full extent of her helplessness, abhorrence and disgust. 'It was awful. I hate him and I hate myself.'

If the individual gets hung up at the recognition stage, they become people who are continually appealing for help and don't know how best to obtain it. 'Somebody please help me. Please don't let it happen again. I feel so helpless.' They tend to be dependent, multi-problem people who search from one agency to the next looking for some type of help.

2. Protest

(a) At this stage the child and parent must be encouraged to explore their angry feelings and determination to change. 'I was a victim but I am not going to be a victim any more. I have been a victim too often. Enough is enough. I have got to solve this problem.'

(b) Protest is then directed at whoever made the child a victim. This means as clearly as possible, visualising that person (using gestalt or role-play) to make the protest as real and direct as possible. 'At last I have a chance to say what I think of you, you dirty bastard.'

(c) A strong protest may be directed at society, particularly police, the opposite sex, law-makers, judges, etc.

Support groups are often stuck at this stage of their incest resolution. They are enraged, conceive of the problem mainly as a power struggle and may become punitive. Although there is considerable help for incest survivors in becoming part of a group, the group may prolong the incest resolution by encouraging them to stay at one stage.

(d) The child is encouraged to protest against that parent who should have protected her when she was most vulnerable. 'Why Mummy? Why didn't you stop him? Dammit, you should have!'

3. Grapple with Guilt

(a) The child and parent must begin to recognise their contribution to the problem, the times that they have been somewhat seductive or willing or at least not protesting as much as they could. 'I know I was frightened but I could have said no. I guess part of me was letting it happen, but after all I was only a child. Why didn't I say no, what's the matter with me?' People at this stage tend to be angry with themselves, may get depressed and possibly suicidal. If not depressed they appear to be puzzled, questioning people who are eagerly attending meetings, reading books and trying to find out what happened. If this stage resolves it becomes possible for them to look at the problem from the other's point of view.

(b) The parent and the child must begin examining the reasons why others who are party to the incest problem become involved. This means they have to begin seeing the aggressor as a victim also. 'There must be something wrong with him but I wonder what and why? He must have had a terrible childhood if all those things really happened.'

(c) The child must begin re-evaluating her anger and begin recognising that almost everyone involved was a victim in some sense. It is pointless to be angry at any one person, and more reasonable to be furious at the circumstances. 'It isn't right, the whole situation was sick, sick, sick.' People stuck at this phase tend to be those who are eager to change society because it is so damaging to children.

4. Deal with Despair

(a) The child and parent need to examine what they expected in their parent–child relationship and what they actually received. They must become aware of how little they obtained of those things that are required for normal nurture and development. 'I never had a decent childhood and now it's too late. Surely there was someone somewhere who could have loved me properly, but I guess not. I can't believe that my parents could have treated a kid this way.' People stuck at this stage tend to become bitter, cynical and lonely. If they are parents they give grudgingly to their children.

(b) The victims must begin to understand how the lack of the essential ingredients from their childhood has distorted the developments of their mind and body. 'I guess I went along with it because I was looking for something, affection, tenderness. I don't know what. If only I had had a decent childhood I might have become an artist.'

(c) They will need to recognise how there are limited possibilities now or in the future of getting what they needed. 'I would like a proper parenting but it's pointless to keep looking for the parents I wished I had.'

(d) They will need to say goodbye to their idealised self, the person they might have been, had they not been cheated of a reasonable childhood. 'I might have been really good at art but I am what I am and that isn't so bad.'

People who get stuck in the despair phase tend to be less depressed then they are apathetic. Some young people are thrill-seeking in an effort to overcome the feeling of despair.

5. Re-evaluate Relationship

(a) The child and parent will have scrutinised their present relationship to determine what are they expecting, what are the chances of getting what they want and whom they can trust. 'I don't think this guy I go out with can ever give me what I need. I don't know why I keep going out with this person.'

(b) The victims will have to evaluate what they are prepared to give, what they are expecting to receive and what they are prepared not to give in any present or future relationships. 'I'm capable of some loving but I'm never going to let anyone treat me like that again. Maybe if I stop expecting so much I will be able to start giving.'

People stuck at the re-evaluation phase tend to be those who are continually questioning the motives of people they associate with and are sometimes not very trusting, even when they are able to relate fairly well.

Table 5.8: Incest Treatment Programme — Suggested Techniques

Techniques	Time	Goal	Suggested Staff
1. Abreaction	2 hr/day 1st 5 days	No difficulty remembering traumas and attached emotions less intense	Primary worker
2. Amorphous Blob	1 hr/wk	Ego identification	Primary worker
3. Anatomy and Physiology Teaching	2 hr/wk	Aware of body and its functions	Resident (registrar)
4. Assertiveness Training	2 hr/wk	Can deal appropriately with put-downs	Primary worker
5. Body Impulse Directing	2 hr/wk	Unafraid to view own body objectively	Primary worker
6. Compliance Training	wks 2–4	85 per cent on request	All staff
7. Delayed Gratification	3 hr/day	Time depending on age, approx. 1 min/6 min	Primary worker
8. Ego Auxiliary	Daily wks 2, 3, 4	Able to deal with stress	Primary worker
9. Family Counselling	2 hr/wk	Able to identify conflicts and communicate feelings	Social worker or registrar
10. Feelings Rehearsal	5 hr/wk	Able to identify and express feelings	Primary worker
11. Individuation	2 hr/wk	An awareness of parent as separate and ability to identify self	Parent and primary worker
12. Mediational Modification	4 hr/wk last 2 wks	Learn how to talk self out of temptation	Primary worker
13. Name Change	3 hr/wk	Feel comfortable with new name and identity	Primary worker
14. Nurturing Child	first 3 days	A greater awareness of needs	Primary staff
15. Play Therapy – Interpretative	3 hr/wk	Insight into major conflicts	Occupational therapist
16. Recreational Introduction	last 3 wkends	Explore at least three new free fun places	Secondary worker
17. Self-esteem	2 hr/wk	A feeling of I'm OK	Primary worker
18. Sex Education	3 hr/wk	Understanding of basic physiology and emotions	Intern
19. Tradition Engendering	2 hr/wk last 2 wks	Establish two happy family traditions	Social worker

6. Reconciliation and Reconstruction

(a) The victim will have to face her abuser. In doing so she should give and then seek an apology. She should suggest restitution, a symbolic payment for a very personal crime. 'You must realise what a terrible thing you did to me. You should pay for it by buying that piano you kept promising. I made it too easy for you, I maybe even have led you on. I'm sorry for my part. I want to hear you say that you're sorry too.'

(b) She should begin to re-establish relationships, old and new, as a person free of the old hang-ups. She will need to be taught how to say hello and goodbye in an adult or appropriately child-like way. 'Hello Mr X. I'm flattered by your attention but I don't think this relationship will work.'

(c) The aggressor by paying is helped out of his guilt. The victims, with an apology and a symbolic payment, find it easier to forgive everybody, including themselves involved. They may want to smash their symbolic payment but they may also want to use it for constructive purposes. The parent must reaffirm the role as a parent being careful to acknowledge:

(i)   the need for privacy, space, body and mind;
(ii) the distinct roles of children and adults;
(iii) the taboos that restrain sexual incursions during times when rational responses are not readily available. 'I can see how different I must be towards my children. I'm going to start now, so help me God';
(iv) the child has learned what her real needs are, what she's yearning for and some techniques of how to and how not to get these needs met.

Key Conflicts

1. Blurring of parent–child role, who cares for whom, who protects whom.
2. The loss of ego boundaries, restraining taboos and privacy.
3. The repetition–compulsion of conflicts from confused feelings and ambivalent impulses.

Problem Behaviours

1. Inhibited expression of feelings.
2. Dislike of male teachers.
3. Distrust of all men.
4. Inappropriate dressing and/or provocative behaviour.

5. Inability to concentrate in school — high level of anxiety.
6. Feared by peers.
7. Strong mixed feelings to parents — disobedient.
8. Disregard for manners and personal hygiene.
9. Intense sibling rivalry.
10. Immature parents.
11. Low self-esteem.

School Phobia Programme

School phobia or school refusal is usually a variety of anxiety neuroses which result in the child's not being able to leave home or cope with life at school. There is seldom one anxiety responsible for the child's school refusal but rather a series of small stresses. The final refusal is triggered by stress such as moving to a new school, a change of teacher, a peer moving away, poor performance in a test, menarche, death, accident or illness in the family, beatings by peers, hazing or severe discipline. Generally, these children are emotionally immature and have a mutually over-dependent relationship with their mother. There is often a passive or absent father.

Closer observation of some adolescent truancy will reveal an actual school phobia with one of the precipitating factors being school diffi- culties or a fear of revealing incompetencies generally disguised as disinterest.

School phobic children require complete IQ and educational assess- ment to determine the presence of learning or perceptual problems. Remedial programmes are to be instituted immediately. Detailed fine and gross motor assessment is necessary to discover areas where the child needs development-structured programmes to assist skill growth in these areas.

Social skills training groups assist with peer relationship and Amor- phous Blob, Feelings Rehearsal and Assertiveness Training assist the development of a stronger self-concept.

The child and the mother need to be involved in the Individuation Technique. This technique should be supported by marital therapy and self-development for the mother as well as relationship-building with the father and child.

If the child has developed somatic symptoms which disappear once the threat of school has been removed, the parents need some help in accepting that the child is not malingering. The child in this instance will require A & P Teaching and Relaxation Training.

The child is required to attend the unit classroom. This may be gradual or as immediate an introduction as appears possible. A gradual introduction could be based on half-hour to one hour segments which build up to a full school day.

The child is given Systematic Desensitisation to single phobias and then Systematic Desensitisation to the school situation. Once the child has been able to visit school in his imagination without undue anxiety, then staff should start practical retraining with him.

A sample of practical retraining follows. All of these are done with the primary worker, secondary worker, or parent.

1. Drive past a school.
2. Walk around an empty school.
3. Drive past the child's school.
4. Walk around the child's school when it is empty.
5. Walk in the halls of the school when it is empty.
6. Visit his empty classroom.
7. Have a meeting in the classroom with the teacher.
8. Walk in halls when school is in attendance and talk to principal.
9. Visit the classroom on an afternoon of pleasant school time.
10. Go to school for the whole day.
11. Get self to school on own from unit after route finding.
12. Get self home from school on own.

Each of these steps is handled and timed individually with each child. Feelings, fears and alternative behaviours are discussed with the child. Levels of the child's anxiety are constantly monitored by staff. Whenever the anxiety levels rise too high, then staff encourage the child to use his 'magic word' to assist in relaxation. The child should be reintegrated into his own school by the beginning of the fifth week of the programme.

Sometimes reintroduction into the classroom is assisted by staff's going into the classroom with the child, but the child may feel this is too embarrassing. His opinion in this matter should be respected. An alternative approach would be to set up a 'buddy system' with the child and one of his classmates. Again, the child is to assess if this would be helpful.

The role of friends, school counsellor and teacher is important in maintaining the child's attendance. Therefore, staff and unit teacher spend time with him building this relationship and assisting with any difficulties he may have after discharge.

Table 5.9: School Phobia Programme — Suggested Techniques

Techniques	Time	Goal	Suggested Staff
1. Amorphous Blob	1 hr/wk	Ego identification	Primary worker
2. Anatomy and Physiology Teaching	2 hr/wk	Aware of body and its functions	Resident (registrar)
3. Assertiveness Training	2 x 1 hr/wk	Can deal appropriately with put-downs	Primary worker
4. Brief Insight-oriented Psychotherapy	3 hr/wk	Some insight into major conflicts	Psychiatrist
5. Conjoint Marital Counselling	2 hr/wk	A working marital relationship	Psychologist
6. Ego Auxiliary	6 hr/wk for 2 wks	Able to deal with stress	Primary worker
7. Family Counselling	2 hr/wk	Able to identify conflicts and communicate feelings	Social worker or registrar
8. Feelings Rehearsal	3 hr/wk	Able to identify and express feelings	Primary worker
9. Individuation	4 hr/wk	An awareness of parent as separate and ability to identify self	Parent and primary worker
10. Limit Challenge	3 hr/wk	Can push limits on realistic assessment	Primary worker
11. Messy Play and Body Painting	2 hr/wk	Lose fear of primitive enjoyments	Occupational therapist
12. Negotiating Guidelines and Consequences	2 hr/wk last 3 wks	A complete working set before discharge	Primary worker
13. Psychological Testing Interpretation	4 hrs	Realistic expectations by parents	Psychiatrist
14. Sex Education	2 hr/wk	Understanding of basic physiology and emotions	Intern
15. Social Skills Training	1 hr/wk	Ability to make and break social relationships	Occupational therapist
16. Systematic Desensitisation	3 hr/wk last 3 wks	Able to approach most fears without anxiety	Primary worker

Key Conflicts

1. Unable to separate from parent and be happily individual.
2. Afraid of own impulses and ambivalent wishes of parent.
3. Unable to relate comfortably with others.

Likely Problems

1. Fear of separating from parent and being independent.
2. Confused about identity, similarities with parent.
3. Afraid of own aggressive feelings.
4. Unable to deal with real or imagined put-downs.
5. Afraid to be messy, untidy or make mistakes.
6. Inordinate desire for approval.
7. Confused about sexual changes and impulses.
8. Parental immaturity and poor communication.
9. Inconsistent family guidelines and/or consequences.
10. Unresolved losses.
11. Parent's heavy reliance on the child for security and gratification.
12. Child's unfamiliarity with own body functions.
13. Poor self-image.

Weight Control Programme

Under normal circumstances the appetite centre of children will regulate their calorie intake according to their calorie expenditure. Their body can accurately tell them not only how much they need to eat but what types of food are good for them. Unfortunately, many parents can't believe this. They think they know better than the child what he needs and when. The net effect of parents who continually admonish their children with, 'Now Johnny, you must finish your carrots before you can have any ice cream', is twofold. It makes the child distrust his own inner perceptions of what he needs and it makes him want ice cream more than carrots. If Johnny cannot trust his hunger centre to guide him, he will have to count calories to monitor his intake and try to estimate energy consumption from the amount of work he does. This is bound to result in conflict as he realises the impossibility of the task. He may try to ease the tension by eating because eating is a common form of relaxation.

If Johnny is brought up in a family that cannot demonstrate affection for each other, Johnny is bound to hunger for it. If the parents can only nurture their children with things to eat, Johnny soon learns that eating his mother's good food is the way he will be loved by her. When he becomes overweight he feels embarrassed and shy. Since he gets little approval from his peers and scoldings from most adults, Johnny becomes more dependent on his mother. In their anxiety his parents now try even harder to regulate his eating habits. To the extent he trusts his parents he will distrust himself. Yet there is something inside him that tells Johnny he should be in control of his body. He resents his parents trying to control his appetite but he cannot trust himself. He may become depressed because of his frustration and anger. He then begins to stuff himself as the displaced object of his hostility. But the fatter he gets the more lonely he becomes. If only someone would show him how to trust and control himself.

This programme is designed to substitute knowledge of weight for the supressed hunger and satiation responses until they come back into play. The first hurdle is to teach the child to be open and honest about his weight. As the child becomes increasingly aware of his body and how it functions he will become better able to trust himself. Thus Limit Challenge, A & P Teaching and Feelings Rehearsal are vital components. To increase his ability to gain peer approval social skills training is necessary. His parents need to learn to trust their own impulses so they can trust their child. It is important to displace the conflict regarding control away from eating into an area like bedtime where child and parents can have a good safe fight.

Key Conflicts

1. Trust: 'Can I trust myself and trust them?'
2. Self-esteem: 'I'm nothing but a fat blob but I hate being this way.'
3. Expression of Aggression: 'I would like to tell my parents where to go but they are my only source of affection.'
4. Independence: 'I should be able to regulate my own eating but I fear I'll just get fatter if I don't do what my parents say.'

Likely Problems

1. Parental rigidity and inability to express affection openly, especially touch.
2. Child's poor self-image, lack of friends, paucity of interests.
3. Family's inability to express feelings, particularly anger. Difficulty in the ability to assert himself appropriately when teased.
4. Child's difficulty with impulse control.
5. Family preoccupation with weight, counting calories, etc.

Other Procedures

Have the child lay down on a large piece of paper and draw his outline. He should then draw inside this outline the way he would like to look. Cut out the drawing, colour clothes on it, do facial features (hair, etc.) and hang up in his room (inside the closet door).

6. Family's difficulty in waiting for basic types of gratifications.
7. Child's problem in accepting hurt or discomfort, particularly hunger.

To help change an obese child's body image teach him relaxation exercises. Have him visualise himself as he wants to be. Have him examine the 'picture' in detail carefully; hair, eyes, facial expression, arms, legs, chest and body proportions.

Talk about styles of clothing, colours, etc. that the child would like. New clothes can be used as reinforcement for weight loss.

Involve obese children in as many activities as possible. Identify deficient areas in skills and sports and work on improving any area by modelling. Help them seek out creative 'isolate' activities such as sewing, knitting, model building, string art, doodle art, that they can do when bored. Compliment him when doing well.

Start a carefully graduated exercise programme. Concentrate on mild regular exercise. While exercising talk about the body protesting about mild stress but benefiting from it.

Every overweight child needs to become objective about his problem. This begins with regular, daily weighing, recording the weight and plotting weight changes on a graph. Explain to the child that daily weight fluctuates slightly without any significant change. You should do spot checks. Help the child take body measurements once a week.

Set small goals of weight loss. Use non-food reinforcement, preferably time together in a really fun activity.

Through modelling teach the child to eat slowly and take small bites, savouring every taste. Do not talk while eating but wait until finished with mouthful, talk, then eat again, slowly. Do not let the child eat while upset. Talk about what the child is upset about first, then when relaxed, eat.

To strengthen the child's ego, pick a staff member to make an identification with. Suggest similarities (hair colour, sense of humour, name, etc.), then have staff talk about similar problem (want to lose weight). The staff member and the child can go on a diet and weight graph together. The staff member can emphasise the pains and joys of dieting.

Table 5.10: Weight Control Programme — Suggested Techniques

Techniques	Time	Goal	Suggested Staff
1. Amorphous Blob	1 hr/wk	Ego identification	Primary worker
2. Anatomy and Physiology Teaching	2 hr/wk	Aware of body and its functions	Resident (registrar)
3. Body Painting	2 hr/wk	Unafraid to view own body objectively	Primary worker
4. Brief Insight-oriented Psychotherapy	3 hr/wk	Some insight into major conflicts	Psychiatrist
5. Conflict Displacement	1 hr/day	Parent's ability to divert conflict away from critical areas	Primary worker
6. Delayed Gratification	3 hr/day	Time depending on age, approx. 1 min/6 min	Primary worker
7. Ego Auxiliary	Daily wks 2, 3, 4	Able to deal with stress	Primary worker
8. Family Counselling	2 hr/wk	Able to identify conflicts and communicate feelings	Social worker or registrar
9. Feelings Rehearsal	5 hr/wk for last 2 wks	Able to identify and express feelings	Primary worker
10. Individuation	2 hr/wk	An awareness of parent as separate and ability to identify self	Parent and primary worker
11. Kangaroo Kort	5 hr/wk	Able to identify personal and group ambivalence and conflict	All staff
12. Limit Challenge	3 hr/wk	Can push limits on realistic assessment	Primary worker
13. Listen to Your Body	Daily	To recognise and trust inner urges	Primary worker
14. Mediational Modification	4 hr/wk last 2 wks	Learn how to talk self out of temptation	Primary worker
15. Negotiating Guidelines and Consequences	2 hr/wk last 3 wks	A complete working set before discharge	Primary worker
16. Recreation Introduction	last 3 wkends	Explore at least three new free fun places	Secondary worker
17. Self-esteem	2 hr/wk	A feeling of I'm OK	Primary worker
18. Sensitivity Exercises	Daily	To perceive and exchange feelings	Occupational therapist
19. Sex Education	3 hr/wk	Understanding of basic physiology and emotions	Intern
20. Social Skills Training	Daily	Ability to make and break social relationships	Occupational therapist
21. Therapeutic Wrestling	2 hr/wk	Not afraid to win, lose or stress body	Primary worker
22. Tradition Engendering	2 hr/wk last 2 wks	Establish two happy family traditions	Social worker

Conflict Regarding Food

Talk about feeling 'empty', bored, unloved and 'filling up' with food. Suggest fasting. First one meal. Talk about feelings and conflicts. Build up fasting to one day a week. Allow any liquids but no solid food during fast.

Plan weekly meal with family and therapists. Observe any conflicted areas, interpret and suggest alternative patterns, model alternative and give the family praise when utilised.

6 PARENT TRAINING SESSIONS

Introduction

Every week on Monday or Tuesday evening the parents whose children are currently hospitalised on the Child and Family Unit, meet for two seminars lasting for a total of one and a half hours. These seminars emphasise the salient points of child development, interpersonal communication and family management. This chapter contains the notes that are handed out at the end of each seminar. They are intended to cover the main points and remind the participants of some of the issues taught and discussed. The seminars are meant to be entertaining, informing and a forum for a discussion which emphasises the importance of knowing about children.

The parents' involvement is crucial. They are expected to attend and, if not, they are taken aside and given a reminder. If they still do not attend or attend sporadically for any other than critical reasons, they are warned that their child may be discharged. If the couple still do not respond the screening committee meets to decide whether the child should be discharged or whether there are mitigating circumstances. If the child is discharged it is not done in anger, rather, with sadness. The parents are told the child will be welcome back when they are ready to participate. There have been very few discharges, approximately 0.4 per cent.

Each seminar with the parents whose children are presently hospitalised, begins with a request for the parents to introduce themselves and mention one or two aspects of the nature of their child's problems. It's followed by a 25-minute talk which uses video, role-play and films to get across key issues and yet keep the attention high. Fifteen minutes' discussion follows including questions regarding how the parents have done on their homework. The homework is gone over in greater detail with the primary therapist. A coffee-break follows the first seminar.

The second seminar ends with, 'Well, who's graduating this week and how has it gone?' This provides a good feedback opportunity for parents who almost invariably, at least at this stage in their experience, have good things to say about the unit. Their positive remarks encourage other parents who are just beginning. The parents are reminded

273

to attend the follow-up sessions which also go on for five weeks.

The follow-up or graduate group seminars are still centred on particular topics but there is much more discussed. The discussion is more personal and aimed at helping parents work out the problems that they are facing now their child is adjusting to being back home. Because the parents know each other much better, they are able to discuss freely how they personally are finding the difficulties and where some of those difficulties arise.

The feedback from parents regarding the evening training sessions is almost always positive. The attendance is high. The first series is designed to emphasise information partly because the parents desperately need to learn some basic facts about children, partly because they are afraid they will embarrass themselves with their inability to communicate and partly because they are anxious not to disclose too much of themselves and their personal problems. They do discuss enough to make it quite apparent that other parents are not alone with the problems they are facing.

Week One
Lesson 1A: How it Got Started – 'Why Me?'

As parents you must often ask 'why?' Why should we, caring, conscientious parents that we are, have children with emotional or learning difficulties when there are so many other parents, who don't seem to care have children who grow up all right? Part of the problem lies in the very fact that you are conscientious. Parents who are more concerned about their children are more likely to report that their children are having difficulties. They tend to be more attentive and more quickly see when problems arise. They have higher expectations and are more quickly disappointed.

Some of you spend too much time trying to instruct your children or try too hard to make them become what the family think they should be. Try to remember that a good portion of children's learning takes place quite naturally without instruction, by imitation. The reasons your family have problems are very complex but they usually include the following.

Temperament
As parents you may wonder why, when you treat all the children in the

same way, one particular child seems to have problems and the others do not. The reason is that children are born with very different constitutional and temperamental characteristics. You just cannot treat them in the same way. They have different intelligence, adaptability, intensity of mood, attention span, sensory threshold, and other characteristics which stay with them throughout their lives. Wise parents quickly recognise the differences in their children and try their best to adapt to the differences.

Parents don't always fit their children, nor do children fit with each other. Some children are born cuddly, others not. A cuddly child fits well with mothers who like to cuddle. Some children are not cuddly and this sometimes hurts the cuddling type of mother. Unless she can adapt to the difference and provide her bouncy, noisy child with a sufficient amount of close contact to establish a bond, by tickling, tossing, etc., problems may arise.

Unconscious Influences

Believe it or not, we all have an unconscious. Because of our unconscious, we sometimes make irrational decisions. We would like to believe that most of our actions are determined by reason. In fact, a great many decisions regarding how we interact with our children are determined by unconscious conflicts. We find ourselves making the same mistakes repeatedly and then wondering why we haven't learned that some methods don't work.

It has been shown that we will tend to re-enact unsolved conflicts from our past. While unconscious problems are being dramatised, we should have the opportunity to remove ourselves from the action and watch what happens. Hopefully we can then understand why one event precipitates another. Unfortunately, while we're involved in the replay, it's hard to step off the stage. Thus we seldom learn and we tend to repeat our mistakes without gaining much insight.

People tend to mate with those who will help them re-enact early problems. Sometimes, children are used as the major characters in a replay, e.g. a mother may react to her teenage daughter as if she was a younger sister with whom she had unresolved jealousy.

Transactions

People make each other behave in certain ways. Each different mixture of people produces different behaviour. Thus no one person can be held solely responsible for whatever they do. The audience makes the speaker talk by continuing to listen. The speaker makes the audience listen by continuing to talk. Both are responsible for each others' behaviour in a lecture. Neither the child nor his parents are totally at fault. Each contributes to the unhappy situation of the other.

It is possible to understand how children and parents affect each other by seeing each individual as made up of partly parent, partly adult and partly child. Some people tend to be much more parent, telling themselves and others what they must do or must not do. Others tend to be mostly children, acting on whims and impulses, unconcerned about how they affect other people. Some are almost totally adult, always calculating what to do next. Hopefully, we all become more adult, but still there should be enough child in us so that our children can see us enjoying doing things impulsively and letting our feelings have free rein occasionally.

Conditioning

Any behaviour may increase or decrease in the frequency of occurrence, depending upon the nature of the event that immediately follows. It is a punishment if that event tends to make behaviours diminish in frequency. It's a reinforcement if it makes the behaviour stronger. We must not have preconceptions because some things we consider rewarding may be punishing.

It has been found that, if mothers or fathers pick up their children when they are crying, the crying tends to become more frequent. Yet parents must respond to the child's crying to determine whether the child is feeling ill, is wet, hungry, or has a pin stuck in him. Thus, parents are in a bind, not knowing whether they should pick up the child and increase his tendency to cry or ignore him and possibly let him suffer. Wise parents soon realise that you must attend to a child, but it's best to attend to a child quickly and if possible between cries. If you let him cry many times, then when you pick him up, you have rewarded him for long periods of crying.

What you notice tends to grow in frequency. Those parents who notice and comment on bad behaviours may find that those behaviours increase because the child gets attention for them. Every child does need attention and tries his best to get it. Without attention, children cannot survive. Attention is very reinforcing (rewarding) because it has survival value. It is your responsibility to provide attention for the right things.

Imitation

Children will imitate the person who is being reinforced or rewarded, is giving out the rewards, or is in control of the situation. Generally speaking, children imitate adults they enjoy being close to. They will imitate the behaviour that the adults obviously enjoy. Thus, if you want your children to enjoy doing dishes, you should whistle and sing while doing them. If children become lazy it may be because often the only thing they hear their parents say about work is how dreary and difficult it is.

Cultural Factors

Many of the things that we and our children do are determined by the behaviour of those around us. Children particularly are sensitive to how their parents treat them compared with how their friends' parents treat their friends. They complain if they have to go to bed an hour earlier than everybody else in the block. We have to have reasonable expectations of our children and these have to do with what society says is normal behaviour.

Every parent has expectations of their children. Sometimes, these are met and both parents and children are happy. More frequently with problem children, both the child and the parents are disappointed. When the parents are disappointed, they tend to criticise their children. This criticism eventually builds an interaction of hostility. Because the child is continually a disappointment to his parents, he tends to become a disappointment to himself. He grows up with a poor self-image and a critical attitude towards others.

Summary

You may have troubles with your children because of all the above factors. On the Family Unit, we hope to provide an opportunity for you to understand and learn to cope with anything that causes you to hold each other back from becoming what you could be.

Homework

1. Describe the temperamental characteristics of your children.
2. Try to remember your first reaction to your child's (a) first fight, (b) first loss.
3. What do you think your children will become when they grow up.

Lesson 1 B: Three Parts of a Person

Transactions

Transactions are changes in thought and behaviour which occur when two or more people encounter each other. You cannot not make people act differently from the way they will be with others. You cannot not communicate. Whether you believe it or not, you are always communicating. Even being silent is communicating, maybe that you do not wish to talk. Your silence, preoccupation or interest in something says something about you. The silence of the other person will indicate to you that your wishes are respected. Your communication affects what people around you do and what they say or do changes how you act and feel. Since we are always changing each other, no one person is responsible for the way we are. The problems in the family are never just the parents' or the child's fault. The complicated ways we affect each other's behaviour are called transactions.

Levels of Transaction

There are three ego states or parts of a person's thinking involved in transactions. Being able to identify these components can help you resolve problematic transactions.

A. The Adult part of you is the rational and responsible part which helps you make rational decisions.

B. The Parent is the nurturing, caring and the regulating, controlling part which is reminding you of your responsibilities and obligations.

C. The Child is best described as the impulsive, creative, fun-loving part that likes to do things on the spur of the moment.

Examples of Transactions

   (i)   Husband: 'Where are my shoes?' (an adult question)
        Wife: 'In the closet' (an adult response) (Figure 6.1)

  (ii)   Johnny: 'Mom, can I have one of the cookies you just baked?' (child to parent)
        Mother: 'No, it's too close to dinner time' (parent to child) (Figure 6.2)

 (iii)   Husband: 'Where are my shoes?' is an adult stimulus.
        Wife: 'Why don't you look after your things, then you'd know where to find them' − parent response to a child (Figure 6.3). This is a crossed transaction that may end up in a fight.

Appropriate or complementary transactions such as the adult to adult, parent to parent, child to child transactions or the parent to child and child to parent transactions between parent and child do not cause problems. Crossed transactions, as in Figure 6.3 can, and often do,

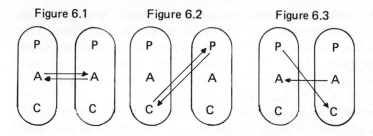

Figure 6.1   Figure 6.2   Figure 6.3

cause conflict because, for the person who begins the transaction, the response feels wrong.

How Much of Which Part?

Children are naturally mostly Child with a little Adult and little Parent growing inside of them. As they are exposed to an increasing number of adult transactions, the Adult in them will develop. Exposure to younger children in school and at play will stimulate the growth of the nurturing Parent. The prohibitive part of the Parent in them develops with correction and criticism. Too much prohibition tends to kill the Child in you. A well-balanced adult has equal amounts of Child, Adult and Parent inside him or her.

If parents become too regulating or controlling the Parent in their children becomes dominant while the Adult can become weaker and the Child at times non-existent.

You must take care that the Parent in you isn't always dominant. The rational, responsible Adult should usually be the stronger, but to understand and enjoy children, the Child part of you must be preserved. If the Child in you has become dormant we want to help you bring it back to life.

The Child in You

Have you ever: stood at the top of a hill across from another hill and shouted for the sheer pleasure of hearing your echo? Did you ever kick a tin can along a beach to see how far it might fly? Surely there were times when you hopped over the cracks in the sidewalk, rolled around on the floor or tickled your spouse, had a snowball fight, played hide and seek with your children? If you are still able to do these silly but delightful things, your Child is showing, and it should. When your Child is showing your children feel very close to you because they can see how you could understand their point of view. Without the silly things in life, it would be a very serious business indeed. If the Child in you is alive, you will understand the joys of being young. You will be able to enjoy your children's fun activities. Children want you to be the Parent and Adult most of the time because they have to count on you, but they love it when you are occasionally silly.

Games

A progressive set of transactions which result in an important payoff are called games. All of us play games. Some of them help us in social situations. Some of them are very destructive. Games are a repetitious way of getting a payoff, usually for an unconscious conflict.

The more destructive games are those which once commenced will elicit a comment such as 'Here we go again', 'Not again', 'I can't stand the way you go on. If you don't shut up I'm leaving.' They begin as offhand comments and end with a threat to break a relationship.

Naming the game is fairly easy, because the name usually comes from the main topic discussed or argued.

Some frequent games are: 'If only I' followed by any number of possibilities, i.e. 'If only I had more money; a bigger house; better job. If only it weren't for my boss . . . this stupid job . . . I could . . .'

'See what you made me do' is a good one. You play it when you have done something you feel badly about, so you want someone else to take at least part of the responsibility.

Identifying the payoff is a little more difficult. The initiator of the game can usually identify what he gets out of it. Often it is an existential payoff, 'Look everyone, didn't I tell you that . . .'

It is important to know the games you're playing because your children will play similar games to get a similar payoff. To be able to identify games helps you to spot the beginning of those you want to stop playing.

Homework

1. Name two games your family play that have an unhappy ending.
2. To understand better the payoff you go after, list the things in your life that are really important.

Week 2
Lesson 2A: How Big is the Problem?

Problems are typically visited upon us in one size — the very big. You tend to overestimate the size of the problems your children have because they bother you so much. 'They're always fighting' usually means you get very upset by your children's hostility. It doesn't mean they fight all day every day. It is important to know how big your problems are because:

1. If there is a big difference between how big you think they are and how big they really are, it should make you want to find out why that problem is so important to you. You'll want more insight.
2. Just measuring the problem will help you assess yourself and your children realistically. You usually find out they aren't so big after all and this helps you change your attitude to yourself and your children.
3. A good measure on problem behaviours gives you a way of knowing if any of the techniques we've taught you are working.
4. Measuring the problem will give you clues about what causes the problem. You'll see when they get better or worse and may be able to make some connections with what was going on at the time.
5. In order to measure you have to watch. When you just watch your children you will discover all sorts of things about them you didn't know. You may discover Johnny is really quite generous or that it's Jane who really starts the fights between them. Seeing all the good things your children do will help develop positive attitudes towards them.
6. An objective measure will give you good evidence with which you can counter any bad assessments of your children given by in-laws, grandparents, teachers or other professionals.
7. Children tend to live up to your expectations. If you expect them to be always fighting that's what you will notice and may inadvertently reinforce with your attention. Your children may say, 'Well, if that's what they expect I'm like, I may as well be that way.'
8. A careful measure, of your own and your children's strengths and weaknesses, will help you all plan your lives.

You will notice that on our unit we are very careful to make measures. That's for all the reasons above plus we want to know if our techniques and programmes are working and if not why not. But making measurements isn't very easy. We suggest you try it this way:

1. Make a list of all your children's problems and good points.
2. Pick two important problems and two good points.
3. Try and guess why it might be hard for you to be objective about

them, e.g. 'That problem reminds me of my oldest bossy sister'.

4. Estimate how often those good points or problems are likely to surface each day or each week.

5. Define and describe all four behaviours so you and your spouse or friend or primary worker will be able to agree when it's happening, e.g. fighting means 'hitting, shouting nasty names and taking the other's toys'.

6. Set aside an observation time when you will be able to concentrate on watching what actually does go on.

7. Observe for the same amount of time each day.

8. Count the number of times one of the good or bad behaviours happen and add them up for a daily total.

9. Plot them on a graph and connect the points with a line. If you have problems, one of the staff will show you how.

10. Make notations on your graph about why any behaviour might be getting worse or better.

If you keep your graph going you can make all sorts of discoveries which you should share with your children. There isn't any reason why couples shouldn't monitor each other's behaviours but try to make your observing not too obvious. As a reminder to everyone in your home of how good and bad behaviours change with attitudes, expectations, conflicts and rewards, you should post your graphs for all to see.

Homework

1. (a) Estimate how often a behaviour you want to see less of now occurs.

   (b) Estimate how often a behaviour you want to see more of now occurs. Count it.

2. List the most important events that shaped your personality.

Lesson 2B: The Child's Perspective or 'The View from Down There'

As adults, you tend to forget how you heard, saw, felt and responded to people, events and objects, when you were children. Perhaps more importantly, you even forget that your experience was simply different. To understand your child's experience of the world around him, you must keep in mind that it does differ from yours. Their reactions may be very irritating to you, unless you remember why they are reacting like they do. They may seem to be frightened for no reason at all, unless you remember that from their point of view everything is much bigger and much stranger than it is to you. They may get extremely excited about what are 'stupid little things' from your point of view, but to them it may be the most exquisitely beautiful object they have ever seen. So the better you understand the world from a child's point of view, the better you will understand why they appear to behave so strangely. One of the ways to see the world as a child sees it is to get down on their level. Another way is to remember what it was like for you as a child at various ages.

Small children live in a world of giants — people, furniture, cars, dogs are all big. They naturally feel intimidated even if the big person or big dog is very friendly. When talking to adults, the child may be talking to knees or belly buttons unless care is taken to make eye contact. Chairs, car seats, theatre seats, are big and uncomfortable. 'It's enough to make a kid squirm!' From the child's perspective every crowd is incomprehensibly huge and every machine moves like lightning. The lack of knowledge and experience makes the world a much newer and stranger place for young children than it is for us.

Initially your children use movement, touch, smell, taste, hearing — all these faculties to obtain information about the environment and themselves. Progressively, with the augmentation of language, learning becomes more 'abstract'. This process is gradual and not all children develop at the same rate. The pace of learning varies from child to child and is different at different times in the child's life. As your children learn, it is important to keep expectations in line with abilities. Expecting more than a child is able to do leads to feelings of frustration and failure. Expecting too little could cause boredom.

Playtime is learning time for children, not simply funtime. Play provides children with everything that education, work, recreation and social life provide adults. It is through play the child learns how to use his body and his skills, how machines work, what is bigger or smaller, cause and effect, before and after, and about how to interact with peers. How children play and what children play with will greatly enhance their curiosity and their intellectual capabilities.

Simple transactions can be quite startling to you if you don't understand how the child's mind is developing. For example, if you pour lemonade into different shaped glasses for two small children, one may protest that he has less to drink than his sister. He has not yet learned that mass can stay constant despite changes in shape.

Your children's lack of knowledge and experience may cause you embarrassment when they reveal some very personal detail of family life to neighbours or teachers. Your child has not yet discovered the difference between what family members can discuss and what can acceptably be told to others. If he hasn't learned what belongs to him, he will not appreciate that taking something belonging to a shop-keeper is stealing.

Emotions

Your young child will tend to be very impulsive and react to situa-tions, 'just the way he feels'. If excited, he may jump around, make lots of noise, laugh, shout or clap his hands. If he is sad, he may cry desperately for no apparent reason. In situations like this, you may be inclined to remark, 'keep quiet, settle down' or demand that he 'stop crying'. Don't discourage your children from expressing their feelings. Rather, teach them the appropriate expression of feelings. When there is a crisis in your child's life, e.g. his puppy is killed, remain with him and assist him in working through the particular emotions of the moment. Adults appreciate it when someone can name and understand the feelings they are experiencing. Your child also feels warm and appreciative when you can name the emotion, and say, 'I know how you are feeling, I feel happy and excited when I'm invited to a friend's birthday party' or 'I felt sad when my dog was hurt'. Your child will feel supported if you go through the emotions with him. He will learn that life can go on when you gradually recover from the vicariously experienced hurt.

One of the most important emotional confrontations, both for children and adults, is death. For a child, the meaning and significance of death is an extremely difficult concept to understand. Generally speaking, it has been found that a child below the age of twelve years is unable fully to comprehend that if someone dies, they will never return; while the older child begins to understand the permanency and implications of death. Young children don't seem to take death seriously while 12-year-olds may become very preoccupied with it.

Homework

To gain a better understanding of your children's point of view try the following:

1. Get down to your children's level and make eye contact when you talk with them.

2. Use active listening. This consists in listening to what a person says, then instead of responding immediately, rephrase the speaker's words to indicate your understanding of what he said. If the speaker and listener agree about the meaning of what was said, the listener may then reply and the process is repeated.
3. Use role reversal – 'OK, you be the Mummy and I will be the little girl'. Keep it up as long as you can.
4. Remember:
   (a) Your first day at school; it seemed like a huge place crammed with mobs of people who all knew what they were doing, until you visited it as an adult then it seemed quite small and familiar.
   (b) The time one of your pets died and how heart-broken you were.
   (c) The day the circus came to town and how excited everyone was.

Week Three
Lesson 3A: How the Problem Gets Larger

How can we understand the fact that many disturbed children we see on the Family Unit have conscientious, loving parents and that the harder the parents try, the worse the child's behaviour gets?

The answer lies in realising that you and your children have at your disposal strong ways for changing each other's behaviour. You unconsciously train each other in a continuous reciprocal interaction. In most cases, the most potent reinforcer (reward) for the child is your attention. The reason is simple. Without your attention to your child's needs and your response to your child's danger, your children could not survive. Thus attention is necessary for survival and is the most powerful reinforcer of behaviour. Similarly, a powerful reinforcer for most of you is peace and quiet, or relief from the child's annoying behaviour.

Consider crying. Crying is one way an infant can use to exert control over its environment to get its needs met. Parents (especially mothers) have a built-in tendency to respond to a child's crying. They can't relax until the child stops crying. Because of their built-in mechanism, the harder the child cries, the more tense the mother feels. This tendency may be intensified in a parent who felt neglected as a child. Responding to an infant's needs is necessary and desirable, but at the same time the parent is unwittingly strengthening the child's tendency to cry.

As your child grows older, you mothers may resolve to stamp out your child's excessive crying, say at bedtime. You sit in the living room trying to watch TV, but feel uneasy because you can hear your child crying in the background. Because his desire for attention is not being met, he may cry longer and louder than usual. If you give in and comfort your child at this point, your child may stop crying and go to sleep. Now you will feel relieved. The catch is that although your child is quiet for the time being, you have unwittingly made the problem worse in the long run. You have rewarded your child for crying harder and louder than before. Ironically, with your attention, it is often you dedicated mothers who fall into this subtle trap. The solution is simple but takes courage. You must withhold your attention until your child stops crying. Otherwise, your child's crying may eventually escalate into temper tantrums, head banging, etc. Worst of all you may begin to dislike your child because he so often makes you uncomfortable and angry.

The same basic principles apply to many annoying behaviours. Some children are so hungry for parental attention that they will settle for any kind they can get, even if it means being yelled at or smacked. Some children can coerce you with annoying behaviour that is very hard to ignore, such as messing, whining or 'bugging'. When you respond with attention of some kind your child settles down temporarily. In the short run, both you and your child are 'paid off'. Your child gets attention and you get quietness, at least temporarily. As the child's behaviour becomes increasingly annoying, parent and child become bewildered by a vicious circle. The remedy is simple but not obvious: the parent must ignore the child's annoying behaviour and give attention only when the child is being good. It is as hard for you to change your bad habit of rewarding your children's obnoxious behaviour as it is for them to change. They have been rewarding you with quietness when you give them attention. You have conditioned each other over a long period. You find you can't change even when you say you won't give in. There is no point in your blaming your child any more than there is in his blaming you.

If you decide to decrease an undesired behaviour by withholding your attention, you must do so totally and consistently. A half-hearted attempt will probably make matters worse. Consider what would happen if you gave in to your child about every fifth time he has a temper tantrum: the child would probably continue having tantrums almost indefinitely, because he would expect you to give in but wouldn't know exactly when. (The same principle explains why, after winning a small lottery 15 years ago, you will probably continue to buy lottery tickets for many years afterwards, without being reinforced again.) Being rewarded for a portion of the wrong behaviours makes those behaviours stick even more firmly.

Penalties and rewards vary considerably according to the age of the child and also from family to family. We would like to make a slight distinction between penalties and punishments. Penalties are most effective when they are basically frustrating to a child. They should be simple and easy to apply, without placing the parents under duress. Punishments, such as spankings, may be necessary as a more serious consequence, but can lose effectiveness if used as a standard penalty. The usual natural reward for a child is your approving smile, a word of encouragement or a pat on the head. There are times when more concrete types of reward are also very useful in helping your child mature.

A child who has the opportunity to learn through the experiences we are describing will begin to like the behaviour patterns that are being encouraged instead of those patterns that are being penalised. Once your child has mastered approved forms of behaviour, they are self-sustaining by the general approval of friends, classmates, etc. Good behaviours give a child pleasure. The sense of mastery is its own reward.

Homework

1. Describe how you may have accidentally strengthened the behaviours in your child that you like least of all.
2. Using the same principles, explain how a peace-loving husband trains his wife to nag at him.

Lesson 3B: Education of our Feelings and Behaviour

The first point to consider is that the basic emotions we experience are chemical events in our body. A moment's reflection on your own experiences with fear and anger and excitement and joy will allow you to notice that there are certain changes occurring within your body. These changes are occurring, not only in your nervous system, but also in your body chemistry. As chemical events, these changes are usually temporary and they will subside on their own account over a period of time. We must pay particular attention to changes that do not subside and tend to become long-lasting, habitual, or unnatural in their frequency.

A second consideration is that emotional states show themselves in certain patterns of behaviour that are part of our way of being. The spontaneous physical expressions of fear, anger, sadness or excitement can be seen in infancy. They tend to develop into more complex behaviour forms as a child grows.

The chemical and physical expressions of feelings happen to everyone. The issue then is how to express these feelings in ways that our community find acceptable. Some expressions of anger can be healthy, others are destructive. Your goal as parents is to help your children to develop verbal expression about life events that cause them to be angry and if they get angry, how to express it in acceptable ways. Out of such encouragement can come the possibility of discussing feelings rather than acting them out.

While you can easily see the emotional states in your children, they may be unaware of what words to attach to what they feel. You may need to tell your child what he is feeling. To know the right words for your feelings makes it easier to express your feelings appropriately. It is not uncommon to see unhappy children who do not know that they are sad or very angry children, who are misbehaving without appreciating that the feeling that is driving them is anger.

Once a child's emotions are known to him, it becomes possible to discuss the behaviours that are generated by strong emotions. It is also possible to point out which emotional behaviours are unacceptable in your family. Simply to stop a behaviour that is a manifestation of a feeling is not enough. To stop one form of angry behaviour often means the emergence of another form equally undesirable.

You must introduce your children to acceptable ways of expressing underlying feelings by showing them the good ways you express feelings. It is important that your children have clear models and understanding of the forms in which emotional expression can be accepted. Once your children have alternative ways to express feelings, it is reasonable to use reward and punishment to shape the right ways.

Children go through stress and distress as they go through different stages or meet different life circumstances. A stress response may be seen in the emergence or return of unwanted behaviours. This does not necessarily indicate a failure of your parenting. It usually means some situation is giving your child difficulty and it is time for a second look at what's happening in your child's life. All children want to discuss their problems. As new problems emerge, the whole process of identifying feelings and behaviour may have to be initiated once again. If anyone cannot express his feelings, the chemical changes may begin to result in physical changes, e.g. a rise in blood pressure, spasm in the gut. If unexpressed feelings go on for too long, the physical changes may become more or less permanent, and that is hard on our health. As parents you must encourage children to express their feelings, model good ways of expressing them appropriately and talk about what are the experiences and problems behind the feelings.

Homework

1. List the strongest feelings and how they are expressed in your family.
2. Think of what might happen if you could never express your feelings.

Week Four
Lesson 4A: Changing Behaviours

There are many ways to change behaviour. On our unit we use most of the good ones to help your family. Our greatest hope is that you will learn enough about your responses that you will be able to take charge of your own lives. We want you to learn how to communicate more directly and more honestly so you can encourage each other. You'll find with reasonable expectations that your spouse and children are more often successful, therefore they try harder and go further. When you can name the games your family play, you can stop them and change them. We teach your children to change their defeatist thought patterns, challenge their limits and develop good ways for socialising. We believe that negotiating guidelines and consequences is a good way to manage the family and learn democracy.

We want you to understand basic behavioural techniques of rewarding or punishing behaviours because we want you to be able to stop small problems becoming big ones. Too often parents resort to physical punishment because they get backed into a tight corner and can't think of other ways of handling their child's irritating or demanding behaviours.

Unfortunately, whenever you hit children you make them both frightened and angry, more of one than the other depending on your relative sizes. The child will seek to express his anger because it hurts to keep it bottled inside. If he lets it out by fighting with his little sister, he's likely to get punished again. In that way, neither you nor your child can win.

Here are some basic principles that may help you:

1. The number of times a behaviour occurs depends on its present consequences.

2. A consequence is punishing if it decreases the frequency of a behaviour.
3. A consequence is reinforcing (rewarding) if it increases the frequency of a behaviour.
4. You can tell what's punishing or reinforcing by counting how often behaviours are occurring.
5. Reinforcing the behaviour you want is more effective than punishing the behaviour you don't want.
6. At least 50 per cent of the consequences you apply should be reinforcing.
7. The sooner you can apply consequences the more effective they are.
8. Use shaping and fading (the staff will explain) and start where the child's at.
9. If there are unconscious reasons why you have been reinforcing the wrong behaviours, you will need someone to help you uncover them before you can be logical with your consequences.
10. He who punishes becomes a punisher a child wants to avoid. He who reinforces becomes a reinforcer children want to be near and want to please.

Consequences which increase the occurrence of behaviour	Consequences which decrease the occurrence of behaviour
1. Giving Reinforcement (a) primary reinforcers: biological satisfiers, e.g. food, water, physical contact, attention, warmth, praise (b) secondary reinforcers: anything consistently paired with primary reinforcers, e.g. tokens, smiles, 'yes', money, feedback — 'that's right'	1. Giving Punishment (a) primary punishers: biological annoyers e.g. loud noises, painful stimulation, spanks, shouts. (b) secondary punishers: anything consistently paired with primary punishers, e.g. frowns, raised arm, 'no', feedback — 'that's wrong'
2. Taking Away — Negative Reinforcement removing a biological annoyer (primary punisher) or a punisher, e.g. stop yelling, quit nagging, no more smacking or criticism	2. Taking Away — Negative Punishment removing a biological satisfier (primary reinforcer) or a secondary reinforcer e.g. grounding, deducting allowance, isolation or time-out
3. Vicarious Reinforcement the child wants to imitate the one who is being reinforced	3. Vicarious Punishment. the child wants to stop doing the behaviour which he sees another child punished for
4. Reinforcing the Opposite Behaviour	4. Extinction no reinforcement

Homework

1. Name the main punishers or reinforcers which influence your working behaviour.
2. Try using a reinforcer on the opposite behaviour of your child that you are punishing.

Lesson 4B: Communication that Uplifts or Puts Down Children

1. Praise, Criticism and Correction

Praise may be defined as expressing warm approval or commending the merits of a person or his behaviour. Criticism means to pronounce judgement on someone or something. It is usually disparaging and fault-finding. Correction implies pointing out errors, faults or defects without embarrassing or humiliating a person.

Similarly, praise and criticism can both be expressed by words alone, but also conveyed by a look, a gesture or a change in expression.

With praise, both the receiver and the giver usually feel good about it, but with criticism, the receiver is apt to feel angry, frustrated, humiliated or just plain dumb.

If a person frequently criticises another, he or she is acting as an aversive, or unpleasant, stimulus. Over a period of time, he or she becomes a conditioned aversive stimulus whose presence alone may elicit the negative responses generated by criticism. Children try hard to please somone from whom they usually receive praise. They avoid people who often criticise them. If the criticism embarrasses or humiliates them, they will have difficulty even hearing the criticiser's instructions.

There is an important difference between criticism and correction. While both imply that judgement is made, criticism generally attacks the person, while correction is directed towards the problem. Correction uses an 'I' statement rather than a 'You' statement. When you correct you say, 'I am uncomfortable driving at this speed.' When you criticise you say, 'You're driving like an idiot. Slow down!'

2. Expectations

Everyone in your family tends to have both legitimate and unrealistic expectations of the others. Expectations should be related to a child's ability and interest, rather than what we would like him to do or to be. We should work on making our expectations appropriate and realistic. Expectations which are unrealistic or too high create the 'need' for criticism because the person being judged never 'measures up'. Expectations which are set too low may cause a child to give up, without really trying. Realistic expectations should be set just above your child's present level of performance. Then there is a good chance you will be pleased with his performance.

Damning with faint praise can be a very destructive form of criticism. An example of such praise is, 'Your hair really looks good for someone who does it herself.' It is more subtle than obvious criticism, but can be equally painful and more difficult to deal with. To a child the sarcasm hurts but is hard to understand.

3. Important Points to Remember

Criticism may produce anger, humiliation, revenge, frustration, destroy incentive and damage self-concept. Eventually we see ourselves as our parents have seen us. If they have frequently criticised us, we will be frequently critical of ourselves. People who are very self-critical may give up easily, demand a lot of others or become depressed. We can correct without hurting someone if we can remember:

(a) it is important that correction be private, not public.
(b) it is essential that the correction be directed at the situation, not at the person.
(c) it is important to avoid derogatory name-calling: stupid, idiot, fat, worthless, etc.
(d) it is essential that the amount of praise and approval outweigh the amount of correction or criticism. Without a large amount of praise and approval, correction can become as harmful as criticism.

Homework

1. Make a list of the 'likes' and 'dislikes' about yourself. (Be honest.)
2. Count the number of times you praise or criticise your spouse or child each day. Try to increase your praise score by one (+ 1) and decrease your criticism score by one (− 1) each day.

Week Five
Lesson 5A: Putting It Into Practice

1. Select and Define Behaviours

To begin with, select one behaviour that you would like to see occur more often, and one behaviour that you would like to see occur less often. Do not attempt to change too many behaviours at once. The fewer the number of behaviours you attempt to change at any one time, the less confusion and the greater the chance of being successful.

The entire family should sit together to complain frankly and list all the changes they would like to see in themselves and each other. Try to agree about the behaviours that are important and those less important. Agreement ensures that everyone will be working together on the same problem. You want to start changing the less important behaviours first because they are usually the easiest to change. Tackle the important, difficult to change ones when you have more confidence in the method.

2. Measure the Behaviours

Before attempting to change the behaviours, obtain a record of how often the behaviour occurs. This record serves as a baseline and allows you accurately to assess your success. We recommend that the behaviours be graphed for about four to five days prior to your attempts to change them. You'll be surprised how often they begin to change just because you are monitoring them more objectively.

3. Select an Appropriate Technique and Negotiate

Many techniques for changing behaviour were discussed in Lesson 4A. The family should agree about the technique to be used.

(a) Wherever possible, reinforce desirable behaviour rather than punishing its opposite, e.g. praise your child for speaking politely rather than criticising him for being rude.

(b) At least 50 per cent of the consequences should be rewarding. Most of our adult behaviours are maintained with rewards and children can see double standards.

(c) Use natural consequences whenever possible, e.g. get them up early when they go to bed late to emphasise the natural result of not going to bed.

(d) Use consequences that are easy to apply and that are clearly in your control. Don't use making the child go to bed earlier the next night if he is late. It creates the same problem only earlier. Waking a child up is something you can do much more easily than making them go to sleep.

(e) Don't try to control a child's behaviour that is really his responsibility and which you can't really govern anyway, i.e. going to sleep, speaking, eating, defecating, urinating, learning. If you try to control these behaviours your child will fight you and neither of you will win.

(f) Give your children a chance to help you change your problem behaviours.

4. Negotiate

(a) Tackle one problem behaviour at a time, beginning with the least important. Negotiate the guideline first. Give your children the first opportunity to suggest what it should be, e.g. 'OK, we've got a problem with Tanya getting to bed by a reasonable hour. What do you think it should be, Tanya?'

(b) Give yourself lots of bargaining room, e.g. 'So you think a 12-year-old like you doesn't need to be in bed until 11 p.m. I think it should be 7.30 p.m.'

(c) Encourage your children to present their best arguments and give them praise for making good points even if you don't agree.

(d) Present your best points carefully and not angrily.

(e) Compromise gracefully, it helps your children accept something less than what they were aiming for.

(f) Don't forget all the finer points of the guideline, e.g. being in bed by 9.30 p.m. includes having your face washed, teeth brushed, pyjamas on, and under the covers.

(g) Once a guideline is agreed upon, give a handshake to cement the agreement and write it down.

(h) Negotiate the consequence in the same way, making sure your child has the first opportunity.

(i) Remember small consequences frequently and consistently applied work best.

(j) Agree on the duration of this contract.

(k) Write out your contract in two columns and get all parties to sign it.

5. Write Down the Guidelines and Consequences

The written contract for your first few guidelines and consequences should be posted in a convenient spot, e.g. refrigerator door. When these guidelines and consequences are working well, get the family together and work on the next most difficult ones. Any that don't work after two or three weeks need to be renegotiated.

6. Try Your Guidelines and Consequences

On the agreed-upon date, try your guidelines and consequences. Once the children have agreed, you should not remind, threaten, bribe or coerce them. If they forget, direct them to where the list is pinned up and for small children read it over twice. After that let the consequences do the reminding. Stick strictly to the terms, no getting off, say, because the child is only two minutes late.

For example:

Guidelines	Consequences
1. If temper tantrum	Then child ignored for ten minutes
2. If no temper tantrum for one hour	Then child allowed to watch television for half an hour
3. If in bed at 8.30 p.m.	Then mother reads to him for 15 minutes
4. If not in bed at 8.30 p.m.	Then will be awakened earlier next morning

Homework

1. Negotiate one guideline and consequence.
2. Think of all the advantages to negotiating the rules that govern your life.

Lesson 5B: Developing Family Strengths and Traditions

In a world where problems get so much attention in newspapers, on the TV and in our daily lives, it is important to focus on your strengths and positive qualities as families and individuals. When you take an inventory it may be surprising to find out how many good qualities your family has.

To make a family strength inventory get the whole family together, explain what you are about to do and have each person make a list of the good things about the family for which he is thankful. Share the lists and talk about why each strength is important to the person presenting it. One member of the family can make a master list.

If you are having difficulty look at this list for suggestions. Try to write what comes to your mind first and then refer to this list for further thought.

Family Strength Survey

1. Family's physical resources — home, health, good food, etc.
2. Good family relationships with each other.
3. The skills of members of the family in outside events: bowling,

swimming, etc.

4. Good recreation and leisure times you've had together.
5. Personal characteristics.
6. Spiritual life and times of stress when family members have helped each other.
7. Creative interests, knitting, writing, etc.
8. Child-rearing practices and discipline.
9. Family's help to others outside the family.
10. Interesting relatives and friends.

Try to gain a more objective view of your family's history. There are sure to be some very funny episodes. Even problem times can be valuable. What value, if any, do problems have? Do they accomplish anything in us? List all the important lessons life has taught your family. What has your family been hoping life would bring? Have you not achieved some of these goals? Have your expectations been too high? Haven't many of the real joys come without a lot of fuss, effort or material things? Is not life a patchwork of joys and sorrows? Do we over-react to problems because of our own expectations, rather than accept them as opportunities to become more mature and wise? Someone has said, 'You have to fall down before you can learn how to get up.'

Often when you look back at the times of struggle you see such growth and change for the better that you appreciate some of the problems you've had. A wise person once said, 'What's important is, not what happens to you but what you do with what happens to you.' If you can only see problems as inconvenient interruptions in your pursuit of happiness, you will resent each one regardless of how small they are. If you can appreciate that in a family the process of growing up is more important than the big events that mark the finishing, you can begin to learn the value of patiently seeing things through.

Traditions are valuable markers to help families remember important events. Traditions also help you cope with stressful times by helping you look forward to that time when you are quite sure you're going to have some fun because you always have. Traditional celebrations are occasions when more distant family members return, old hurts are put away and everyone tries to contribute to a good time for everyone. There are big traditional get-togethers but there are also small funny ones that keep families together, like the mother who, on the Sunday following any one of her children's birthdays, would take the family for a drive. The child who just had the birthday could point to any side road he or she wanted and the mother would drive along it as far as she could or until it was time to go home. Silly though it may seem, the children — young and grown up — of another family, all insisted on hanging up their stockings at Christmas at the fire place or any reasonable facsimile such as a barbecue, if where they were living didn't have a fire place, because it was traditional.

Homework

Make a list of your family's traditions. If you don't have many, invent a few. A family tradition needs these features:

1. It is a something you do regularly, even if it isn't frequent, come what may.
2. Everyone in the family should come and come determined to make it enjoyable for everyone else.
3. Even if it's a serious occasion it must have some funny or light-hearted aspects.
4. It should be an occasion when everyone can regress a little, be comfortable, act a little childish. You can tell when it becomes a tradition when you hear your children saying, 'Do you remember last . . .?' or 'Just wait until next . . . then we will really . . .'

Follow-up Lesson 1: Consistency

Consistency is the key to many problems. Children badly need it. Without it they are unable to predict the effects of their behaviour on you as parents. They never know when they slam a door in anger whether you are going to ignore them or blow up. When the outcome of something is unpredictable, everyone becomes anxious and many can in time become neurotic. When a child can be less anxious about the results of his behaviour, he is more secure and free to devote his energies to constructive activity rather than testing your limits. We clearly see as we observe child behaviour that when the situation is uncertain, a child must test to find out how far he can go before he has the security of a limit. Too often you give in just when the child is expecting that limit. This makes the child more anxious and more likely to test you again in order to see just how far he can go before you will stop him.

What kinds of consequences work best? An automatic predetermined consequence provides the greatest consistency and therefore the greatest security for the child. It is important to set up guidelines first so that you know what to do each time. Being consistent with natural consequences is the easiest way. Don't try to be consistent with something that takes all of your effort because you won't be able to keep it up.

Another factor is agreement between parents. Parents should be able to agree on what is and what is not happening with their child so that they can be consistent in their approach.

Research indicates that unless a rule is enforced at least 80 per cent of the time it has very little effect on behaviour. Of course, 100 per cent reinforcement is desirable but with humans almost impossible, taking into account our changing emotions. As parents are able to control their child's behaviour more easily, the relationship between them and the child will improve.

In our follow-up discussion we discuss how consistent you are able to be at home with the guidelines that the unit has suggested during the five weeks of admission. In other words, are they workable in the home situation? We will also consider how consistent you are able to be with your actions and what is making consistency hard to achieve. All children need to be able to count on their parents. When they are pretty sure you are predictable, they believe you know what you are about and, therefore, they rely on you. When they trust you, they want to obey because they feel you are in the best position to get them what they need. The problem is that it isn't easy to be predictable when you don't know why you react so strongly to some of the things your children do. Basically you react strongly to the things you don't like and you don't like those behaviours that create struggles with old conflicts inside yourself. A parent who has difficulty controlling his or her anger quickly reacts to children fighting. He tries to stop the fighting which makes him angry because it threatens the shaky control he has of his own anger. In a similar manner, parents who over-react and are inconsistent with tidiness, homework, punctuality, etc., are struggling to control some aspect of their personality that is very important to them but not yet easily managed. Try to think of the personal reasons which cause you to over-react to some of your children's behaviour.

Follow-up Lesson 2: Techniques for Change — Problems in Control

During the child's stay on the Family Unit, a considerable variety of techniques are used in attempting to bring about acceptable change in behaviour, with the hope that you will continue to use those techniques which prove to be effective. Although many children complain about these rules, on our unit they expect and hope they will have something similar at home. As the atmosphere in the family improves and as the techniques become accepted as being appropriate and reasonable, the rigidity about them can be gradually relaxed.

1. The Child's Parents

One of the most important characteristics of the new controls, is that both parents agree on how they will be applied. Then the child learns promptly that he cannot appeal to one parent over the decision of the other. We emphasise not only what the child can expect if he fails to measure up, but the good things that he can enjoy as his behaviour improves and as you see again so many attractive things about him. Some investigator has demonstrated to his satisfaction that, in order for progress to be made, there have to be almost three times as many positives as negatives. One 'put down' from an important adult in the child's environment can only be neutralised by three or more pleasant, reassuring or complimentary responses.

2. The Family as a Whole

You should not be surprised to discover that there are problems with other members of the family which seem almost to be worse while another child is away. Some siblings are resentful of all the attention the hospitalised child has received. The new pattern of controls applied to the child who's been a patient in hospital will work only if similar expectations are made of the other children.

3. The School

We hope the child's regular teacher will stress the child's special abilities and how to challenge him to reveal them, rather than dwell on his failures. This is why it is so important for us to determine the child's learning ability, to make sure he isn't placed in an environment where he is chronically failing. Some parents discover that a few teachers of the child don't seem to be as convinced of the importance of 'positive reinforcement' as our staff are. It may take a lot of tact to get this message across. Generally we have been impressed with the desire of most school teachers to bring out the best achievement in children. Unfortunately, they have more children to teach than our unit teacher, so be patient. Offer to be helpful. Our teacher has already been in contact with the child's regular teacher and given him some tips.

4. The Community

Sometimes your child has become labelled in the neighbourhood as a 'problem'. It's necessary for all of you to demonstrate by the way you interact that things have changed. There are still some people who look with disfavour on the idea of hospitalising a child with problems. Parents sometimes communicate their negative attitude to their child's friends. In anticipation of any teasing about being on our unit, we have suggested and practised with your child a number of appropriate assertive responses. Keep an eye and ear open for any teasing and try to back your child up by quietly encouraging him.

5. Medication

Medication is necessary with some children who have convulsive tendencies, those who have difficulty with attention and impulse control or those who have bizarre, confused ideas, which make it hard for them to decide what is real and what is fantasy. We do not use medication as a means of control. Do not discontinue the medication without discussing it with your psychiatrist or family doctor. Your general practitioner has been sent a copy of the results of our investigations and our recommendations.

6. Self-control

Self-control is the chief aim of our therapy. If we didn't believe that children can grow to acquire an awareness of their needs for control and learn how to manage without reminders from others, we wouldn't be interested in working with children at all. Children learn to control themselves by modelling your well-controlled behaviour, having insight into what makes them react, communicating your feelings and conflicts and thinking through alternative ways of responding.

Follow-up Lesson 3: How to Make the Weak Part of Ourselves Stronger

We are all partly a parent, an adult and a child. Depending upon our upbringing and our experience, we are more one than the other. The balance of these components will determine who we relate to our children.

Someone who is almost entirely a parent may only see what a child should or should not do. They cannot see the creative qualities in their children or enjoy playing with them.

Someone who is mostly a child may relate only to the sensitivity of a child and try never to hurt them, always protect them and encourage their uniqueness. They may neglect to teach the child that they must become responsible for themselves and considerate of others.

Someone who is predominantly an adult may only be able to relate to a child's calculating, rational qualities. They may neglect to teach the child occasionally to say no to themselves or impulsively to enjoy themselves.

It we want our children to grow into well-rounded individuals, then we need an even distribution of the various components in our own personalities. Occasionally we need to be child-like; to crawl on the floor, engage in a pillow fight, whoop when we are excited. We need to be a model as an adult, carefully and quietly thinking an issue through. We need to be strict with ourselves, saying no to our own impulses and consider what is best for others dependent upon us.

We all recognise that there are deficits or weaknesses in various parts of our personalities. How then do we make those weak parts stronger?

1. Objectively assessing ourselves, how much are we one part or the other? Rate yourself as to what percentage is parent, what percent adult, what percent of you is child.

2. Recapture some of those old feelings that you have since repressed. Try and remember what it was like to be a child, to become excited about something or very disappointed. Try to remember the times when you have had to say no to yourself or when you needed quietly and carefully to calculate.

3. Say goodbye to that parent inside of you. You must differentiate between who you are and who they were. Use one of our individuation forms to see how you differ from your parents. Write a letter to your parents telling them how you perceive them and how you differ from them.

4. Practise strengthening that weaker part. Say no to yourself if it's hard to be like a parent. Think quietly and carefully if it's hard to be adult-like. Horse around, crawl on the floor and let yourself get excited if it's hard to be a child.

5. Try it out on your family.

Follow-up Lesson 4: Forgiving and Forgetting

Often the method used in our own rearing, the neglect, the painful punishments, the inconsistencies, have made it difficult for us to use more appropriate methods with our own children. Sometimes we are so intent on doing things better that we end up only doing them differently. Our children are just as confused and angry at us as we were with our parents. Sometimes, family traditions as to behaviour or goals in life or beliefs, have coloured our upbringing and perhaps made us rebellious and resentful, sometimes in a way that affects our response to any authority figures, whether they be representatives of the law, school or school agencies. Sometimes, our parents are still far too much involved in trying to tell us how tc .aise our children and far too quick to make negative judgements as to what we are trying to do (even like having the children admitted to the Royal Jubilee Hospital for its programme).

If there is a lot of marital disharmony, if one partner deserted after having been badly used by the other and if the child in question resembles in some way the offending partner, the child may come to bear to brunt of our resentment against his other parent. Sometimes this is the case even when parents stay together. The situation can be aggravated if there is chronic disagreement between the parents as to how the children should be handled.

Usually if a child is seriously disturbed enough to be admitted to the Family Unit, there has been a great deal of heartache in the family. Often the whole family has come to see the hospitalised child as the major and only problem they have. As a result, he is reacted to negatively by everyone. It begins to appear to him as if there is nothing good in him and all that interests the rest is his misbehaviour.

We even recognise that there are times when parents feel resentful towards the staff of the hospital unit. This may be because they seem to be taking the side of the child against the parents. (We do make a real effort to be neutral. We avoid blaming either side and seek, rather, ways of improving the relationships in the family.) If the recommendations given parents as to how to change the handling of the child are to be used optimistically and effectively, it is important that negative feelings about the staff be faced up to, and dealt with by forgiving and forgetting too.

Each parent must deal in a similar way with feelings of responsibility for the trouble that's developed. In order to be able to marshall your strengths, to get on with more appropriate methods of coping, you must stop blaming yourselves for the unhappy situations. For some parents this is the most difficult of all the steps to take. Yet a reasonable approach to the situation and a capacity to enjoy the new relationship with the child are unlikely to be gained without it.

When problems in your family get severe, when nothing you try seems to make anything better, when no one appreciates your efforts, when your family grabs more than gives, strong hurt and angry feelings grow. It becomes increasingly hard to let go of these feelings because they have become part of you. But to start again you must forgive and forget. It isn't easy. It feels like letting down your guard and someone may take advantage of you again. On the other hand, what have you got to lose? Why not try it once again, like this:

1. Identify the old, unresolved hurts. Remember them as clearly as you can.

2. Recognise all your feelings for each event and what might have happened if you had not controlled them.

3. Understand your own ambivalence about those involved and how you may have contributed to each unhappy situation.

4. Take these memories, feelings and contributions and discuss them openly with one family member who was most involved.

5. Ask for his/her forgiveness for your part in it.

6. If you are forgiven, say you would like to forgive him/her also. Hopefully they will have done steps 1-3 also.

7. Go over each event in detail, releasing your feelings and granting and getting forgiveness many times over.

8. Ask him/her how you can make restitution. Insist on something even if it's mainly symbolic.

9. When he/she asks you, be as specific as you can.

10. Make a contract to cut into any reoccurrence of a similar painful situation with some words like, 'Let's not do this again, remember we have forgiven each other'.

11. When real forgiving has occurred, the forgetting will begin to happen quite spontaneously.

Follow-up Lesson 5: Corrective Feedback

To provide top quality care for children we must have corrective feedback, i.e. accurate measures on how children and families respond to our treatment programmes. Therefore, we measure children's behaviours and emotional responses frequently.

We also need your subjective reactions to our programmes. What have you found most helpful or most difficult? What brought about the biggest change in your family?

As much as we need accurate feedback, so do you. You need to know from your children what they find difficult or helpful about your help and guidance. Make a regular time to discuss with the whole family the way they assess your parenting. They are going to think it even if they don't tell you. If you listen you may find you're doing much better than you thought.

We acknowledge that we have sometimes hurt you in order to make changes. If we have been unnecessarily hurting we want to know. If we have been helpful we would like to know that too. Many of the staff work far beyond the call of duty because they really do care. Please tell them, they're human too.

7 GENERAL INSTRUCTIONS AND SPECIFIC EXAMPLES

A. Discharge Summary and Recommendations

Introduction

All primary care workers spend considerable amounts of time working out a summary of their patient's progress during both the inpatient and follow-up period. They know they will be required to present these both in a written and a verbal form, and they take great care summarising the problems, the techniques, the amount of improvement and the explanations which tie it all together. They include the dynamic, transactional, behaviourial, social and existential components to their explanations. The need to be able to explain what happened and why, is part of the motivation to understand the family's problems as thoroughly as possible.

The final recommendations are based on the trial recommendations used for the child's two weekends at home during admission. As you will see from the examples, they are very individual and represent both the different workers' style and the different problems. There are recommendations for the family and for the child. After a careful explanation, the summary of recommendations are sealed in an envelope and handed over. Copies are sent to the family physician and whenever the child is a ward of the state, to the responsible social worker.

A review of all the professional reports and lab findings and further explanation of the treatment is written by the consulting psychiatrist or registrar. This report has to be comprehensive and short, so it is useful for the busy family physician. The family physician is made aware that if he wants more complete information he can obtain it on request. The family is made aware of what is in all the reports at the discharge conference. If they have any reason to wish some of the information be withheld, they are entitled to make that known. If we feel someone should know what went on, we will bargain, but the family has the final say.

Each of these summaries are from real cases but names and ages have been altered to preserve confidentiality. The techniques described have been age-adjusted.

Discharge Summary: Mark Fisher

23 August 1983
Ward 24

Dr G.F. Desmond
33 Somerset Avenue
Christchurch

Dear Dr Desmond,
Mark Fisher, Christchurch, aged 9 years
Your patient was admitted to Ward 24 on 27 June 1983 and discharged
on 29/7/83 to be followed up for five weeks as an outpatient.

Presenting Problems
Mark had previously been in the ward for a 48-hour emergency admission on 11/5/83. This was due to three episodes in the previous 2½
months involving hanging. On each of these occasions, although it was
difficult to ascertain exactly what Mark's intention was at the time, it
was clear that Mark was putting himself increasingly into dangerous and
life-threatening situations. It has also appeared that Mark had been difficult to handle at home and that he had been oppositional to his parents'
wishes. He was having trouble at school, particularly with teasing and
bullying and seemed to be withdrawn and unwilling to communicate.

Psychiatric Diagnosis
296.2 Major depressive order.

History of Presenting Problem
You will note from Mark's previous discharge summary of 19 May
1983, that Dr Erickson gives a fairly clear background to the history.

Background
Mark is the middle of three boys, Carl, aged 10, Mark, aged 9 and
Christopher, aged 6. They live with their parents in Rangiora where
father has a job as relief teacher. They apparently have been in Rangiora for five years. Mark sees himself in direct competition with his
two brothers. Particularly at school, Mark has not been achieving
and has been the butt of a lot of jokes and bullying. He finds this very
hard to take and has had difficulty in defending himself. At home he
constantly tries to compete with his brothers but does not do so very

effectively. Mark normally tries to please his brothers or his parents, usually at his own expense. Mark's problems, as he perceived them, were that he had few friends and felt very lonely. He denied any suicidal ideation and seemed rather surprised at any insistence on our part about questioning him regarding suicide. However, it was presumed early on that Mark was experiencing a fairly strong unconscious drive towards self-destruction even if he was not aware of it.

Communication, or lack of it, is not an unusual thing in this family as I think the parents discovered during Mark's admission here. They are not a family to discuss problems outwardly and hence this probably contributed to Mark's feeling of isolation before his admission.

Progress in Hospital
Mark's presenting problems were listed as the following:

1. Self-destructive acts.
2. Sadness and depression.
3. Anxiety.
4. Sibling rivalry.
5. Sensitivity to teasing.
6. Underachieving at school.

We therefore devised the following treatment goals:

1. To help Mark gain insight into his anxieties and how to cope with them.
2. To help develop awareness and appropriate expression of feelings.
3. To help develop his body awareness (being able to identify limits for himself).
4. To desensitise Mark to teasing and increase his assertiveness.
5. To help Mark enhance his social and communication skills.
6. To help Mark learn new ways of having fun.
7. To review Mark's academic abilities and enhance his appreciation of school.

While on the ward Mark participated in the following treatment programmes:

1. Nurturing and abreaction of the past.
2. Feelings rehearsal and expression.
3. Self-esteem.

4. Amorphous blob.
5. Messy play and body painting.
6. Relaxation.
7. Teasing desensitisation and assertiveness training.
8. Therapeutic wrestling.
9. Limit challenge.
10. Guidelines, limits and consequences.
11. Ego auxiliary at school.
12. Body awareness.

The parents and siblings also participated in family sessions which included relaxation, sensitivity games, communication, co-operative play, constructive activities, woodwork and guidelines and consequences. Janet and Gary had several sessions on their own talking over problems at home. Mark was also seen in individual psychotherapy.

Initially Mark's progress was slow. There was a definite reluctance to share his feelings with others, partly through unwillingness but partly one suspected, through an inability. As previously stated, Mark is clearly not practised in expressing himself verbally and when required to do so on the ward, had major difficulties. However, in his play and in other therapies, he was able to explore some of his difficulties regarding his own self-esteem, his sensitivity and some of his more confused thoughts regarding family and family relationships. This was particularly important with regards to his parents' relationship over which Mark had certain doubts. One important occasion on the ward was when Janet and Gary sat down and took time to reassure Mark that their relationship was a stable one and that he should stop worrying about it. By the third week on the ward it became fairly clear that Mark's depressive symptoms were probably as much a barrier to his progressing as anything. Although his dexamethasone suppression test for depression was normal, this did not deter us from making the diagnosis of depression on clinical symptoms alone. Consequently Mark was started on the tetracyclic anti-depressant, Maprotyline and is taking 25 mg at night. Mark has responded very favourably both to the therapies on the ward and to his anti-depressant medication.

Physical Condition
Mark was physically well on admission and routine blood testing, including a dexamethasone suppression test, proved normal. Since there had been some question about Mark's hearing, he attended the audiology clinic. Pure tone audiometry showed Mark's peripheral

hearing to be within the normal limits. Further tests were carried out regarding his central auditory perceptual function. The chief clinical audiologist felt that Mark showed a short-term auditory memory problem. This condition is known to be associated with some behavioural problems in children, but the significance of this finding in Mark's individual case is unclear. It may be that it is a contributing factor to the overall picture.

Follow-up and Prognosis
Mark's depressive symptomatology and subsequent response to antidepressant medication leads us to believe that he was suffering from a major depressive disorder. Consequently we feel that this carries a good prognosis for Mark and would like to see him maintained on antidepressants for at least three months before consideration is given to terminating it. As stated previously, the role of the central auditory processing deficit in Mark's problems is unclear. There is no doubt, however, that there is a significant social contribution to Mark's problems, not only from school but also from within the home setting.

If Mark is to be able to maintain some of the gains he has made on the ward, then equally his parents will have to continue to make the same efforts that they are at present, to make the environment at home better for him. Mark certainly made great strides in improving his own self-image and self-esteem and it seems that the lifting of his depression has enabled him to defend himself more effectively even though I suspect it has led him to get into a couple of scrapes at school, because he is no longer willing to sit back and take it.

It is with some misgivings that I see that the parents are moving to Wanaka, although hopefully this will not complicate the recovery period for Mark. Since Maprotyline is not on general release, we will liaise with the general practitioner in Wanaka regarding supply of the drug until it is decided to try to withdraw it.

In general, we feel that Mark has made enough gains to prevent him from repeating his dangerous behaviour in the near future but a lot is dependent upon the attitude of his parents towards maintaining the lines of communication that have been established.

Yours sincerely   Child and Family Unit, Ward 24

Dr Doug Brindad   cc. Ms M. Harlow
Psychiatric Registrar   Public Health Nurse

Child and Family Unit, Ward 24
Therapists' Discharge Summary – Mark Fisher

Admitted: 27/6/83
Discharged: 29/7/83

Presenting Problems
1. Self-destructive acts.
2. Sadness/depressed demeanour.
3. Anxiety.
4. Low self-esteem/negativism.
5. Sibling rivalry.
6. Sensitivity to teasing.
7. Underachieving at school.

Key Conflicts
1. Self-expectations – to succeed or fail?
2. Control – how/when or whether to be self-responsible.
3. Trust and communication – to confide or not?
4. Confusion/mysteries – i.e. what is not understood, secrets.

Treatment Goals
1. To help Mark gain insight into his anxieties and how to cope with them.
2. To help develop awareness and appropriate expression of feelings.
3. To help develop his body awareness (being able to identify limits for himself).
4. To desensitise Mark to teasing and increase his assertiveness.
5. To help Mark enhance his social and communication skills.
6. To help Mark learn new ways of having fun.
7. To review Mark's academic abilities and enhance his appreciation of school.

Review of Treatment Programme: Individual
1. Nurturing/Abreaction of the Past. Mark appeared to really enjoy the intensity of 'fussing' attention during this intensive three-day period of bedside nurturing, as an introduction to ward therapies. Yet he was

clearly anxious of each new experience, until it occurred as non-threatening. However, this anxiety certainly inhibited age regression or abreactive work, though the latter was achieved to a limited degree, non-verbally. (3 days)

2. Feelings Rehearsal and Expression. At an early stage Mark demonstrated an understanding of a broad range of feelings and readily related them to his own experience at a fairly superficial level. He was also able to correlate (in pictures) many facial expressions with appropriate feelings. Beyond this, Mark has been resistant to revealing or discussing deeper emotions, except briefly on a couple of occasions when fear, anger and grief were related to a therapist. (5 sessions, 4 hours)

3. Self-esteem. Measures were taken throughout admission of Mark's positive self-statements (unsolicited). Frequent praise, modelling and reflecting Mark's abilities to him, has been the standard procedure throughout his stay. Focus has been placed on encouragement to extend his abilities — particularly at a physical level, where he responds more readily to praise. The increase in recorded self-praise was principally related to Mark's recognition of his own efforts to apply himself in gymnasium activities.

4. Amorphous Blob. These graphic depictions of his self-awareness, completed at weekly intervals, reflect fluctuations in his concentration and co-operation during the sessions, yet a positive overall development is also apparent. Mark seemed to find this process of reviewing his self-concept quite threatening. (5 sessions)

5. Messy Play/Body Painting. Mark chose to be painted (or paint himself) in different guises on three occasions — choosing to become the 'Incredible Hulk', a happy clown and a black clown in each case. Although revealing himself was difficult, his confidence quickly developed. He preferred not to act out the characters unless supported by similarly garbed children. Additionally, Mark undertook other messy activities, occasionally observing that he preferred not to be grubby, though this very frequently occurred in fact. (4 sessions, 4 hours)

6. Relaxation. Initially introduced successfully during nurturing and again in family therapy sessions, relaxation exercises latterly were used to prelude therapy sessions where Mark showed anxiety or resistance.

Although a deep state of relaxation was not accomplished at all, he usually responded to treatment more willingly after these exercises.

7. Teasing Desensitisation/Assertiveness Training. This is a definite area of concern to Mark. After his initial denial of the problem, we established a list of 17 offensive teases. Periodically our sessions broke down when discussion of the topic drove Mark to use oppositional stances to protect himself, inhibiting his abilities to effectively 'parrot' the teases. Presently Mark is still sensitive in this area, even though he has shown he can cope in sessions. His capacity has varied according to his self-esteem and attitude on different days. (7 sessions, total 2 hours)

8. Therapeutic Wrestling. Despite his early assertions that he 'didn't like fighting', i.e. hurting or being hurt, Mark showed a ready inclination to sort our peer problems by 'punching heads in', so that our concept of 'controlled contest of strength' became a useful alternative to his normal response. As he developed more confidence in his capacity Mark demonstrated significantly greater self-restraint in fighting. Therapeutic ward wrestling was also a useful variation which helped increase assertiveness. (6 sessions, 2 hours)

9. Limit Challenge (Physical and Mental). A series of developmental exercises were planned in the gymnasium to encourage Mark to challenge, test and extend his capacity, over the period of admission. At first Mark tended to underrate his strengths at the same time exhibiting recklessness in attempts to beat himself. With one-to-one encouragement, he developed remarkable determination and self-control in every exercise, dramatically extending his ability. In such cases he was clearly proud of his gains — in strength as well as self-esteem. Regrettably, when not under firm one-to-one supervision, Mark rarely stuck to the established programme, correspondingly his gains in self-appreciation tended to fluctuate. (13 sessions, approx. 10 hours)

10. Guidelines, Limits and Consequences. Initially, while clearly attempting to please, Mark tended to leave tasks uncompleted, preferring to move to a different activity, usually claiming that to be more appropriate. Gradually this tendency broadened to frequent inappropriate assertion, resulting in many contraventions of ward rules, thus involving 'natural' consequences. Mark's frustrated attempts to manipulate his way out of consequences presented him with a new

experience – firmly consistent limits. This appeared to have a valuable therapeutic effect. While continuing to test the limits, Mark has gradually responded more readily to the self-regulated option of 'staying in play'.

11. Ego Auxiliary. Mark's efforts at school fluctuated, without a pattern of application becoming apparent. On occasions, when supported in school by an ego auxiliary, his work was exemplary. This was latterly monitored by a teacher who reflected appropriate courses of option to Mark. (4 sessions, 7 hours)

12. Body Awareness. Two sessions, conducted by the house surgeon, in anatomy and physiology and sex education. (2 sessions, 1½ hours)

Group Therapies
1. Sensitivity/awareness group (approx. 12 hours).
2. Peer/social skills group (approx. 6 hours).
3. Kangaro Kort, dramatic role-plays of everyday experiences (approx. 8 hours).

Family Therapies
1. Family Sessions. Included relaxation, sensitivity games, communication, co-operative play, constructive activities, woodwork, guidelines and consequences. (approx. 10 hours)

2. Parent/Couple Therapy. Included participation and observation of preliminary sessions with Mark. Individual and conjoint abreactive and reflective discussion with Janet and Gary. (approx. 8 hours)

Summary
Mark's reluctance to share his feelings with others is a continuing problem. His conflicts are still largely a mystery of secrets and he sometimes seems overwhelmed by a confusion he can't communicate about. Yet he has made positive, if cautious, moves towards sharing with and trusting others as well as having moved a significant way towards accomplishing the treatment goals originally set.

Steven Lee
Primary Therapist

29 July 1983
Ward 24

To: Mr and Mrs Fisher

Child and Family Unit, Ward 24
Discharge Recommendations — Mark Fisher

These also include Carl and Christopher.

1. Firm limits are a necessary security barrier for Mark's psychological and physical well-being. Within them he will respond more self-responsibly if he understands where your limits give him room to make his own day-to-day choices.

Consistent adherence to the attached guidelines and consequences will help create a mutually co-operative family routine, though it will undoubtedly need some working at before it runs like clockwork. Don't give up!!

2. Mark always likes to be appreciated when behaving in a pleasing way (and don't we all?). Knowing you are appreciated means being told. Please try to make the effort and be clear — say what (and why) you appreciate about each other; it will soon pay off. You'll be amazed how much more you'll like yourself this way as well!

3. The boys are very different in temperament, needs, abilities and capacity. They need to be respected and treated individually as people, in order that they can grow up as THEMSELVES. Make it a habit to settle them separately — invest the extra time in a 'special' story each, to reward that 'special individuality'. They will be greater companions to you and each other if they don't have to compete for your time always.

4. Family Activities. Make it a feature of your routine to plan and complete a joint venture each week. If you each took turns to choose one outing/activity/venue each week, you would all probably enjoy broadening your horizons . . . (even if you are not fussed about someone else's choice or idea, give it a try). This can be a positive consequence for appreciated behaviours as well.

5. Time Out for Mum and Dad. A vital investment for your present and

future happiness. Don't be slaves to work. (Remember how, without any play, work only made Jack a dull boy?) So, come on — discuss it and plan it, but do it. Have a regular time out. Make a night of it.

Janet and Gary, you have both put a lot into the Ward 24 programme for Mark, as well as yourselves. But now is just the start . . .

I have enjoyed working with you all and am very keen to help in any way I can over the next five-weeks' follow-up. I will be in frequent phone contact and I hope you will be down for some of the parent evenings.

Don't hesitate to phone me any time you have queries or concerns.

With best wishes to you all.

Steven Lee
Primary Therapist

Heather Thomas
Charge Nurse

To Mark
Mark, I know you have got a mixture of memories to take home from Ward 24 with you . . .

Like: You know that you can make friends easily. Isn't it easier to do so when you learn a bit about the person before you decide you don't like them? Yes, Linda, Stuart, Andrew and the others all like you too (not to mention me).

And: How many weights could you pull? 123 wasn't it? How does that sound? And remember, you began with only 41. Amazing!

And: Who's the woodwork expert?

And: Who's firm (but fair) and doesn't 'do deals'? But I'm sure you don't need too much reminding about who can decide to keep you in play and how to do it.

And: When they tease you, look 'em in the eye and always add 'YOURSELF'.

Guidelines and Consequences — Mark Fisher (and Carl and Christopher)

Day	Time	Daily Routine	If Does (+)	If Doesn't (—)
Mon/Fri	8.00 a.m.	Rise 'n' shine (means up, dressed, washed, hair brushed, shoes on, bed made, room tidy, TIME AT BREAKFAST TABLE)	Gets brekkie	Doesn't
Mon/Fri	8.45 a.m.	Gets self off to school	Bike to school	Walks to school
Mon/Fri	3.30 p.m.	After school — 'Keep cool routine': Home by 3.30 p.m. unless permission given	Gets afternoon tea	No afternoon tea
		Pocket money jobs:	Earns weekly comic subscription	Weekly subscription cancelled
		Mark — cut wood		
		sweep garage floor		
		feed animals in evening		
		Christopher — set table, breakfast		
		set table, tea		
		milk bottles out		
		Carl — stack wood		
		mow lawns		
		feed animals in morning		
		Carl and Mark to dry dishes		
		All to clean bathroom after they use it.		
Mon/Fri	5.30 p.m.	Tea time (must be on time/hands washed, etc.)	Gets tea	Bed one hour early that night
Sun/Thurs		Bath 'n' bed (means shower or bath at appointed time — in bed on time ALONE)	Gets bedtime story	No story
	7.00 p.m.	Bath — Christopher		
	8.00 p.m.	Bed — Christopher		
	7.30 p.m.	Bath — Mark		
	8.30 p.m.	Bed — Mark		
	8.00 p.m.	Bath — Carl		
	8.45 p.m.	Bed — Carl		
		Stays in own bed	Lots of hugs and praise	In own bed one hour earlier next night

Other Guidelines

		Swearing	Praise	Time-out one minute
		Fighting/aggression	Praise	Time-out ten minutes
		Home by 4 p.m. after school		Bed straight after tea

And: Who doesn't need to 'get tough' when he knows he's already strong enough?

And: We sure will miss you . . .

And lots more.

Love from Steve

Discharge Summary: John Trenton

25 May 1983
Ward 24

Dr P.K. Harris
Fairfax Medical Centre
Christchurch

Dear Dr Harris
John Trenton, Christchurch, aged 8 years
John was admitted to Ward 24 for a five-week arranged admission on 13/1/83. He was discharged on 15/2/83 for a five-week follow-up period as an outpatient before final discharge.
    The presenting problems were:

1. Episodic stealing and lying.
2. Feelings of insecurity and inadequacy in keeping up with social and academic demands.
3. Temper tantrums, verbal abuse to both Mum and others.
4. Lack of communication of inner feelings to anyone.
5. Episodes of soiling and wetting.
6. Unable to deal with teasing by children at school.
7. Chronic non-compliance.
8. Low self-esteem.

Formal Psychiatric Diagnosis
296.2   Major depressive episode.
312.10   Conduct disorder, under-socialised non-aggressive.
V61.20   Parent/child problem.

Summary of Background History

Mr and Mrs Trenton's marriage broke up about three years ago following an affair Mr Trenton had with Mrs Trenton's younger sister, Wendy. Since that time, Peter, aged 10, has been living with Dad and John, aged 8, has been living with Mum. John apparently has always been a difficult child but his behaviour has been particularly worse since the break-up of the marriage and includes those things listed above. Since the marriage break-up, Mrs Trenton has observed that John has become quite socially withdrawn and has very few friends. In the month or so before admission he seemed to be particularly unhappy, was noticed to be eating continuously between meals; lollies, ice cream, biscuits, etc. and seemed to be putting on weight. Mrs Trenton also noticed that he was becoming very hard to rouse in the morning and seemed sleepy during the day. In the three weeks prior to admission he was becoming more and more difficult to get to school and apparently, when he attended, was getting into a lot of trouble with other children and finally refused to go. In several weekends when he went to see his father, a considerable amount of money was stolen by John. It was thought, diagnostically, that John had a depressive illness or a long-standing conduct disorder, basically involving non-aggressive, deviant behaviour in the context of social isolation and a chronic problem of John to make friends. A dexamethasone suppression test was positive and confirmed our clinical impression of a depressive illness.

Progress in Hospital

John was involved in a multi-faceted therapeutic programme with five key conflicts:

1. John's struggle for security by trying to be in control.
2. Being a ventilator for his mother's feelings.
3. Trying to cope with school in the face of stressful home circumstances.
4. To attempt to satisfy unmet needs by stealing.
5. Grief over the loss of Dad and older brother.

Specific therapeutic programmes included three days' nurturing, feelings rehearsal, assertiveness, a trust programme, compliance, self-awareness, delayed gratification, individuation, therapeutic wrestling, limit challenge, social skills and wood-working, self-esteem programme. It was felt that progress was particularly helped by the nurturing programme. It was felt that he would be trustworthy only if the situation was not stressful. His compliance varied greatly according to how he was feeling at the time. John was also involved in individual therapy which turned out to be an uphill battle. Discussion focused on the difficulties he has with control, particularly his being controlled by rules.

In view of his depression, John was started on an anti-depressant. He was begun on 37.5 mg of Maproptyline. This was increased to 50 mg and it was noticed that after about two weeks of being on the drug, John showed a clinical response to medication. His mood brightened and his behaviour around the ward turned him from being a rather obnoxious, sneaky and extremely negative individual, into a more normal, mischievous, active boy. Serial blood screens are part of the protocol for the use of this drug. John will be followed up by Professor Ney at the Child and Family Guidance Centre following discharge from the ward, to continue the monitoring of his clinical state as well as ongoing observation for untoward side-effects.

June Trenton, who has an ongoing treatment with Graham Smart of the Crisis Team, continued to have individual sessions with him during the five-week therapy programme. In addition to this she was involved in a three-day nurturing programme on the ward. It was found that she was able to open up and share painful experiences, particularly those involving her feeling extremely victimised. The primary therapist concluded that June does have the necessary strength to deal with John. There were some family sessions involving June's parents as well as her separated husband. The meeting with June's parents was particularly helpful. June was able to voice to her parents her loneliness which she hadn't been able to before. A closer bond now appears to be present between them. A better understanding between June and her husband has been established and there is greater continuity of John's care in the two different households.

Prognosis and Follow-up

In the follow-up period John will be seen at home by the primary therapist to consolidate the therapies. Graham Smart of the Crisis Team will continue to see June and John at the Child and Family Guidance Centre with Professor Ney, relating to the Maproptyline. John seems to have made a clinical response to medication and it is anticipated that there will be a positive shift in his behavioural disturbance. If Mrs Trenton is able to maintain a secure nurturing control of John for an ongoing period of time and parental access is securely established on a smoother level, there is definite hope that John will emerge from childhood as a fairly normal individual. Probably the best indication of this will be evidence of more appropriate socialisation and making some good friends in the next few years.

More details relating to this admission are available from the Ward 24 file on request.

Yours sincerely

Dr Doug Brindad
Psychiatric Registrar
Child and Family Unit, Ward 24

cc. Graham Smart
    Crisis Team

Child and Family Unit, Ward 24
Therapists' Discharge Summary – John Trenton

Admitted: 13/1/83
Discharged: 15/2/83

Key Conflicts
1. Attempting to be in control during stressful situations when his more basic need is security.
2. Ventilating his mother's frustrated feelings and then being punished for it.
3. Struggling to cope with school, academic and social demands.
4. Stealing for excitement to dispel gloomy thoughts and loneliness.
5. Incompleted mourning for the loss of his father and brother.

Presenting Problems
 1. Depressed, unhappy feelings.
 2. Episodic stealing and lying.
 3. Feelings of insecurity and inadequacy.
 4. Temper tantrums, e.g. verbally abuses Mum and others.
 5. Does not communicate inner feelings, shuts himself off.
 6. Episodic soiling and wetting.
 7. Teased by children at school.
 8. Non-compliant to mother.

9. Low self-esteem.
10. Rejects father.

Goals

1. To enable John to deal with painful past experiences and loss of father.
2. To show John appropriate ways of controlling his aggression and anger.
3. To teach John how to assert himself appropriately.
4. To improve John's self-esteem.
5. To improve interfamily relationships through better communications.
6. To establish a sense of positiveness with current and future plans.

Therapies

1. Nurturing and Abreaction. John responded well to this. He could recognise his needs by allowing himself the role of nurtured child. Abreaction occurred with talking and encouraging John to deal with painful past experiences. (3 days)

2. Feelings Rehearsal. John has a good insight into his feelings but has difficulty communicating them to others. He is afraid to acknowledge and take responsibility, particularly the painful ones, as they evoke bad memories from the past. Rehearsing the expression of feelings made it possible to feel more comfortable communicating them to others. (8 hours)

3. Assertiveness Training. A hierarchy of names he is teased with was established. John is now responding appropriately most of the time but sometimes reverts to aggression, depending on whom the insult comes from. (18 hours)

4. Trust Programme. John will be very trustworthy if the situation is not stressful. On two occasions he regressed to stealing money when he wasn't coping with an underlying conflict. (15 hours)

5. Compliance. Varied from 20–100 per cent depending largely on how depressed John was. It gradually improved and his mother knows what to reinforce. (72 hours)

6. Amorphous Blob. John found it easier to write his feelings down on

paper so this proved a useful exercise. He is now aware of inner self. although a little unsure of how others see him. (5 hours)

7. Delayed Gratification. At first he was impatient but now John is comfortable to wait 10-15 minutes. (10 hours)

8. Ego Auxiliary. We implemented this the first three weeks as school holidays interfered with the last two weeks. John coped well with our school, partly because he liked the less regimental approach but also because I taught him how to cope under pressure. I feel he may still be rather apprehensive about his present school setting. (30 hours)

9. Individuation with Mum. This technique was aimed at acknowledging the similarities and differences of John and his mother and helping them accept their own identity. Both were reluctant at first but learned a lot from the experience. (16 hours)

10. Therapeutic Wrestling. We taught John how to use his strength appropriately. Eventually he learned to control himself really well. He tended to be a wee bit boisterous with the smaller children. It was important for John to feel he was one of the 'toughest and strongest' on the ward. He also learned how to accept winning and losing. (10 hours)

11. Social Skills Training. He participated spasmodically but towards the latter weeks became a good leader. He continues to experience 'conflicts' if unsure how to cope with a particular situation. (10 hours)

12. Limit Challenge. He has a reasonable knowledge of his limitations and capabilities, both physically and mentally. He worries about how smart he is but by setting his own goals will try harder. (15 hours)

13. Kangaroo Kort. At first he contributed only when asked, but became more spontaneous towards the latter weeks. (15 hours)

14. Woodwork for Self-esteem. He was full of constructive ideas and enjoyed this. He now knows he is pretty good with at least one skill. (6 hours)

Sessions with June Trenton
Nurturing and Abreaction. June had the 'flu' during nurturing so she

enjoyed a lot of tender loving care. She abreacted really well. I felt it was a relief for her to open up the past and have some supportive people listening to her. On many occasions she felt she was the 'victim'. June tends to introspect on a destructive level. Due to her depressive states her positiveness and self-esteem were lacking. She could not provide John with a good model. John, I feel, needs more security and support within his relationship with Mum. Her coping mechanisms are improving but June remains quite dependent on others to get her through the critical stages in both the past and the present. (80 hours)

Summary
I feel progress has been made with both John and his mother, June. The next five weeks will be important to assess whether June's coping mechanisms will provide John with a more stable and positive future. John's happier outlook will help June feel her mothering has its rewards.

Michelle Greenslade
Primary Therapist

20 May 1983
Ward 24

To: Mrs Trenton
Child and Family Unit, Ward 24
Discharge Recommendations, John Trenton
June, to review our time spent with John, we will start with the problems which referred John to the ward. These being:

1. Unhappy mood.
2. Episodic lying and stealing.
3. Feelings of insecurity and inadequacy.
4. Temper tantrums involving verbally abusing you and others.
5. Not communicating his feelings and thoughts.
6. Couldn't cope with teasing by other children at school.
7. Disobedient, refusing to do things when asked.
8. Feeling not very important and bad about himself.

Our aims were to assist John to cope with these anxieties and

Guidelines and Consequences for John Trenton

Guideline	Consequence
1. Making bed and doing chores on time	Give 'best bed' award, praise
2. In control with no fights or temper tantrums	A special treat or daily surprise if possible
3. Encourage John to wait for something he wants, do this daily	Praise for being patient and give him whatever you promised
4. For being compliant when asked to do tasks	Praise him by expressing how happy it makes you feel when he does as he's told
5. Encourage John to talk to you if he has a problem	Listen attentively, give him feedback on how well you understand, offer support and advice
6. Send John on trust mission daily, e.g. to the shop	If correct change and correct quantity of goods, praise for being trustworthy
7. Stops fighting with his brother within two minutes after being warned	Praise him for being a good sport. If they don't stop, send both to bedroom for ten minutes' cooling off

Recommendations
When things are not going well these suggestions may be helpful:

1. Swearing	Time-out for five minutes
2. Temper tantrum or physical aggression	Encourage John to count up to ten. Offer to have a pillow fight. Listen or ask what is bothering him. Time-out if absolute refusal and no other alternatives available
3. Stealing	Encourage John to speak the truth. If he has been caught stealing John is to return the goods to the person concerned and they are to negotiate the terms of restitution
4. Lying	Praise John when he tells the truth. He needs more positive praise to learn that he can get attention through doing good things
5. Teasing	If John reports he's being teased at school or by others, encourage him to talk about how the situation arose; you could encourage him to say the insult back

problems. This involved fourteen therapies in which we listened, then showed John appropriate ways of dealing with his inner and environmental conflicts.

The success of our therapy, especially over the last fortnight, has become more apparent. John, I feel, has become more aware of what is socially acceptable by identifying with his own feelings. He is slowly learning what others expect from him.

Management of John after discharge is going to be really important. For continuity please follow the attached guidelines and consequences on a daily basis.

Many thanks for your participation over the last five weeks, June. I have admired your fight and strength during this period. Take each day as it comes, naturally some days will be better than others. Stability and a positive outlook on life for both of you will be necessary.

We have appreciated your regular visits and attendance at meetings and therapies. My time with you will consist of another five weeks which we call follow-up. This involves home visits weekly, where we can talk about any problems and concerns you have. Parent meetings will continue for another five weeks, on Monday night at 7 p.m.

All the best for the future,

Michelle Greenslade
Primary Therapist

Discharge Summary: Susie Boyd

Royal Jubilee Hospital
Victoria, BC

To: Dr G. Andrews
From: Dept of Nursing, EMI 6-A

Discharge Summary of Nursing Programme — Susie Boyd, aged 13 years

Admitted: 21/5/76
Discharged: 26/6/76

Key Conflicts
1. Susie's conflict re control — can she trust herself?
2. The three-generation conflict — Mum over-identifies with Susie's hurts.
3. Communication with Dad. Susie is intensely close to Mum.
4. Susie is torn over her identity as a woman.

Measures

The following measures were recorded throughout Susie's hospitalisation to indicate to staff how Susie was progressing:

1. Decision-making. Susie was given ten choices per day and allowed 30 seconds in which to make a choice. At first, all that was required was a simple 'yes' or 'no'. The choices became more complex in time. If she decided within 30 seconds, then her choice was rewarded with verbal support. She was not allowed to change her mind about her first decision. If no choice was made within 30 seconds, then the staff decided for her (usually the least desirable). However, she had some difficulty when parents gave her the choice. Perhaps this was because she may have been embarrassed or reproached for past mistakes.

2. Weight. Susie was allowed complete freedom in the area of eating and vomiting. No staff watched her, and she responded by saying that she felt less pressure in these critical areas while living in hospital. In order to give Susie feedback on how she was doing in controlling her eating and vomiting, staff weighed her daily in a non-committal fashion.

3. Spontaneous Expressions. Susie was observed for all expressions. Staff noted that towards the end of her five-week hospitalisation, she was much more relaxed and allowed herself to show her emotions.

Individual Programme

Susie's first conflict was identified as her difficulty with control – she doesn't trust herself. Our goal was to teach Susie to be more carefree and to trust herself.

Susie appears to subordinate herself and frequently is a conformist. We could hypothesise that guilt feelings have helped her find this role. In any event, our aim was to help her relax. The following aids were used to facilitate this end:

1. Using the decision-making technique as described under Measures above.

2. A weigh-in daily with no hassles (as described under Measures above).

3. Feelings Rehearsal — staff modelled for Susie by verbalising to her how they were feeling, e.g. 'I'm feeling angry because the noise level in

this room is so high that I'm finding it difficult to talk to you', or by asking Susie at random, to state how she was feeling at the moment (e.g. there was a fight between two male patients, and Susie was asked during the ruckus what her feelings were at that moment).

4. Role-playing — the staff modelled for Susie by verbalising at the dinner table their ambivalence about enjoying eating but not wanting to take too much food and thus become fat. Staff completed the modelling by verbalising the compromise of taking enough to satisfy most of the urge to take a lot and still leaving some food behind in order not to gain weight. On discharge, Susie continued either to eat huge quantities of food (and quite possibly vomit), or not eat at all.

5. Susie was taught to assert herself. Prior to hospitalisation she had been supported for willingness to conform and had tried very hard to please others (in fear of disapproval). Once again, role-playing was used by staff, and role-training for Susie was done. She responded well to going through the motions physically of asserting herself, although it was difficult to know if she gained much insight into her former behaviour.

6. Susie models herself after her mother. Mum has very high expectations and is compulsive. Staff asked Mother to role-model for Susie a more relaxed form of dress and attitude towards things in general. Both parents bought jeans, and Mother did try to seem more relaxed. Susie's good clothes were exchanged for less formal ones — e.g. jeans and T-shirts for the remainder of her stay in hospital. Susie said she was extremely happy that her parents had finally become 'with it', as jeans are in style now. Dad's help has been elicited too. He is to take both Mum and Susie out in the canoe and dump them in the water.

7. To aid Susie in her effort to relax, staff helped her to do some cooking of desserts such as cakes and cookies. Staff modelled for Susie that it was OK to snack on the goodies (such as chocolate chips, nuts and raisins) that went into the baked foods. Susie did not snack on the goodies. As noted above, Susie either did not eat or ate huge quantities. She identified this as her main area of concern, i.e. her lack of control when it came to eating.

8. Susie was given many difficult tasks which made her feel frustrated. Staff attempted to teach her that it was OK to fail. This also tied in

with her own high expectations as well as helping her both to assert herself in stating that the job was too difficult, and verbalise how she felt at the time (as in Feelings Rehearsal above).

9. A word association test was done to see if Susie's response to a charged word such as 'vomit' would be connected to anger. Staff also talked with Susie about vomiting's being a form of anger, as in, 'piss on you'.

10. Susie will be taking creative dancing and playing more active sports with Dad. These will be to help her loosen up and relax.

11. During the last week of Susie's admission, it was noted that Susie was extremely emotionally involved in her own therapy and sometimes perceived her problems in an inaccurate way. She was told to stop analysing herself, as her efforts to know herself completely were fruitless. After these directions were given, Susie seemed really to relax and enjoy herself.

12. Susie seemed uncomfortable with her emotions. She tried to intellectualise in order to cover up these emotions. She also procrastinated and was often heard to say, 'I just know I'll be better (or different) next week'. Staff did not protect her from her emotional expressions such as anger and sadness. For example, after one particularly trying discussion between the staff member, Mother and Susie, Susie tried to seclude herself in her room. Mother supported the idea and told Susie she needed 'time to recharge her batteries'. Staff did not allow Susie the seclusion she desired and forced her to participate in group activities where she was not able to cover up her emotions.

On Susie's two weekend passes, the parents were given guidelines which incorporated many of the items listed on the 'Recommendations to Parents' which they received at the discharge conference. To help the parents be aware of how they are doing with Susie, we have asked that, during the five-week follow-up, they continue being in tune with their own feelings at a specific time after dinner.

Susie's second conflict was identified as the three-generation conflict. Mum over-identifies with Susie's hurts. Our goal was to help Mum deal with her own mother and with Susie.

Mum had many insecurities in her own childhood and tries desperately to protect Susie from a similar experience. However, whenever Mum talked about her childhood, Susie said that she felt guilty for enjoying things in life. Both Susie and Mum were concerned for the maternal grandmother as she is dying of bone cancer. To deal with these conflicts, staff:

(a) Had both Mum and Susie symbolically say goodbye to the maternal grandmother. Susie verbalised on a tape, and Mum wrote a letter. Both were instructed to remember all the good and bad experiences they had had with the maternal grandmother. They both expressed feelings previously denied or distorted. This 'saying goodbye' gave each of them insight and increased self-understanding.

(b) Mum had a number of areas she had yet to deal with with her own mother. With encouragement, she wrote to her mother about these things. Susie expressed a feeling of relief that Mum had finally stopped talking about these areas and had done something about them.

(c) Staff got Susie and Mum together and instructed them that they should no longer talk about the past but should talk about happy things. Susie was then told to tell her sad experiences to Dad. Mum was told to discuss her sad experiences and past insecurities with either Dad or some professional.

The third conflict identified was that of poor communication between Dad and the rest of the family. As there had been an alliance of Mother and children against Dad, it was our objective to shift relationships within the family, thereby opening up new channels of communication.

Father had always been viewed as the strong one who showed no emotion and who was hard to become close to. This was a position Mr Boyd had been forced into as a young man, and it continued into his own family situation. It was necessary to help the family see Father as a sensitive person with feelings and to help desensitise Father to highly emotional, dependent women such as Susie and Mrs Boyd. In order to facilitate this objective, the following steps were taken:

(a) Establish a Closer Relationship Between Susie and Dad. Upon her admission to hospital, Susie was given two days of bed rest and placed in a position of being dependent upon staff for food and social contact.

When a nurturing relationship was established, Father alone was asked to visit and carry on this nurturing. This involved bringing gifts and taking Susie on rewarding outings. Staff then helped Father to establish emotional contact with Susie by getting him to talk of his younger life while Susie was present. It soon became evident to Susie that Father was not made of stone. As Father revealed more about himself, Susie became confident enough to express to him her anger and disappointments about his lack of involvement with the family in the past.

(b) Marital Counselling and Parental Psychotherapy. Mr and Mrs Boyd had arrived at a point in their relationship where tension was high and communication was low. One partner would expect the other to be aware of one's needs without any verbalisation and also would assume motives for some action on the other's part. There had been a long history of conflict with Mr Boyd being very involved at work and in hockey, to the exclusion of his family. Mrs Boyd is very dependent and, as the husband was unavailable for communication, she turned to Susie to confide all her sorrows and hurts.

Communication between the parents was established by having them talk about the past and about their individual perceptions of different episodes. This proved quite revealing to both partners as they had both tended to assume the other's state of mind rather than asking.

Mr Boyd had to leave home to play hockey while in his teens and never really got to know his father. His father had committed suicide while Mr Boyd was away, and he returned home to take over as head of the family even though he was not the eldest. His mother and sister went to pieces during this time, and he had to be the strong one even though he resented their dependence. When Mrs Boyd and Susie present themselves as very emotional and dependent, the scene is re-enacted and his reaction is to back away. Mrs Boyd and Susie were shown to be stronger than Mr Boyd had estimated. Dad had to learn that he can be broad-shouldered without being smothered.

(c) Establishment of New Patterns of Communication. Mother was advised to share her problems with Dad or a therapist but not with Susie.

Susie was encouraged to talk about sad feelings with Dad, not Mum. Mother was advised not to force son John to communicate.

Each family member practised expressing their emotions with the person involved rather than dumping on someone else. Father was encouraged to express his emotional needs within the family rather than waiting and becoming frustrated until someone guessed his desires.

Susie's fourth identified conflict was her confused identity as a woman. Our goal was to help her deal with her feelings about growing up.

Upon admission, Susie made a self-portrait by lying on a piece of paper and having her body outlined. She then added her features and hung the picture on her bedroom wall. Just prior to discharge, she was asked to evaluate the drawing. She stated that it was a young stranger and no longer a picture of herself. A new drawing was made and compared, and Susie was pleased with her more mature self.

Another technique used for helping Susie assess her personal changes during her five-week stay, was the use of the Amorphous Blob. She wrote down all the traits and attributes she possessed upon admission. Staff then drew a line to enclose all her attributes inside the blob. Outside the line she listed the characteristics she would like to attain. The blob was assessed regularly and updated by deleting the attributes no longer characteristic of Susie and including those attributes previously outside. Over the course of time the blob acquired a more human shape.

Susie was given encouragement to explore her childhood and the painful moments of the past — the things Susie and Mother talked of frequently. Susie was helped to express her fears and anger. As Mrs Boyd had had no one else for emotional support, she confided in Susie, not as her young daughter, but as an adult. These confidences made Susie feel very important but, at the same time, she was very frightened by the pain and responsibilities of adulthood and recoiled from growing up. Susie was then asked to write down all her childhood recollections, to put them into a bottle and sink the bottle at sea as a dramatisation of gently saying goodbye to childhood. It was also agreed that Susie and Mother were not to talk about the past.

Susie was able to achieve a more realistic appraisal of growing up and was therefore more able to accept her changing status.

The following is a list of recommendations given to Mr and Mrs Boyd at the time of Susie's discharge:

Mr and Mrs Boyd, you have both worked very hard during your time with us, as has Susie. This hard work has paid off. The following recommendations are to help you sort out what has happened here and to give you support, should you need it:

As you communicate and share, so your children will follow your example. You have both begun to work towards a method of compromise in your communication. Many of your own difficulties have stemmed from unverbalised needs and from giving the partner incorrect motives for some action.

In the future we would encourage you to put your own feelings into words rather than expect your partner to anticipate your needs. Go out together more often in unstructured settings.

The lines of communication in the family have been established so that things go through Dad. Judy, don't allow Susie to suck you back into your former role; refer her to your husband.

Susie needs to be treated as normally as possible. She is not as fragile as you have been led to believe. In so far as eating is concerned, arrange your meals in self-serve fashion. Don't be upset if Susie misses a meal and if she heads off to her bedroom afterwards. The two of you should do something pleasant together, perhaps including Susie, so as not to become involved in any scene with Susie. There is no need to encourage her to eat or restrict her diet or comment on her weight. Rather, communicate to her that you are pleased with her as she is, that what she does in private does not affect your estimation of her or take away from the family's happiness.

To give you some immediate feedback on how you are doing, please keep a record for the next five weeks on the following:

(a) How each of you feels right after dinner is finished.
(b) Who is present at the time you are tuning in to your feelings.

Judy, keep looking for something to challenge your mind outside the home. You have a bright, searching mind and should turn it to some constructive use. Remember that mistakes are inevitable, but these won't alter the changes that have been made for the good. All of you, as a family, have the resources to meet any eventuality as long as you continue to communicate effectively. Good luck.

The following is a list of recommendations given to Susie at the time of her discharge:

Susie, in the past few weeks, you have made a great deal of progress. The following recommendations are to remind you of the ground we have covered and to give you some further advice if you should ever need it.

In the past, you and your Mother have shared many intimate secrets and have burdened one another with your problems. It is not your responsibility to solve your Mother's misfortunes and, in some instances, you can be responsible for yourself. Forget the past and share the good things of the present and future with your Mother.

For some time you felt uncomfortable with your Father as his emotional involvement with you was somewhat limited. Now you have discovered that he is a sensitive, responsive person to whom you can turn to share your troubles or your joys. He is responsible for the family and is capable of handling anything that may arise.

One of the more important lessons you have learned is how and when to be assertive. This goes hand in hand with expressing your feelings as they occur rather than stifling or ignoring them. Expressions of how you really feel at a given moment are never expressed as a put-down of someone else but are verbalised as your perceptions of the moment.

We all make mistakes, and you're just like everyone else. The trick is to focus on the things you are doing right, to remember that a mistake won't bring your world crashing down and to remember that you must pick yourself up and carry on. Keep your attention focused on a goal rather than trying to figure out all the ins and outs.

You've worked very hard since you've been in hospital, Susie, and you can be proud of yourself as it has paid off. You are more assertive; you are more able to say what you feel; you are more aware that you are not responsible for everyone else's problems; your family is more open; Dad is more involved and can understand you.

We hope this summary will be of some assistance to you in the future care of Susie and her family.

Mrs H Donaldson
Head Nurse
6th Floor Family Unit

Prepared by: B. Martin RN
               N. McKenzie BA

Discharge Summary: Julie Warner

Royal Jubilee Hospital
Victoria, BC

To: Dr T. Jones
From: Child Psychiatric Department

Discharge Summary of Nursing Programme — Julie Warner, aged 10
years

Admitted: 6/9/76
Discharged: 8/10/76   .

Key Conflicts
1. Is mother able to provide the care needed by Julie?
2. Mother's depression, hopelessness and guilt.
3. Has mother accepted Julie's mental deficits?
4. Poor peer relationships.

Problem Behaviours on Admission
1. Non-compliant.
2. Fights with siblings.
3. Teases.
4. Physical aggression.
5. Compulsive eater.
6. Occasional bedwetting.
7. Tantrums — sometimes destructive and mean.

Our Goals
1. Assess need for placement outside home.
2. Ensure that mother's expectations are realistic. Explore with mother
   her own feelings.
3. Assess Julie's abilities and make recommendations.
4. Teach social skills.

Measures
1. Compliance. In order to assess Julie's ability to respond to requests
made to her, she was put on a compliance programme. Ten requests
were made of her each day and the number with which she complied in
ten seconds were recorded as a percentage. She was praised appropriately

when she responded positively and, when the response was negative, she was ignored for ten minutes. Asking Julie to do something often met with resistance. She responded well to being given time limits — i.e. you have five minutes to clean your room, then its school, or whatever. Also, while doing something (i.e. getting her coat), Julie liked to be timed as to her speed. This was done by clapping hands and counting out loud.

Compliance Averages %
1st week 35
2nd week 50
3rd week 37
4th week 48 (on medication during this week)
5th week 70

2. Temper Tantrums. These became apparent when Julie was given the consequences of breaking set rules. These tantrums decreased in number and intensity as Julie began to accept the rules and saw that she got no attention for a tantrum (being matter-of-factly isolated for five minutes or until she was quiet).

Tantrum Frequency No.
1st week 5
2nd week 3
3rd week 6
4th week 5
5th week 0

Individual Programme
1. Feelings Rehearsal. Modelling, role-playing and cueing were used to help Julie express and deal with her feelings in an open and appropriate manner. Julie responded to this fairly well and quickly, as every positive incident was responded to with praise and a hug which she really enjoyed receiving.

2. Training in Assertion. Julie had trouble holding her own ground and tolerating teasing or pressure. Appropriate responses to situations were suggested and modelled. Then Julie was involved in role-playing. She was also desensitised to names she was teased with, such as 'Fatty' and 'Dummy'. Julie picked up on this quickly and used what she learned fairly well. She particularly enjoyed being able to respond to teasing in

a way that would stop it — 'I'm not getting into fights!' Again Julie was motivated to use what she had learned, as each time she did, she was met with praise and a hug.

3. Hitting Out, Grabbing People and Throwing Things. Julie was not aware of her strength and did not understand how she could really hurt someone. These incidents were considered unacceptable. When they occurred, Julie would be told, 'That's not acceptable' and isolated for five minutes. Afterwards, alternatives to hitting were discussed and rehearsed.

4. Self-image. Initially, Julie's self-image was poor. She could readily say she was fat, bad, plus give a list of negative behaviours. She was not able to give many positives about herself. This changed over the five weeks as all of Julie's positives were frequently reinforced (her nice hair, eyes and smile, her helpfulness, etc.) and encouraged. Her desire to help and do things for people was strongly supported and very rewarding for her.

5. Wetting Programme. During Julie's third and fourth weeks, there were quite a few incidents of her being wet during the day. This was handled in a matter-of-fact manner confirming that Julie was wet and having her change and clean herself. She was then responsible for gathering together and doing her washing. When Julie did not wet herself during a shift, she was praised. During the fifth week, there were no further incidents of wetting.

6. Personal Hygiene. Initially, Julie's personal hygiene was poor. Her comb, toothbrush and toothpaste, and some sweet-smelling soap which she was taken to buy, were all placed in a kit. She began to take more interest in her hygiene and was lavishly praised. By the end of her stay, Julie was taking care of her personal needs fairly consistently.

7. Weight Programme. Julie felt she was fat and didn't like the teasing she received. She was put on a programme that involved taking and recording her weight daily (a 'happy face' chart was used so that every day that she lost weight, she received a happy face), and counting every mouthful using a counter. During the first week, Julie was encouraged to slow down when eating and count mouthfuls. Following this, she was encouraged to try reducing the number of mouthfuls. Julie really enjoyed this programme and was pleased with the small weight loss that

did occur. She was encouraged to carry on with this following discharge.

Therapy with Julie's Mother
Time with Mrs Warner was limited as she was only able to be on the unit for two 3-day periods (at the beginning and at the end of the programme). The first period was spent encouraging her to talk about herself, Julie, the family and their problems and what she felt should be done about them.

Mrs Warner was very open in talking about everything, as she felt she was being 'really listened to'. She expressed a lot of sadness and guilt in not being able to manage Julie, but she also felt that the resources in Prince George, especially those regarding Julie's education, were not adequate. It was made quite clear that Mrs Warner felt she could not manage Julie and that this was affecting everyone in the family and not helping Julie. Over a number of years she had decided that Julie should be placed outside the home and came to the unit to state this and get assistance with finding a placement that could properly manage Julie and provide her with the best possible education.

During the second period, Mrs Warner could see definite improvement in Julie. She felt that was due to their being consistent, skilful management. This made her feel that given some direction and support, she could continue Julie's programme and improvement. Mrs Warner was given material to read, and time was spent teaching her parenting skills that she found helpful in the management of her other two children.

The following is a list of the recommendations given to Mrs Warner at Julie's discharge:

1. Compliance. When Julie responds to a request within ten seconds, give her appropriate praise and share your appreciation. When she does not respond, ignore her for ten minutes. Do not get caught up in talking about it.

2. Temper Tantrums and Disruptive Behaviours. When Julie has a tantrum or is disruptive, isolate her in her room for ten minutes or until she has quietened down. This is to be done matter-of-factly. Do not respond in an angry way — be firm, but softly spoken. Afterwards give Julie an opportunity to talk about what happened.

3. Praise. It is important for everyone to be praised, and Julie really needs this. When you observe a positive behaviour in Julie, acknowledge it. These behaviours will then increase. Julie really responds well to a hug.

4. Criticism. This should be avoided if possible as Julie is sensitive to it. If there is something you don't like, respond by talking about it and giving alternatives, i.e. when Julie baulks at doing dishes or other chores, say something like, 'You seem to have difficulty settling into doing the dishes. Maybe we could set aside a certain time each evening and I could help you get started.'

5. Expressing Feelings. Julie requires assistance in this area, particularly with regard to expressing frustration, anger and hurt. Pick up on cues and share them, i.e. 'You look angry. Would you like to talk about it?' Also be available to listen when Julie does want to talk. Another way to help is through modelling. If you express and deal with your feelings, Julie will follow suit.

When Julie is obviously tense and doesn't want to talk about things, do not push. Painting or pounding a pillow has been found helpful and should be encouraged.

6. Bedwetting/Wetting During the Day. This should be handled in a matter-of-fact manner. When Julie's bedding or clothing is wet, she is to be responsible for changing it. There is no need for discussion. When bedding or clothing is dry, praise her and show your approval.

7. Weight Programme. Julie has been started on a weight programme and should be encouraged (but not pushed) to keep the number of bites per meal down. She has worked really hard on this, and praising her helps.

8. When Things Get Tense. If, when dealing with Julie, you find yourself getting frustrated, angry and/or tense, it is time for a break. Send Julie to her room for a set period of time; then sit down and get yourself together. You should explain to Julie that the break is to benefit both of you.

9. Remember Mum, when you have concerns and questions, turn to your social worker and/or doctor. They are there to listen to you and offer whatever assistance they can. Say how you feel, and do not try

to interpret how they might respond to you — that is their responsibility.

We hope this summary will be of some assistance in your future care of Julie.

Mrs H. Donaldson
Head Nurse
6th Floor, Family Unit

Prepared by: N. McKenzie BA
                        L. Simons RN

Discharge Summary: Jane Whittle

1 September 1983
Ward 24

Dr L.M. Norris
Greendale Medical Centre
Christchurch

Dear Dr Norris
Jane Marie Whittle, Christchurch, aged 12 years
Your patient was admitted on 25 July 1983 and discharged five weeks later to be followed for a further five weeks as an outpatient.

Presenting Problems
Jane was referred by Dr Larry James who, as you know, has been seeing her off and on for some time. The major problems were:

1. Fighting. Jane constantly fights with her 9-year-old sister Emma. The parents feel that Emma and Jane have never got on and the situation is slowly getting worse.
2. Jane's opposition. Jane is rarely compliant with the parents' wishes and this frequently provokes conflicts between her and her parents.
3. Jane is said to have a very short concentration span and is very impulsive.

Psychiatric Diagnosis
Conduct Disorder, 312.23, socialised aggressive.

History of Presenting Problems and Background
Mr and Mrs Whittle see Jane's problem as life-long. Jane is adopted and, at the time, Mr and Mrs Whittle had been trying for seven years to have a child, before discovering that they would have to accept that they were an infertile couple. Mrs Whittle literally gave up work in the morning and picked up Jane in the afternoon on the day of her arrival. Mother said that they had problems from then on with her. Jane was three weeks of age at the time of her adoption, her developmental milestones proving normal. Despite her normal development, Jane has been a constant problem to her parents in other ways. Emma is also adopted.

Jane's continual opposition from an early age to her parents' wishes, her wakefulness, restlessness and high levels of energy and activity, have all worn her parents down. She has, in the past, been diagnosed as hyperactive and treated with methylphenidate with only limited effect.

The way in which this long-term problem has now crystallised, is that the family see more than their fair share of arguments and uproar. The usual scenario is a fight or argument between Emma and Jane. Mother then intervenes and generally takes the side of Emma since it seems that Jane provokes more arguments than her sister. This leads to a two-day screaming match between mother and Jane and finally father can take no more and intervenes himself in loud fashion. This has really caused a strain on all the interpersonal relationships within the family.

Progress in Hospital
The problems seen, therefore, that needed attention on the ward were:

1. Sibling rivalry.
2. Non-compliance.
3. Short concentration span.
4. Impulsiveness.
5. Jane's general sociability and peer relationships.

While on the ward, Jane participated in the following therapies:

1. Amorphous Blob.
2. Compliance.
3. Delayed Impulse and Self-control.
4. Feelings Rehearsal.

5. Limit Challenge.
6. Nurturing.
7. Relaxation.
8. Trust Programme.
9. Red and Green Button Programme.
10. Family interaction.
11. Sessions with herself and her sister.

It seems that Jane's behaviour over the years has alienated her more and more so that she felt very much on the outside of this family. She has not really known how she could change the situation and so the *status quo* has prevailed. Jane is certainly a girl who is full of energy but her impulsiveness, attention and concentration span, and ability to finish tasks, all improved while on the ward. This, we felt, pointed against the diagnosis of hyperactivity and placed her more appropriately into the diagnostic category of conduct disorder.

Much appears to have been gained from the involvement of Emma and the parents during Jane's admission to the ward. While her relationship with Emma has not improved enormously, the parents have realised that their children do not fall into quite the good and bad camps that they previously thought. Many of the positive aspects of Jane's character have been emphasised to them and Jane feels far more positive about herself and her relationship with her parents. At the same time, the balance has been redressed in terms of the parents realising that they need to be a little more critical of Emma and not side so much with her. Mr and Mrs Whittle also had some issues to sort out individually regarding their own relationship and their long wait for parenthood. All of these things seem to have progressed really well with the Whittles and we feel generally that this has been a very positive admission.

Physical Condition
Jane proved to be perfectly fit and healthy during her stay on the ward. All routine blood testing including a dexamethasone suppression test for depression, proved negative. She had no medical problems while on the ward.

Follow-up and Prognosis
Jane will be visited by her primary therapist during the next five weeks. Jane and Emma will continue to be seen together during the five-week follow-up period, but Mr and Mrs Whittle will not be followed further

unless they feel they need to contact us on the ward. We feel generally that the prognosis for Jane is good in that we have managed to break the cycle of family interaction which was leading them nowhere fast and merely increasing the tensions between individual members. Jane appears to feel far more positive about herself and her relationship with her parents, and her parents have also been able to form a much closer bond with their daughter. Assuming that the Whittles do not fall back into their previous pattern of interactions, we feel that they probably will not require further counselling after their involvement here.

Kind regards.

Yours sincerely

Dr Doug Brindad
Psychiatric Registrar
Child and Family Unit, Ward 24

cc. Dr L. James

Child and Family Unit, Ward 24
Therapists' Discharge Summary – Jane Whittle

Admission: 25/7/83
Discharge: 26/8/83

Key Conflicts
1. Jane versus Mum (is Mum picking on Jane?).
2. To be friends with Emma or not?
3. Jane – a part of the family or a separate unit?

Presenting Problems
1. Sibling rivalry.
2. Non-compliance.
3. Short concentration span.
4. Impulsiveness.
5. Doesn't make friends easily.

Individual Therapies

1. Amorphous Blob. This was done to help Jane get in touch with her inner feelings. Each week I got Jane to draw a blob, or amorphous shape, that depicted how she was feeling. She co-operated well with this, but showed a lack of insight regarding not so good qualities. She could label concrete attributes, e.g. good at . . ., but very few personal characteristics. The third and fourth amorphous blobs were the most productive. Jane would like to change most of the relationships within the family (somewhat unrealistic). (2½ hours)

2. Compliance. This was measured each morning and afternoon. We gave Jane five tasks to do and converted the amount completed into a percentage. The consequence for doing the task without moaning was praise. Jane was very compliant on the morning shift, but in the afternoon found it difficult to obey requests. This was possibly due to having more contact with other children in the afternoon. Average compliance was 77 per cent. (each shift)

3. Delayed Impulse and Self-control. It was noted on Jane's arrival to the ward that she was very impulsive in her words and actions when aggravated. Throughout the five weeks I have shown her appropriate ways of reacting in these situations, i.e. to stand back and count to ten before doing anything, then voice her feelings. (1 hour each shift)

4. Feelings Rehearsal. During these sessions, Jane and I explored different emotions, and the way we felt at different times. We also discussed the way you hold your body and talk at these times. Jane was very perceptive in this area, but found it hard to discuss her own emotions. We talked at length about anger and jealousy — both are things that I think Jane feels quite often. Lately, Jane has been able to withdraw from a situation and graph the intensity of her anger — hopefully illustrating to her that this anger she feels is variable and therefore controllable. (6 hours)

5. Limit Challenge. This therapy was done each night to see how well Jane could assess her physical capabilities. In most cases, in the activities she chose, Jane bettered her estimation. I feel that Jane underestimates her capabilities and requires plenty of praise, and positive comments regarding her achievements. (each afternoon).

6. Nurturing. Nurturing was done in the first week of Jane's stay in the

ward. During this time, I attempted to relax Jane and establish a good working rapport. I was very impressed with Mrs Whittle's participation in this therapy (a total of seven hours). I noticed that, alone, Mrs Whittle and Jane interact very well, and become demonstrative and affectionate towards each other. (3 days)

7. Relaxation. During Jane's stay on the ward I taught her some useful exercises to do before she went to bed. An alternative to this was to have a back massage. At first Jane remained rigid and tense but soon learned how to loosen up. We discussed physical ways of telling how relaxed you are. I think that Jane has a good idea of relaxation and that she needs to continue this after discharge. (each night)

8. Trust Programme. In order for Jane to gain confidence and responsibility, a trust programme was commenced. This was divided into three stages:

First Stage – doing errands, e.g. posting letters, going to the shop on her own, with a time limit of ten minutes, and a certain amount of change to bring back.
Second Stage – going for bike rides on her own, and walks in the park with a time limit of 20 minutes.
Third Stage – bus trips into town with me at first, then on her own.

Jane reacted very well to this programme, and accepted the responsibility in a mature way. I think she found this gratifying and hopefully will continue to take some responsibilities at home. (7 hours)

9. Red and Green Buttons Programme. Jane's inappropriate behaviours often frustrate and irritate others around her. To increase her awareness of the things she does that others don't accept, we drew up some lists of 'red' and 'green' buttons. When Jane does something to annoy someone, or make them angry, she is pushing their red buttons. If Jane is making others happy, she is pushing their green buttons. Jane had a container into which the staff put either a red or green token. This was a concrete way of showing which behaviour was appropriate and which was not. Jane's reward was a fishing trip for having no red buttons on one shift. Jane is now back to verbal reminders of this, and I hope Mr and Mrs Whittle will continue this, encouraging all the good behaviours with positive comments and praise. (each shift)

10. Family Interaction. Jane and her mother get on quite well with each other, when there is no one else around. Jane tends to be selfish with her mother or father's attention if Emma is around. As Emma has been an easier child to bring up, Mum has bonded more satisfactorily with her, while Jane has been rather a handful. Both girls are aware of this, and act accordingly. Mr Whittle is fond of both girls and seems to relate well to both. There is much work to be done in this area during follow-up. The family were involved as a whole in negotiating guidelines, and generally in group activities during the evening.

11. Emma and Jane. Jane and Emma spent two hourly sessions per week doing a project with the charge nurse. During this time, Jane treated her sister quite unfairly and with obvious animosity, but it was also noted that some of Emma's behaviours were irritating. Throughout the five weeks the relationship has not really improved, but the conflict that Jane obviously feels, requires time and patience to resolve. This will be a major focus in follow-up. Jane is willing to accept that she would not mind other people doing the same things that annoy her about Emma. (I feel this is part of Jane's inability to accept the negative points about herself and therefore in others.) However, Jane and Emma have not fought while at home on the weekend together, and I see this as a step in the right direction.

Summary. Jane has learned and practised many new ways of coping with her impulsiveness and anger. I have put many ideas forth regarding this, some of which Jane did not choose to discuss at the time, but I feel may act on them nevertheless. Jane needs a lot of praise and encouragement for behaviour that is acceptable and strict consequences for unacceptable behaviour. From observation, Jane needs more practice with sharing and co-operating with others in a group situation. She is very much an individual and independent and I hope will be able to take responsibilities on at home which will assist her in her struggle for maturity.

I have really enjoyed working with Jane and the whole Whittle family. We will have sufficient to work on during the follow-up five weeks.

Suzanne Campbell
Primary Therapist

26 August 1983
Ward 24

To: Mr and Mrs Whittle

Child and Family Unit, Ward 24
Discharge Recommendations — Jane Whittle

During this five weeks, when Jane has been on the ward, you have participated in everything requested, and I congratulate you on the effort you have put into the programme. I realise that you may feel disheartened at this stage, but I would like to stress that there is a five-week follow-up in which time I will be visiting you twice weekly.

Recommendations for You
1. It is important for you, as parents, to be consistent in setting guidelines and giving consequences. There will, of course, be times when you will not agree on an issue, but children pick this up quickly, so the fewer times, the better!

2. You need time alone yourselves. In order to be able to cope with the girls, you need your relaxation and peace and quiet. Try giving yourselves an hour together at the weekend, when the girls are doing something else.

3. Jane is a very independent little person and responded very well to our trust programme. She is able to take responsibility and in fact, enjoys this. Being 12, she is on the threshold of adolescence and will be looking for a little more freedom, which I hope you will be able to give her in time. I also hope you will celebrate Jane's adolescence with her, being a positive and delightful advance when and as it comes.

Recommendations for Jane and Emma
1. Both Jane and Emma have very separate identities and as such find it very difficult to co-operate. Please encourage them to work on activities, whilst at the same time realising their age differences. It is important that they learn to work side by side, before any more progress can be expected.

2. Each girl needs a specific time with you Mrs Whittle, so the girls get their attention fairly.

3. As Jane is the elder daughter, she requires chores around the home that carry a greater degree of responsibility than those which Emma does. When chores are set each girl must carry them out, or take the consequence.

4. Remember the procedure for negotiating? i.e. if one of the girls wants something, you can say that they are not to mention this again until a certain time. This will hopefully control nagging and give you a clear break to think about the request. It also gives the child another chance to negotiate.

Jane
1. Please praise Jane when she uses her self-control.
2. Please remind Jane when she is pushing red or green buttons for you.
3. Encourage her to be open about her feelings, because then she can work them out, rather than bottling them up.
4. I think it would be a good idea to encourage Jane's relaxation.

I have enjoyed working with you very much and I am sure you will use your new knowledge to the greatest extent.

Suzanne Campbell
Primary Therapist

Heather Thomas
Charge Nurse

26 August
Ward 24

To: Jane

You have really worked hard on Ward 24 and learned lots of new ways of working things out.
　　Here are some things to remember:

1. If something/someone bugs you, step back, count to 10 and then tell them how you feel. I have seen you do this, so I hope you will continue

when you are at home.

2. Please think about which buttons you are pressing for Mum, Dad or Emma. Remember — green stands for good (= go, it will get you further).

3. Through the trust programme I know you are a very trustworthy person, and can be responsible for yourself.

Good luck, Jane, I have enjoyed being with you.

Love from Susie

Guidelines and Consequences for Jane and Emma

Guideline	Consequence
Girls make their beds before breakfast	Praise — 'You did a good job'
Quiet while news is on	Chips on Saturday night
Temper tantrums	Send child to bathroom (without a word) until calmed down
Do an assigned chore	Stay up ten minutes later
Have a bath, brush teeth and hair and be in bed on time	Praise
	If not in bed — take the amount of time off the following night's bed time

B. Example of a Child's Weekly Programme

Introduction

We have found that many of the admitted child's acute symptoms and his high levels of anxiety diminish rapidly when the child is admitted to the hospital unit. This is often because the unit is a very supportive and very predictable place to be. The predictability is enhanced by making sure the child is given a copy of the timetable of all the appointments and treatments that he will have for the week. This is worked out by the primary therapist with the child and his family by the end of the preceding week. The child has a copy in his room, the parents have a copy at home and the staff have a copy in the nursing station.

It becomes obvious that with a wide variety of staff doing different treatments there has to be a careful co-ordination of treatment times. This is the responsibility of the primary therapist. If there is any over-lap of appointments, for example, between the time when the registrar would like to see the family and the occupational therapist see the child, the primary therapist makes the decision which is in the best interests of the child.

The treatment plan for the whole admission, with a careful deter-mination of who is doing what with whom and how often, is put together at the admission conference. Decisions on changes in the treatment programme are made at the weekly conference. These conferences are strictly regulated to ensure that every child is discussed and each discus-sion has the same amount of time. With reports on the results of 10-20 techniques, it isn't hard to imagine that there is seldom enough time to discuss each child as much as they could need. However, the primary therapist reviews the work, the teacher's reports and those of any other therapists are included. There is usually time to discuss major questions and make decisions to change the procedure or direction when progress is too slow. The day-to-day management of the hospitalised child is the responsibility of the primary therapist. If there must be a major change in direction before the weekly conference is held, the primary therapist organises a mini-conference with any of the family's other therapists. Decisions are usually made by consensus, but sometimes the Unit Director must decide.

Table 7.1 gives an example of a timetable for the third week of a child's therapy.

C. Staff Skill Inventory

Introduction

One of the best features of our programme appears to be the effective utilisation of frontline staff time and talent. This depends on:

(1) Using describable, measurable techniques.
(2) Maximising staff motivation by:
    (i) giving them the prime responsibility which inclines them to want to work to reduce the child's suffering and to learn in order to be effective therapists;
    (ii) frequent measures providing the staff with feedback.
(3) Determining staff skills.
(4) Matching individual staff members with various types of prob-lems.

Table 7.1: Aaron Steiner — Week Three

Time	'Normal Routine'	Monday	Tuesday	Wednesday	Thursday	Friday	Saturday	Sunday
07.00								
07.20	Clean up	Rise & Shine	Rise & Shine	Rise & Shine	Rise & Shine Swimming	Rise & Shine		
07.45	Breakfast	Clean up	Clean up	Clean up	Clean up	Clean up		
08.00		Breakfast / Wizard Chart Monitor Consumption	Breakfast / Wizard Chart Monitor Consumption / Parents to Don Quick	Breakfast / Wizard Chart Monitor Consumption	Breakfast / Wizard Chart Monitor Consumption	Breakfast / Wizard Chart Monitor Consumption	W E E K E N D	
08.30	Group Sensitivity	Group Sensitivity	Group Sensitivity	Group Sensitivity	Group Sensitivity	Group Sensitivity P L A Y		L E A V E
09.00	School	Typing Lessons with Cheryl 9.00-9.45	Typing Lessons with Cheryl 9.00-9.45	Typing Lessons with Cheryl 9.45-10.00 Morning Tea	Typing Lessons with Cheryl 9.45-10.00 Morning Tea	Typing Lessons 9.45-10.00 Morning Tea		
09.30	→ Morning Tea	9.45 Mental Limit 10.15 Challenge – Jan 11.00 ↓ with Jan Isherwood	10.00 O.T. Gym 11.00 Group	10.00 with Colleen	10.00 11.00 Group Social Skills			
10.15/10.45 11.30	(Morning Break) →		Social Skills Colleen	Audiology				
12.00	Lunch	Lunch / Wizard Chart Monitor Consumption	Lunch / Monitor Consumption	Lunch / Monitor Consumption	Lunch / Monitor Consumption	Lunch / Monitor Consumption		
13.00	Group Recreation	Group Recreation	Group Recreation	Group Recreation / Mental Limit Challenge	Group Recreation	Group Recreation		
13.30	School	Anatomy & Physiology – Peter F / Typing Lessons with Cheryl	Mental Limit – Janine Challenge / Typing Lessons with Cheryl	Weight	Mental Limit 13.30-14.30 Challenge app. Carol / Typing Lessons with Cheryl			
14.00	→			Typing Lessons with Cheryl				
14.30	(Afternoon Break)		→ Cooking with Colleen					
15.00	Free Period	Therapy with Dr Jan Isherwood		Assertiveness Abreaction	with Dr Jan Isherwood Assertiveness	Watch video of play Farewell Poster PARTY		
15.30	Kangaroo Kort . . .							
16.30	Gym/Pool	KK Gym – / Limit Challenge	KK Gym – / Limit Challenge	KK Gym – / Limit Challenge	KK Gym – / Limit Challenge			
17.00	→	Pool Dinner	Pool Dinner	Pool Dinner	Pool Dinner	Pool Dinner		
17.30	Dinner Time	Monitor Consumption	Monitor Consumption	Monitor Consumption	Monitor Consumption	Monitor Consumption		
18.00	Group Activities (GA)	GA	Construction GA Project	Construction GA Project	Construction GA Project	Construction GA		
18.30	Therapy 6 yrs + under 7 p.m.	→	Individuation	Cooking	Cooking			
19.00	Bedtime 7 yrs 7.15 p.m. 8 yrs 7.30 p.m.	Assertiveness	Assertiveness Training	→	→			
19.30	Bedtime 9 yrs 7.45 p.m.	Free Time						
20.00	Bedtime 10 yrs 8.00 p.m. 11 yrs 8.15 p.m.	Shower – Bed / Story	Shower – Bed / Story	Shower – Bed / Story	Shower – Bed / Story			
20.30	Bedtime 12 yrs 8.30 p.m. 13 yrs 9.00 p.m.							
Therapist of the day	A.M. P.M.	Jan Tim	Janine Tim	Jan Tim	Lois Tim	Lois Chrissy	– –	Chrissy

On the inventory of techniques and procedures, all our staff are asked to check what they are most interested in learning and what they feel they are capable of doing well. An interest may indicate they would like to be taught a particular technique because it is required in their work or they feel they have a particular talent in that area.

We have found that staff quickly discover what techniques they are best able to use. The staff who would like to learn a particular technique can organise a group instruction period. This is slotted into the weekly inservice instruction time or otherwise an individual can obtain individual instruction from the staff member they think is best able to teach a particular skill.

When the staff feel that they are good at a technique they ask a small committee of peers, who are expert in that technique, to watch and evaluate their work with a child. Most of the initial evaluations were done by us but now staff are aware of the experts among themselves, who are often just as able and often more available to evaluate them and correct any mistakes.

The Child and Family Unit uses a consultation rather than a supervision model. This means that the primary responsibility is with the primary workers. They function much like general practitioners, who maintain the responsibility for the patient and determine who should be the consultants and when they should be asked for consultation. If a primary worker feels that they are having difficulty there are a number of more experienced staff who are available to talk with them about their lack of skill or personal problems. The staff do not have mandatory supervision times but can seek consultation when they feel they need it most and with the person who is best able to provide it and at the most opportune time. There is a certain amount of monitoring which allows those responsible for the operation of the ward to know if certain staff members are not seeking consultation frequently enough. If someone never bothers to get a consultation they are asked why and they may be requested to provide a time to be evaluated.

D. Ward Milieu

Introduction

If treatment is going to go anywhere in five weeks, it is essential that the staff have as much time as possible to engage in treatment. This means that they cannot spend a great deal of time controlling group behaviour. We have found that with a minimum of consistency adhered

Table 7.2: Staff Skill Inventory Technique

	AB		AT		BD		BP		CD		CF		DIR		EA		FR		MM		NC		SG	
Skills	I	S	I	S	I	S	I	S	I	S	I	S	I	S	I	S	I	S	I	S	I	S	I	S
Staff																								
Mary Potter																								
George Gray																								
Greg Harrison																								
Margaret Fife																								
Bill Benett																								
Gill Green																								
Wendy West																								

Notes:
I = Interest in.
S = Skilled at.

to guidelines and consequences there is a good supportive ward milieu. Occasionally the staff or the patients will object to certain guidelines and then it is discussed in a management-type meeting.

The guidelines attempt to emphasise the need for the children to take responsibility for their own life. In this way the consequences are as natural as possible. For example, if the child goes to bed late, the natural consequence of feeling tired is emphasised by getting him up early. As much as possible, we use consequences which can be easily applied in the parents' home.

The ward guidelines and consequences in this book have been tried and tested in three Child and Family Units. You can be very sure that there have been many revisions. We have tried to make them acceptable to most families. It is very important that the families see how they work, adapt them for their homes and use them with a minimum of hassle. It seems children from a wide variety of backgrounds have little difficulty adjusting to these 'rules' as long as the staff are consistent.

We keep a monthly graph of the amount of time-out used. It is a fairly sensitive barometer of the level of tension on the ward. If at all possible, we teach children to put themselves into time-out. If a child becomes wildly uncontrollable and dangerous, we will use an intramuscular injection of a tranquilliser. It is such a rare event, the staff may forget the guidelines for its use.

Time-out

If a child yells, swears, kicks or thumps in time-out, he must be quiet for at least a minute before the door is opened. Children who are totally uncontrolled or can't respond to these consequences probably require individual medical treatment.

Timing of Consequences

If at all possible, enforce a consequence immediately. Praise a child immediately he exhibits desirable behaviour. Ask him to leave the table immediately following a display of bad manners. Wherever possible, use a natural consequence and one that fits the behaviour. At least 50 per cent of consequences should be reinforcing desirable behaviours rather than punishing undesirable ones.

If difficulties arise with undesirable behaviour at or after bedtime, it is preferable to institute immediate consequences, e.g. running up and down stairs, rather than leave a consequence to be carried out next morning. We try and use guidelines that are appreciated in most homes; but we find children can adapt quickly if our standards are

354   *General Instructions and Specific Examples*

Table 7.3: Child and Family Unit Guidelines and Consequences

Guidelines	Consequences
Up at 7 a.m., wash hands, face, get dressed, shoes on, brush hair	No breakfast until all ready. Go to group in PJs if not dressed. Tidiest room gets 'award'
Set tables in turns	No meal if tables not set. Group applause for setter when done well
Make beds by 8.30 a.m.	If not done strip bed and fold bed-clothes. Commendation for neat bed
Put belongings away by 8.30 a.m.	Any item left out is confiscated for 48 hours, or do extra chores to retrieve each item
Meal quantity selected 1 hour before meal	If refused, gets 'standard' food
Must eat what requested, a little of everything on the menu	If not, no seconds and no dessert. Remove meal if child complains. Do not push eating. Praise if tries new food
Reasonable table manners, depending on age	If unacceptable standard for individual, child must leave table without food for five minutes. If child hasn't been taught manners, he remains at table and appropriate behaviour is demonstrated. Commend publicly best-mannered child
No hitting staff with intent to injure	Time-out for one minute per year of age. Encourage child to put self in time-out to cool down
No hitting other children with intent to injure	Time-out for one minute per year of age. Commend appropriate expressions of aggression
No spitting at people	If hit, wipe spit back onto child's arm. Time-out. Show child picture of bacteria in spit
Leave ward only if given OK	If unauthorised leave, notify as described. Put into PJs and must earn clothes back. Loss of all privileges, i.e. no pool, no outings, no outside activities at lunchtime for three hours. 'Incident form' to be filled out by child
No swearing (staff included) (Check list for approved expletives)	Time-out for one minute each time
Do not pull fire alarms	Time-out two minutes per year of age. Personal apology to Fire Chief and hospital switchboard and administration. Given lectures on dangers
Attendance at school during usual school hours is required	If not, do cleaning chores until ready to return. Make up lost time at lunch and after school. Best weekly attendance child is 'teacher's pet' for the day

Table 7.3 (contd.)

Attend therapy sessions promptly	If refuses, given choice of cleaning chores until agrees. Sweets and commendation for participation, as required
In bed on time, washed, teeth brushed, etc.	If on time — story read to. If late without adequate reason — awaken the equivalent amount of time earlier the next morning
May read or talk quietly until asleep	If noisy and disruptive, ten minutes after lights out, child gets up to exercise for 15 minutes, repeat until sleepy
No taking things from someone else's bedroom	If losses, bedrooms of both children concerned to be locked for day
Child must not damage hospital or personal property	Any breakages child cleans up, apologises to superintendant and negotiates with family to repair or replace according to their means
No running away	If leaves hospital, into PJs. Clothes confiscated and earned back in increasing lengths of time at each run away, e.g. first time — one day
Must get out of pool when asked	If not, equivalent time taken off swim next day

different from those to which they are accustomed. If their parents strongly object, refer them to the management committee. Use your clinical judgement for behaviours not covered here but don't over-react. You can trust children more easily if you trust the child inside yourself. Remember to model good behaviour and commend each other.

E. Ward Procedure

1. Community Care

Community care is defined, for the purposes of this manual, as any care or assessment that takes place outside of the hospital or inside of its confines before or after admission. Some aspects of community care involvement do occur during the hospital stay, in terms of participation by the child in community activities, and contacts with the community agencies by personnel.

Pre-admission Home Visit. Community care begins before the child is admitted. Home visits are arranged with the parents and should be at a time when the family are most likely to be together. The visiting staff must include the primary worker who will be caring for the family during admission.

Purpose of the Visit.
1. To establish rapport with the child and his family.
2. Assess the physical environment, e.g. does he have a room of his own, or does he share? Does he have toys? If so, what type, what is his favourite object? What are his favourite haunts and places he avoids?
3. Reassure the parents and child about the pending admission.
4. Get a data base on health; note any allergies or disabilities.
5. Get a data base on how the child perceives reinforcing and aversive stimuli.
6. Determine how the child perceives his problems and the problems of his parents and siblings.
7. Assess the potential for changes in the home.

The Family Unit nursing assessment form should be used to collect the data base and the clinical record progress note should be used to write other observations and interpretations of the home and family. The data base and notes are kept in the child's folder until the clinical record is commenced on admission. The progress notes made prior to admission become the first page of the clinical record.

Home Visit – Inpatient. Home visits may be planned during the child's stay in hospital. Unless the programme says there shall be no further visiting, it will remain a nursing judgement as to how many and how frequently, home visits are made.

2. Discharge Conference and Summary Report

During the last week of admission, a well-defined nursing summary and guidelines for parents must be prepared for each child, regardless of continued visiting. Use the trial guidelines and consequences used for the previous weekends. These summaries are sent to those doctors participating in the child's care. The recommendations for parents may be given to parents only, or if a ward of the court, to the guardian authority. A photocopy of the summary is kept on file for use during the follow-up phase of community care.

At the discharge conference, plans are made with the parent for the first home visit, post-discharge. During the conference the plan of care will be discussed with the parents, and their continual support and co-operation sought for the continuing care of the child. It is important that an accurate picture be presented of what the parental expectations of the child should be.

3. Follow-up Care

Purpose.
1. To ensure that the plan of care is maintained or modified to achieve the desired response.
2. To continue teaching the parents management and communication skills.
3. To give reassurance, support and guidance to the family, school or agency.
4. To teach the child to cope with those situations that appear to be unchangeable.
5. To seek the assistance of the social worker, when other resources may be necessary to continue care.
6. To introduce and assist other agencies when their involvement is sought.
7. To work co-operatively with other agencies involved.
8. To keep an ongoing clinical record.

4. Guidelines for Confidentiality and Non-employees Present on the Unit

Only employees of the hospital are allowed access to data related to patients. The term 'employee' is further defined as being those employees directly concerned with providing care. On the Child and Family Psychiatric Unit, special arrangements have been made for the teachers, consultant psychologist and other nursing students to have access to data on a need-to-know basis.

Visiting professional and lay people involved with care of a patient, including prior to and during hospitalisation, may not have access to written material, the chart room or charts. Participation in therapeutic activities should be related to the identified patient. Participation in group activities will be allowed when a defined purpose is established.

When arrangements are made to spend time on the unit, the above guidelines should be outlined and our professional concerns regarding confidentiality shared with them as necessary to the effect that any information relating to the patient or his family is strictly confidential. Hospital policy demands that the confidentiality is maintained.

Areas of participation will be outlined to them by a member of senior staff, i.e. social worker or head nurse. They will determine the proposed purpose and extent of involvement.

Very extensive involvement and those persons seeking to fill educational needs will have to gain the written approval of the hospital or nursing administrator.

It is the responsibility of all professional staff to maintain good relationships with persons visiting the unit and to ensure the above guidelines are followed.

You may discuss the family problems with:

(a) The family itself.
(b) The psychiatrist, general practitioner or area clinician.
(c) If the child is a ward of the court information can be shared with the guardian or guardian authority.

Refer questions from:

(1) Human resources — to the social worker.
(2) School teachers — to the unit school teacher. You may share information regarding behaviour modification techniques found to be helpful in the home, and on the Unit. Do not get into any discussion of the child's family and their problems.

A clinical record must be kept on post-discharge contacts with the child, the family and others. The progress notes made during this period of time will be sent to medical records for inclusion in the child's record at the end of the follow-up period.

5. Staff Tasks

Remember that you are part of a team and what you do and how you plan your day affects others. Please arrange duties away from the unit and 1:1 interactions at other than conference or staff training times. Make sure that your time away from the unit leaves the unit well staffed.

1. Sign in on hours sheet.
2. Make provision for compulsory group activities.
3. After checking the child's weekly timetable, start the appropriate treatment with your patient promptly.
4. Check up on patient needs for the following day and provide for them or leave a note for someone else to do so.
5. Arrange time for follow-up visits with team leader, and put in

appointment book.

6. Make appointments with parents and put in appointment book.
7. Attend conferences as assigned.
8. Chart as things happen. Leaving this duty until the end of the shift contributes to erroneous reporting.
9. Have kardex completed by one hour before the shift change. Small additions can be made later if indicated.

6. Patient Care Plans

The format of the care plan has been designed to: identify the behavioural repertoire of the child; the conflicts which generate the behaviour; resources to check on the frequency or change in the behaviour; goals to resolve the conflict; and an individual plan of care-listing approaches to use in reaching the goals.

Key Conflicts. These are not goals and not behaviours. Usually they are related to family, community or school. When deciding what the conflicts are, ask yourself why the behaviour exists, what happened or happens to provide this behaviour.

Example: Poor Self-concept. Lack of own identity. This is the patient's conflict, but when listing this, one should also look at what is happening to the child to produce this feeling. The answer might be that father puts the child down a lot. This is a behaviour so you need to look at why he does this. You may find that father, himself, was put down a lot as a child. In that case the father has an unresolved conflict with his own father, and this would be the key conflict you would record.

Put simply, the Key Conflict answers the 'whys'.

Goals. It is important that these be as reachable as you can predict. They may need revision as more is known of the family dynamics and personalities involved.

Goals are a statement of expectation and relate to resolution of the Key Conflicts.

Behaviours. These are things the child does or says that are unacceptable to the parents, community or school. These may be added to when or if the child identifies behaviours of his own that he would like to change. You may identify unacceptable behaviours yourself. These should also be added to the list. Many of the behaviours identified relate to non-compliance; these can be combined under the one heading. It is helpful to find out which behaviours are most distressing; these may then become the primary behaviours upon which we would concentrate effort.

Measures. These are a record of the number of times a behaviour occurs. These may be behaviours as previously outlined, but are more frequently opposite behaviours, i.e. instead of counting the number of times a child is non-compliant, we count the number of times he is compliant. These then become a measure of improvement. Measures may be unrelated to the identified behaviours, i.e. a pulse rate may be counted as a measure of the child's anxiety.

Therapists. The primary therapist should be the RN who, by virtue of medical and psychiatric training, is better able to assess the overall needs of the patient. The secondary therapist can be an orderly or an RN. This person is on a different shift to the primary therapist. Aspects of care may be divided or shared, depending upon availability of parents and the special skills of the therapist. The primary therapist is responsible for the discharge summary and guidelines, but it is an expectation that the secondary therapist will contribute to them. There is, however, much flexibility in the performance of this duty and it may be that the secondary therapist can, and is able to, take full responsibility, based on the relationship developed with the family.

Individual Programme. These are tailored to fill the specific needs of the patient and his family (please see Chapter 5). It is the responsibility of the therapists assigned, to update this information frequently and to initiate graphs and token systems.

Individual Psychotherapy. This is specific to the patient's needs. In general, deal with how the child feels about himself, his environment, siblings, parents, peers and school. This aspect of care requires considerable skill, an ability to 'get into a child's thinking process', a non-judgemental attitude, interpretative skills, and the ability to project a warm, understanding and supportive feeling to the child.

7. Use of the Nursing and Medical Care Plans

Care plans should be brief, up-to-date, legible and understandable. Remember that an on-call worker should be able to follow them with as